MARQUEE SERIES
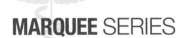

Using COMPUTERS in the Medical Office

Microsoft Word | Excel PowerPoint® 2013

with Windows 8.1 and Internet Explorer 11

Audrey Roggenkamp

Ian Rutkosky

Denise Seguin

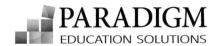

PARADIGM
EDUCATION SOLUTIONS

St. Paul

Director of Editorial: Christine Hurney
Developmental Editor: Sarah Kearin
Director of Production: Timothy W. Larson
Production Editor: Carla Valadez
Cover Designer: Jaana Bykonich
Design and Production Specialist: Sara Schmidt Boldon
Indexer: Ina Gravitz
Director of Marketing: Lara Weber McLellan

ISBN 978-0-76385-241-2 (Text)
ISBN 978-0-76385-242-9 (Text + CD)

Internet Resource Center: www.ParadigmCollege.net/MedicalOffice13

© 2015 by Paradigm Publishing, Inc.
875 Montreal Way
St. Paul, MN 55102
Email: educate@emcp.com
Website: www.ParadigmCollege.com

Brief Contents

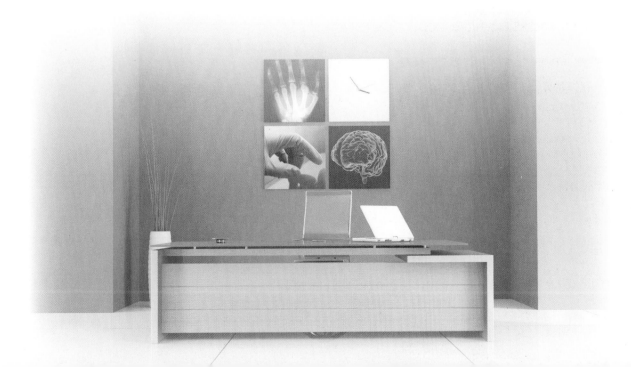

Contents

v

Preface

Using Computers in the Medical Office: Microsoft® Word, Excel, and PowerPoint 2013 prepares students to work with Microsoft Office 2013 in medical office settings. Medical offices are fast-paced environments that require proficiency with a variety of duties specific to the healthcare setting. Many of these duties require skill in using the Microsoft Office suite of programs. This text teaches the key computer competencies needed and provides practice in applying the skills in realistic healthcare scenarios.

Throughout *Using Computers in the Medical Office*, authentic medical documents provide the context for learning essential computer tasks performed in the medical office. Students prepare documents, reports, and presentations for two medical clinics and a hospital. Cascade View Pediatrics is a full-service pediatric clinic that provides comprehensive primary pediatric care to infants, children, and adolescents. North Shore Medical Clinic is an internal medicine clinic, and the healthcare providers in this clinic specialize in a number of fields including internal medicine, family practice, cardiology, and dermatology. Columbia River General Hospital is an independent, not-for-profit hospital providing high-quality, comprehensive care. All of the computer skills are taught in the context of preparing materials to support the services provided by these three healthcare settings.

In Word, students are asked to:
- produce an x-ray report
- create and maintain medical records and chart notes
- edit and format informative documents for patients about appointment scheduling, disease prevention, and education opportunities
- prepare envelopes, mailing labels, and documents for mailings
- create patient questionnaires and forms for gathering patient information

In Excel, students are asked to prepare the following:
- a report calculating the average standard cost for cardiac surgery patient stays
- purchase orders and statistic calculations for costs of exam room supplies
- invoices for medical services
- inventory reports
- a lab requisitions billing report
- a radiology requisition form
- a bypass surgery report
- a dermatology patient tracking worksheet
- cardiac nurse call lists
- revenue summary reports

Students are also asked to create PowerPoint presentations to inform patients about clinic and hospital services, cholesterol, fibromyalgia, sickle cell anemia, and chicken pox. Through these engaging projects, students learn Microsoft Office skills in the context of caring for patients while working as a valuable member of the healthcare team.

Using Computers in the Medical Office is divided into five units. In Unit 1, students are introduced to Windows 8.1 and the basics of using this operating system to display and manage information. In Unit 2, students are introduced to navigating the Internet using Internet Explorer 11. Skills taught in this section include using URLs and hyperlinks, searching, and downloading resources. In Unit 3, students work with Word. Basic skills, as well as more advanced functions such as using layout and design features and creating and editing forms, are taught in the context of the medical office.

Unit 4 focuses on using Excel to present and analyze types of data used in the medical office. In Unit 5, students learn how to create engaging and effective presentations using PowerPoint.

Within each section, activities present computer program features in a highly visual, project-based manner. Each activity introduces a topic, presents a short paragraph or two about the topic, and then guides the student through a hands-on computer project. The book offers several additional elements to enhance student learning, including:

- In Addition—Sidebars offer extra information on key features and subfeatures.
- In Brief—Bare-bones summaries of major commands and features provide instant review and a quick reference of the steps required to accomplish a task.
- Features Summary—Commands taught in the section are listed with button, ribbon tab, Quick Access toolbar, and keyboard actions.
- Knowledge Check—Objective completion exercises allow students to assess their comprehension and recall of program features, terminology, and functions.
- Skills Review—Additional hands-on computer exercises reinforce learning. These review activities include some guidance, but less than the section activities.
- Skills Assessment—Framed in a workplace project perspective, these independent assessments evaluate students' abilities to apply section skills and concepts in solving realistic problems. They require demonstrating program skills as well as decision-making capabilities and include Help and Internet-based activities.
- Marquee Challenge—Culminating assessments test students' problem-solving abilities and mastery of program features.

An Integrating Programs section follows both Unit 4 and Unit 5. These sections include projects demonstrating how to share data between programs within the Microsoft Office suite. Projects include practice with copying, exporting, linking, and embedding data. These sections emphasize the ability to integrate data seamlessly among programs and thus allow students to learn how to most efficiently manage data in the medical office.

System Requirements

This interactive text is designed for the student to complete section work on a computer running a standard installation of Microsoft Office Professional Plus 2013 and the Microsoft Windows 8.1 operating system. To effectively run this suite and operating system, your computer should be outfitted with the following:

- 1 gigahertz (GHz) processor or higher; 1 gigabyte (GB) of RAM (32 bit) or 2 GB of RAM (64 bit)
- 3 GB of available hard-disk space
- .NET version 3.5, 4.0, or 4.5
- DirectX 10 graphics card
- Minimum 1024 × 576 resolution (or 1366 × 768 to use Windows Snap feature)
- Computer mouse, multi-touch device, or other compatible pointing device

Office 2013 will also operate on computers running the Windows 7 operating system.

Screen captures in this book were created using a screen resolution display of 1600 × 900. Refer to Windows 8.1, Section 2, pages 41–42, for instructions on changing the resolution of your monitor. Windows 8.1, Section 2, page 42, illustrates the Microsoft Word ribbon at three resolutions for comparison purposes. Choose the resolution that best matches your computer; however, be aware that using a resolution other than 1600 × 900 means that your screens may not exactly match the illustrations in the book.

Resources for the Student

The Student Resources CD that accompanies this textbook contains pretyped documents and files required for completing section activities and end-of-section exercises. A CD icon displayed on the opening page of a section indicates that the student needs to copy a folder of files from the CD to a storage medium before beginning the section activities. (See the inside back cover for instructions on copying a folder.) The Student Resources CD also contains model answers in PDF format for guided section activities so students can check their work. Model answers are not provided for the Knowledge Check, Skills Review, Skills Assessment, or Marquee Challenge.

The Internet Resource Center for this book at www.paradigmcollege.net/medicaloffice13 provides additional material for students preparing to work in the medical office. Here students will find the same PDF files of intra-section model answers as are on the Student Resources CD along with study tools, web links, and other resources specifically useful in the medical office.

Resources for the Instructor

Instructor resources are available on the password-protected instructor side of the Internet Resource Center for this title at www.paradigmcollege.net/medicaloffice13. Besides providing access to the materials on the Student Resources CD, the Instructor Resources section offers PDF and live model answer files for all section activities and end-of-section exercises.

Other Medical Office Resources

In addition to *Using Computers in the Medical Office: Microsoft Word, Excel, and PowerPoint 2013*, Paradigm Publishing offers several resources to support job-training for the medical office. Titles include:

- *Applied Anatomy and Physiology: A Case Study Approach*
- *Emergency Preparedness for Health Professionals*
- *Essential Healthcare Terminology for English Language Learners*
- *Exploring Electronic Health Records*
- *Health-Care CareerVision Book and DVD: View What You'd Do*
- *Keyboarding in the Medical Office: Sessions 1–60*
- *The Language of Medicine CD*
- *Medical Terminology*
- *Medical Transcription*
- *What Language Does Your Patient Hurt In? A Practical Guide to Culturally Competent Patient Care*

For a complete listing of these and other titles, visit www.paradigmcollege.com.

About the Authors

Audrey Roggenkamp has been teaching courses on keyboarding, skill building, and the Microsoft Office programs in the Business Technology department at Pierce College Puyallup since 2005. In addition to co-authoring *Using Computers in the Medical Office: Microsoft® Word, Excel, and PowerPoint 2013, 2010, 2007*, and *2003*, she has co-authored the Benchmark, Signature, and Marquee series on Office 2013, 2010, and 2007; *Paradigm Keyboarding and Applications I: Using Microsoft® Word 2013*, sixth edition, *Sessions 1–60* and *Sessions 61–120*; and *Computer and Internet Essentials: Preparing for IC3*.

Ian Rutkosky teaches business technology courses at Pierce College Puyallup. In addition to co-authoring *Using Computers in the Medical Office: Microsoft® Word, Excel, and PowerPoint 2013* and *2010*, he has co-authored the Benchmark, Signature, and Marquee series on Office 2013 and 2010; *Computer and Internet Essentials: Preparing for IC3*; and the SNAP 2013 training and assessment software content.

Denise Seguin has served in the Faculty of Business at Fanshawe College of Applied Arts and Technology in London, Ontario, since 1986. She has developed curricula and taught a variety of office technology, software applications, and accounting courses to students in postsecondary information technology diploma programs and continuing education courses. Seguin has served as program coordinator for computer systems technician, computer systems technology, office administration, and law clerk programs and was acting chair of the School of Information Technology in 2001. Along with co-authoring *Using Computers in the Medical Office Microsoft® Word, Excel*, and *PowerPoint 2013, 2010, 2007*, and *2003* she has also authored Paradigm Publishing's *Computer Concepts and Computer Applications with Microsoft® 2013* and the 2000 to 2013 editions of *Microsoft® Outlook* and co-authored *Our Digital World* first, second, and third editions; *Benchmark Series Microsoft® Excel 2007, 2010*, and *2013*; *Benchmark Series Microsoft® Access 2007, 2010*, and *2013*; and the 2000 to 2013 editions of the *Marquee Series Microsoft® Office* books.

Acknowledgments

The authors would like to thank the editorial team at Paradigm Publishing, Inc. as well as the following list of reviewers and contributors for their expert advice and opinion on how to make this an effective and realistic learning tool.

Jerri Adler, CMA, CMT
Eugene, Oregon

Tracie Fuqua, BS, CMA
Wallace State Community College
Hanceville, Alabama

Debbie Gamracy, BEd
Fanshawe College
London, Ontario
Canada

Connie Lieseke
Olympic College
Bremerton, Washington

Linda Maatta
Davis College
Toledo, Ohio

Tanya Mercer, BS, RN, MA
Fayetteville, Georgia

Donna Reynolds
Cascade Eye & Skin Centers
Puyallup, Washington

Using WINDOWS 8.1 *in the* Medical Office

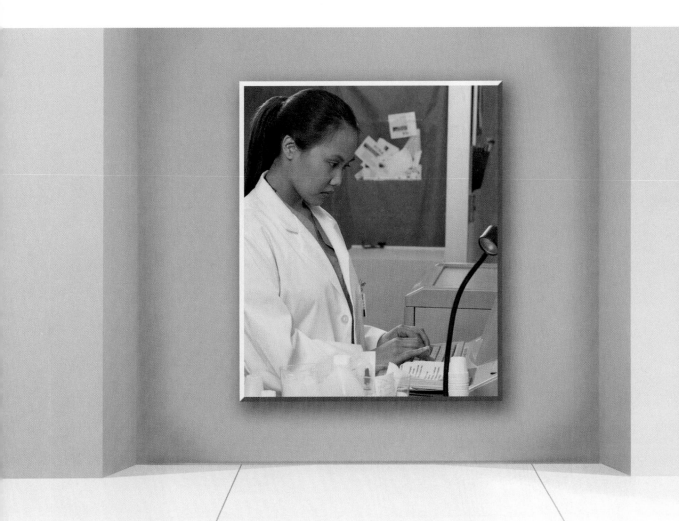

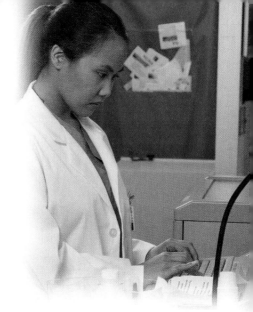

Windows 8.1 SECTION 1

Exploring Windows 8.1

Skills

- Navigate the Windows 8.1 Start screen
- Navigate the Windows 8.1 desktop
- Perform actions using the mouse, including point, click, double-click, and drag
- Start and close a program
- Open and close a window
- Shut down Windows 8.1
- Move a window
- Minimize, maximize, and restore a window
- Stack and cascade windows
- Use the Snap feature to position windows on the desktop
- Change the date and time
- Use the components of a dialog box
- Adjust the volume using the Speakers slider bar
- Customize the Taskbar
- Use the Windows Help and Support feature
- Turn on the display of file extensions

Projects Overview

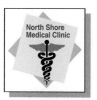

North Shore Medical Clinic has received new computers with the Windows 8.1 operating system. You will explore the Windows 8.1 Start screen and desktop; open, close, and manipulate windows; open a program; customize the Taskbar; explore online help resources for Windows 8.1; and turn on the display of file extensions.

Activity 1.1

Exploring the Windows 8.1 Start Screen

When you turn on your computer, the Windows 8.1 operating system loads and the Windows 8.1 Start screen displays on your monitor. The Start screen contains tiles you can use to open programs or access features within Windows 8.1. By default, the Start screen displays tiles for the most commonly used applications and features. Display all of the applications installed on your computer by clicking the button containing a down-pointing arrow at the bottom left side of the Start screen. Windows 8.1 includes a Charm bar with five buttons you can use to access features and options such as searching apps, sharing apps, and shutting down the computer. Display the Charm bar by hovering the mouse over the upper or lower right corner of the screen.

Project

You work at North Shore Medical Clinic, and the clinic has just received new computers with Windows 8.1 installed. You decide to take some time to explore the Windows 8.1 Start screen to familiarize yourself with this new operating system.

1. Complete the step(s) needed to display the Windows 8.1 Start screen.

   Check with your instructor to determine the specific step(s) required to display the Windows 8.1 Start screen on your computer at school. You may need a user name and password to log on to the computer system. When Windows 8.1 is started, you will see a Start screen similar to the one shown in Figure WIN1.1. Your Start screen may contain additional tiles or have a different background.

2. Move the mouse and notice how the corresponding pointer moves in the Windows 8.1 Start screen.

   A *mouse* is a device that controls the pointer that identifies your location on the screen. Move the mouse on your desk (preferably on a mouse pad) and the pointer moves on the screen. For information on mouse terms, refer to Table WIN1.1, and for information on mouse icons, refer to Table WIN1.2.

FIGURE WIN1.1 Windows 8.1 Start Screen

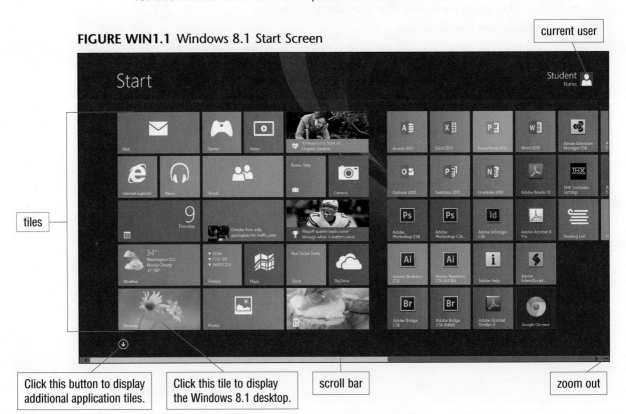

current user

tiles

Click this button to display additional application tiles.

Click this tile to display the Windows 8.1 desktop.

scroll bar

zoom out

TABLE WIN1.1 Mouse Terms and Actions

Term	Action
point	Position the mouse pointer on the desired item.
click	Quickly tap the left mouse button once.
right-click	Quickly tap the right mouse button once.
double-click	Tap the left mouse button twice in quick succession.
drag	Press and hold down the left mouse button, move the mouse pointer to a specific location, and then release the mouse button.

TABLE WIN1.2 Mouse Icons

Icon	Description
I	The mouse appears as an I-beam pointer in a program screen where you enter text (such as in Microsoft Word) and also in text boxes. You can use the I-beam pointer to move the insertion point or select text.
	The mouse pointer appears as an arrow pointing up and to the left (called the arrow pointer) on the Windows desktop and also in other program Title bars, menu bars, and toolbars.
	The mouse pointer becomes a double-headed arrow (either pointing left and right, up and down, or diagonally) when performing certain functions such as changing the size of a window.
	Select an object in a program, such as an image, and the mouse pointer becomes a four-headed arrow. Use this four-headed arrow pointer to move the object left, right, up, or down.
	When you position the mouse pointer inside selected text in a document and then drag the selected text to a new location in the document, the pointer displays with a gray box attached, indicating that you are moving the text.
	When a request is being processed or a program is being loaded, the mouse pointer may display with a moving circle icon beside it. The moving circle means "please wait." When the process is completed, the moving circle disappears.
	When you position the mouse pointer on certain icons or hyperlinks, it turns into a hand with a pointing index finger. This image indicates that clicking the icon or hyperlink will display additional information.

3 Click the Desktop tile in the Start screen.

> The desktop is the main screen in Windows 8.1. Different tools and applications can be opened on the desktop, similar to how different tools, documents, and items may be left out on the surface of a desk.

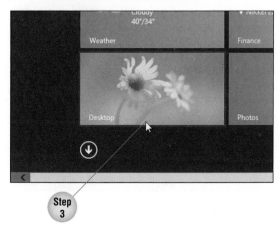

Step 3

continues

4 Click the Start button ⊞ located in the bottom left corner of the screen to return to the Start screen.

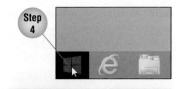

5 At the bottom of the Start screen, click the button containing a down-pointing arrow.

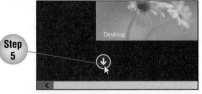

> The Windows 8.1 Start screen displays the most commonly used applications and features. Display all applications (grouped in categories) in the Start screen if you cannot find a desired program.

6 Click the Calculator tile that displays in the *Windows Accessories* category.

> Clicking the Calculator tile causes the Calculator tool to open and display on the desktop.

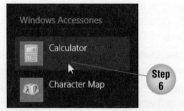

7 Close the Calculator by clicking the Close button ⊠ that displays in the upper right corner of the program.

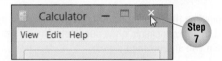

8 Click the Start button to return to the Start screen.

9 Click the Internet Explorer tile.

> Certain applications, such as Internet Explorer, can be opened in the Start screen as well as the desktop. Applications opened in the Start screen have been optimized to be used on touchscreen devices.

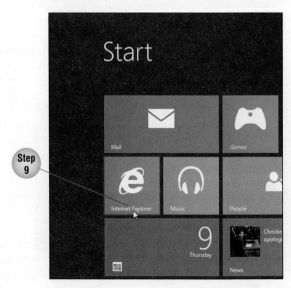

10 Close Internet Explorer by positioning the mouse pointer at the top of the screen until the pointer turns into a hand, holding down the left mouse button, dragging the mouse pointer to the bottom of the screen, and then releasing the left mouse button.

Closing applications in the Start screen is different than closing applications on the desktop. Dragging an application window down to the bottom of the screen will close it, while dragging an application to the left or right portion of the screen will resize the application window and position it on the side to which it was dragged.

11 Display the Charm bar by positioning the mouse in the upper right corner of the screen and then click the Settings button on the Charm bar.

The Settings button contains options for changing Windows 8.1 settings. It also contains the controls to shut down the computer.

12 Click the Power tile located toward the bottom of the Settings panel.

13 Click *Shut down* at the pop-up list that displays.

The Power tile contains three options. *Sleep* will turn the monitor and hard drives off to conserve power. *Shut down* will turn off the computer, and *Restart* will turn off the computer and then restart it.

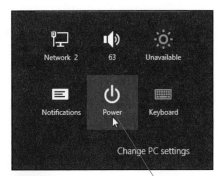

Step 12

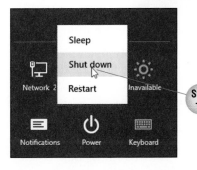

Step 13

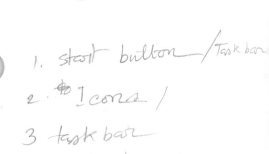

Need Help?

Check with your instructor before shutting down Windows 8.1. If you are working in a computer lab at your school, a shared computer lab policy may prevent you from shutting down the operating system. In this case, proceed to the next activity.

> **In Brief**
> **Start Program**
> 1. Display Start screen.
> 2. Click desired program tile.
>
> **Shut Down Computer**
> 1. Display Charm bar.
> 2. Click Settings button.
> 3. Click Power tile.
> 4. Click *Shut down*.

In Addition

Putting the Computer to Sleep

In Windows 8.1, Sleep mode automatically saves your work and turns off the monitor and hard drive, placing the computer in a low power state. A light on the outside of the computer case blinks or turns color to indicate that Sleep mode is active. Reactivate the computer by pressing the Power button on the front of the computer case or by moving the mouse. After you log on, the screen will display exactly as you left it when you activated Sleep mode. Note that if you shut down the computer rather than putting it to sleep, you will need to manually save your work, since Windows will not automatically do so.

Activity 1.2

Exploring the Windows 8.1 Desktop

The Windows 8.1 desktop can be compared to the top of a desk in an office. A person places necessary tools—such as pencils, pens, paper, files, calculator—on his or her desktop to perform functions. Similarly, the Windows 8.1 desktop contains tools for operating the computer. These tools are logically grouped and placed in dialog boxes or windows that can be accessed using the icons located on the desktop. The desktop is the most common screen in Windows 8.1 and is the screen in which most applications and tools will open and run.

Project You decide to take some time to explore the Windows 8.1 desktop to familiarize yourself with this important screen of the operating system.

1. If necessary, turn on the power to your computer to start Windows. At the Windows 8.1 Start screen, click the Desktop tile.

   When the Windows 8.1 desktop displays, it will look similar to the image displayed in Figure WIN1.2. Your desktop may contain additional icons or have a different background.

2. Move the mouse pointer to the bottom right corner of the desktop, where the current day and time display at the right side of the Taskbar. After approximately one second, a pop-up box appears with the current day of the week as well as the current date.

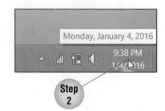

Step 2

3. Position the mouse pointer on the Recycle Bin icon and then double-click the left mouse button.

   Icons provide an easy way to open programs or documents. Double-clicking the Recycle Bin icon displays the Recycle Bin window.

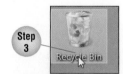

Step 3

FIGURE WIN1.2 Windows 8.1 Desktop

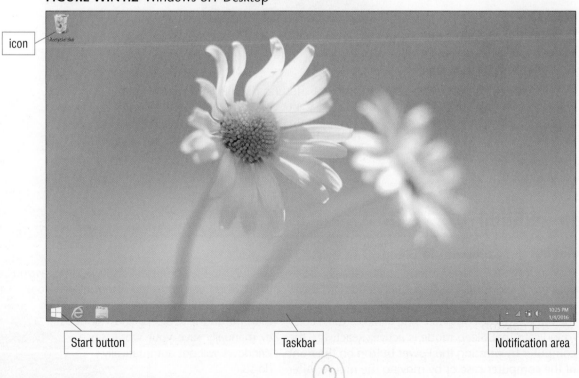

icon

Start button   Taskbar   Notification area

4 Close the Recycle Bin window by clicking the Close button in the upper right corner of the window.

5 Position the mouse pointer over the Start button and then click the right mouse button.

> When you right-click the Start button, a shortcut menu displays with various options. You can use these options to access computer and operating system management tools such as the Control Panel, Task Manager, and Device Manager.

6 Click *System* at the shortcut menu to display information about your computer in a new window.

> Your computer's information will appear in the System window. This information can be useful when determining if your computer is capable of running advanced software, or when you want to upgrade hardware such as RAM or a processor.

7 Close the System window by clicking the Close button in the upper right corner of the window.

8 Right-click a blank area of the desktop (not on an icon or in the Taskbar).

> A shortcut menu displays with various options you can use to manage files and change the way the desktop appears on your monitor.

9 Click *Personalize* at the shortcut menu.

> The Personalization window opens, containing options for customizing the desktop background, color, and screen saver.

10 Close the Personalization window by clicking the Close button in the upper right corner of the window.

In Brief
Display Windows 8.1 Desktop
Click Desktop tile.

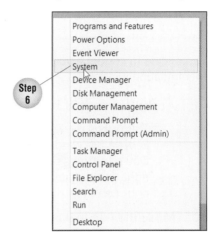

Step 6

Programs and Features
Power Options
Event Viewer
System
Device Manager
Disk Management
Computer Management
Command Prompt
Command Prompt (Admin)

Task Manager
Control Panel
File Explorer
Search
Run

Desktop

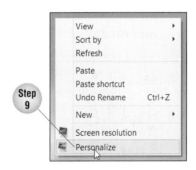

Step 9

View ▸
Sort by ▸
Refresh

Paste
Paste shortcut
Undo Rename   Ctrl+Z

New ▸

Screen resolution
Personalize

In Addition

Changing the Appearance of Windows 8.1

You can change the appearance of Windows 8.1 with options that display when you right-click a blank area of the desktop. Click the *Personalize* option at the shortcut menu if you want to change the Windows theme, desktop background, color, sounds, and/or screen saver. You can also change how the desktop icons and mouse pointer display. Click the *Screen resolution* option at the shortcut menu if you want to change the screen resolution, the monitor orientation, and/or the size of text and other items. The Screen Resolution window also contains controls for setting up multiple displays. Customizing how Windows 8.1 appears on your monitor can make using Windows easier by increasing the size of certain elements and creating more contrast among colors.

Activity 1.3

Opening and Manipulating Windows

When you open a program, a defined work area, referred to as a *window*, appears on the screen. You can move and change the size of a window on the desktop. The top area of a window is called the Title bar. The right side of the Title bar generally contains buttons for closing the window and minimizing, maximizing, or restoring the size of the window.

More than one window can be open at a time and open windows can be cascaded or stacked. The Snap feature in Windows causes a window to "stick" to the edge of the screen when the window is moved to the left or right. When a window is moved to the top of the screen, the window is automatically maximized, and when a maximized window is dragged down, the window is automatically restored down.

Project

You decide to continue your exploration of the Windows 8.1 desktop by opening and manipulating windows.

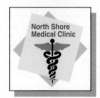
North Shore Medical Clinic

1 At the Windows 8.1 desktop, double-click the Recycle Bin icon.

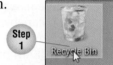
Step 1

This opens the Recycle Bin window on the desktop. If the Recycle Bin window fills the entire desktop, click the Restore Down button, which is the second button from the right (immediately left of the Close button) in the upper right corner of the window.

2 Move the window on the desktop. To do this, position the mouse pointer on the Title bar (the bar along the top of the window), hold down the left mouse button, drag the window to a different location on the desktop, and then release the mouse button.

3 Position the mouse pointer over the File Explorer button on the Taskbar and then click the wheel on the mouse once. *Note: If you do not have a wheel on your mouse, position the mouse pointer over the File Explorer button, right-click, and then click* **File Explorer** *at the shortcut menu.*

Clicking the mouse wheel opens a new File Explorer window with the text *This PC* in the Title bar. If the This PC window fills the entire desktop, click the Restore Down button. You now have two windows open on the desktop: This PC and Recycle Bin.

4 Make sure the Title bar of the Recycle Bin window is visible (if not, move the This PC window) and then click the Title bar of the Recycle Bin window.

Clicking the Title bar makes the Recycle Bin window active, moving it in front of the This PC window.

5 Minimize the Recycle Bin window to the Taskbar by clicking the Minimize button (located immediately to the right of the Restore Down button at the right side of the Title bar).

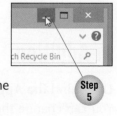
Step 5

The minimized Recycle Bin window is positioned behind the File Explorer button (displays as a group of file folders) on the Taskbar. Notice that the File Explorer button now appears with another button stacked behind it.

6 Minimize the This PC window to the Taskbar by clicking the Minimize button at the right side of the Title bar.

7 Move the mouse pointer over the File Explorer button on the Taskbar.

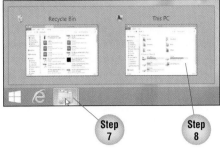

The two minimized windows (Recycle Bin and This PC) are stacked behind the File Explorer button. Resting the pointer on the File Explorer button causes a thumbnail preview of each window to display.

8 Click the thumbnail preview for the This PC window to redisplay the window on the desktop.

9 Rest the pointer over the File Explorer button on the Taskbar and then click the thumbnail preview for the Recycle Bin window.

10 Drag the Title bar for the Recycle Bin window to the top of the desktop and then release the mouse button.

The Snap feature allows you to resize a window by dragging the window to the edge of the screen. Dragging a window to the top of the desktop causes the window to automatically maximize when you release the mouse button. You can also maximize the window by clicking the Maximize button (displays as a square) next to the Close button at the right side of the Title bar.

11 Drag the Title bar for the Recycle Bin window down from the top of the desktop to restore the window to its previous size before it was maximized.

12 Right-click a blank, unused section of the Taskbar and then click *Show windows stacked* at the shortcut menu that displays.

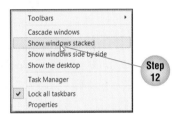

The Taskbar shortcut menu provides three options to display windows: *Cascade windows*, which places each window in a fanned stack with the title bars of each open window visible; *stacked*, which places windows in a horizontal stack with a portion of each window visible; or *side by side*, which places open windows next to each other.

13 Drag the Recycle Bin window off the right edge of the screen and then release the mouse button. When you release the mouse button, the window resizes to fill one-half the width of the screen.

14 Drag the This PC window off the left edge of the screen and then release the mouse button. When you release the mouse button, the window resizes to fill the remaining width of the screen.

15 Close each of the two windows by clicking the Close button at the right side of each Title bar.

In Brief

Move Window
1. Position mouse pointer on window Title bar.
2. Hold down left mouse button.
3. Drag window to desired position.
4. Release mouse button.

Stack Windows
1. Right-click unused section of Taskbar.
2. Click *Show windows stacked* at shortcut menu.

Cascade Windows
1. Right-click unused section of Taskbar.
2. Click *Cascade windows* at shortcut menu.

In Addition

Sizing a Window

Using the mouse, you can increase or decrease the size of a window. To change the width, position the mouse pointer on the border at the right or left side of the window until the mouse turns into a left-and-right-pointing arrow. Hold down the left mouse button, drag the border to the right or left, and then release the mouse button. Complete similar steps to increase or decrease the height of the window using the top or bottom border. To change the width and height of the window at the same time, position the mouse pointer at the left or right corner of the window until the pointer turns into a diagonally point-ing double-headed arrow and then drag in the desired direction to change the size.

Activity 1.4

Exploring the Taskbar, Charm Bar, and Dialog Box Components

The bar that displays at the bottom of the desktop is called the *Taskbar*. The Taskbar is divided into three sections: the Start button, the task button area, and the Notification area. Click the Start screen button to display the Windows 8.1 Start screen. Open programs display as task buttons in the task button area of the Taskbar. The Notification area displays at the right side of the Taskbar and contains the time, date, and program icons for programs that run in the background on your computer. You can right-click a blank, unused portion of the Taskbar to display a shortcut menu with options for customizing the Taskbar. The bar that displays at the right side of the desktop when the mouse pointer is positioned in the upper or lower right corner of the desktop is called the *Charm bar*. Click buttons in the Charm bar to access common operating system features. Some features are accessed through a window called a *dialog box*. Dialog boxes contain features such as tabs, text boxes, and option buttons that you can use to change settings.

Project

As you continue exploring Windows 8.1, you want to learn more about the features available on the Taskbar. You also decide to experiment with using the Charm bar.

1. At the Windows 8.1 desktop, click the current time that displays at the far right side of the Notification area of the Taskbar and then click <u>Change date and time settings</u>.

   Figure WIN1.3 identifies the components of the Taskbar. Clicking <u>Change date and time settings</u> causes the Date and Time dialog box to display. Refer to Table WIN1.3 for information on dialog box components.

2. Check to make sure the correct date and time display in the Date and Time dialog box.

   If the date is incorrect, click the Change date and time button. At the Date and Time Settings dialog box, click the correct day in the calendar box. If necessary, use the left- or right-pointing arrows to change the calendar display to a different month. To change the time, double-click the hour, minutes, or seconds and then type the correct entry or use the up- and down-pointing arrows to adjust the time. Click OK to close the dialog box when finished.

3. Click the Additional Clocks tab located toward the top of the Date and Time dialog box.

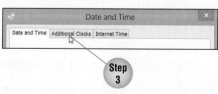

   At this tab you can add the current time for a second clock. This time will display when you click or hover the mouse pointer over the current time in the Taskbar. For example, you could show the time for Cairo, Egypt, in addition to the current time for your time zone.

FIGURE WIN1.3 Taskbar Components

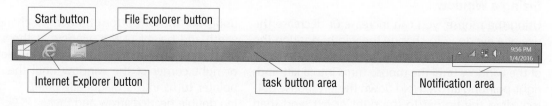

TABLE WIN1.3 Dialog Box Components*

Name	Example	Function
tabs	Date and Time | Additional Clocks | Internet Time	Click a tab to access a different set of options within the same dialog box.
text box	2:54:04 PM	Click in a text box to type or edit the contents. A text box may contain up- or down-pointing arrows so that you can choose a number or an option instead of typing it.
option box/drop-down list	M/d/yyyy M/d/yyyy M/d/yy MM/dd/yy MM/dd/yyyy yy/MM/dd yyyy-MM-dd dd-MMM-yy	Click the down-pointing arrow at the right side of an option box to display a drop-down list with a variety of choices. Click an option to select it.
list box	Windows Asterisk Calendar Reminder Close Program Critical Battery Alarm Critical Stop	A list box displays a list of options. Click an option to select it, or use the scroll bar and/or up- and down-pointing arrows to view more options in the list box.
check boxes	Desktop icons ☐ Computer ☑ Recycle Bin ☐ User's Files ☐ Control Panel ☐ Network	If a check box contains a check mark, the option is active; if a check box is empty, the option is inactive. In some cases, more than one check box in a dialog box section can contain a check mark.
option buttons	○ Smaller - 100% (default) ● Medium - 125% ○ Larger - 150%	Click an option button to make it active. Only one option button in a dialog box section can be selected at any time. An active option button contains a dot in black or another color.
command buttons	OK | Cancel | Apply	Click a command button to execute or cancel a command. If a command button name is followed by an ellipsis (...), clicking the button will open another dialog box.
slider bar	Slow ——◻—— Fast	Using the mouse, drag the slider button on a slider bar to increase or decrease the number, speed, or percentage of the option.

Note: Each component will not be present in every dialog box.

continues

④ Click OK to close the Date and Time dialog box.

⑤ Position the mouse pointer on the Speakers button 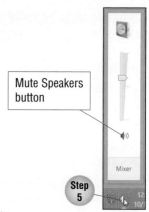 located toward the right side of the Taskbar and then click the left mouse button.

> Clicking the Speakers button causes a slider bar to display. Use this slider bar to increase or decrease the volume. Click the Mute Speakers button at the bottom of the slider bar if you want to turn off the sound. If the Speakers button is not visible on the Taskbar, click the up-pointing arrow located near the left side of the Notification area. This expands the area to show hidden icons.

Mute Speakers button

Step 5

⑥ After viewing and adjusting the Speakers slider bar, click in a blank, unused area of the desktop to close the slider bar.

⑦ Right-click a blank, unused section of the Taskbar and then click *Properties* at the shortcut menu.

> This displays the Taskbar Properties dialog box with the Taskbar tab selected. Notice that the dialog box contains check boxes. A check mark in a check box indicates that the option is active.

⑧ Click the *Auto-hide the taskbar* check box to insert a check mark.

⑨ Click the Apply button at the bottom of the dialog box.

⑩ Click OK to close the Taskbar Properties dialog box.

> Notice that the Taskbar is no longer visible.

⑪ Display the Taskbar by moving the mouse pointer to the bottom of the desktop.

⑫ Right-click a blank, unused section of the Taskbar, click *Properties* at the shortcut menu, click the *Auto-hide the taskbar* option to remove the check mark, and then click OK.

⑬ Position the mouse pointer in the upper right corner of the desktop to display the Charm bar.

> The Charm bar displays as a transparent bar until the mouse pointer is moved over any area of it, making it active. When the Charm bar is active, it changes from transparent to black and a box with the current time and date displays in the lower left corner of the screen.

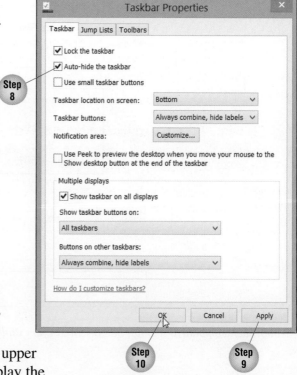

Step 8

Step 10

Step 9

14 Make the Charm bar active by moving the mouse over the bar. Once the bar is active, click the Search button.

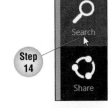

> Clicking the Search button will open the Start screen with a search text box active. You can search for applications, settings, or files by clicking the desired option below the search text box.

15 Type **snipping tool** in the search text box.

> Notice that Windows 8.1 actively narrows the search results below the search text box as you type.

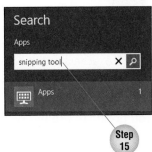

Step 15

16 Press the Enter key on the keyboard.

> Pressing Enter opens the Snipping Tool in a new window on the desktop. If the search does not return a match for what you typed in the text box, a list of possible results will display.

17 Close the Snipping Tool window by clicking the Close button in the upper right corner of the window.

18 Make the Charm bar active and then click the Settings button.

19 At the Settings panel, click the *Change PC settings* option.

> When you click the *Change PC settings* option in the Settings panel, the PC settings screen displays. This screen contains a variety of options for changing the settings of your computer. These options are grouped into categories that display at the left side of the PC settings screen.

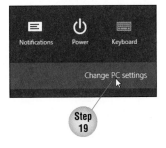

Step 19

20 Close the PC settings screen by positioning the mouse pointer at the top of the screen until it turns into a hand, holding down the left mouse button, dragging the screen downward until it dims, and then releasing the left mouse button.

> In Windows 8.1, certain applications and tools open in the Start screen instead of in a window on the desktop. To close applications or tools that open in the Start screen, drag the top of the screen downward until it becomes dim and then release the mouse button.

In Brief

Display Date and Time Properties Dialog Box
1. Click current time in Notification area of Taskbar.
2. Click Change date and time settings.

Display Speakers Slider Bar
Click Speakers button on Taskbar.

Display Taskbar and Start Menu Properties Dialog Box
1. Right-click unused section of Taskbar.
2. Click Properties at shortcut menu.

In Addition

Managing Devices Using the Charm Bar

The Charm bar contains the Devices button, which you can use to manage devices plugged into your computer. Click the Devices button in the Charm bar and a Devices panel displays at the right side of the screen. Devices plugged into your computer display as a list in the Devices panel. Click a device in the Devices list to display options for that particular device. Devices that are commonly listed in the Devices panel include monitors, projectors, and other peripheral devices that may be plugged into your computer.

Activity 1.5

Getting Help in Windows; Displaying File Extensions

Windows 8.1 includes an on-screen reference guide, called Windows Help and Support, that provides information, explanations, and interactive help on learning Windows features. The Windows Help and Support feature contains complex files with *hypertext*, a term used to describe words and phrases that can be clicked to access additional information. Display the Windows Help and Support window by right-clicking a blank area of the Start screen, clicking the All apps button, and then clicking the Help and Support tile. You can also press F1 at the desktop to display the Windows Help and Support window with information on your current task. At the Windows Help and Support window, you can perform such actions as choosing a specific help topic, searching for a keyword or topic, or displaying a list of topics.

Project

You decide to use the Windows Help and Support feature to learn how to pin an application to the Taskbar. You also want to turn on the display of file extensions to prepare for the next section, which deals with file management.

North Shore Medical Clinic

1. Display the Windows 8.1 Start screen and then click the down-pointing arrow button in the lower left corner of the screen.

2. Use the horizontal scroll bar at the bottom of the screen to display the *Windows System* category and then click the Help and Support tile.

3. At the Windows Help and Support window, with the insertion point positioned in the search text box, type **taskbar** and then press Enter.

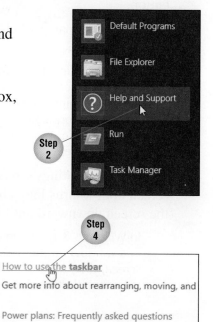

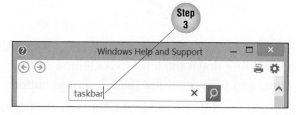

4. Click the <u>How to use the taskbar</u> hyperlink in the search results list.

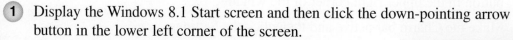

5. Scroll down the Windows Help and Support window and then read the information under the heading *Pin an app to the taskbar*.

   You will open and then pin the Snipping Tool application to the Taskbar in the following steps.

6. Open the Snipping Tool by using the Start screen or the Charm bar to initiate a search for the Snipping Tool application.

7. Return to the Windows Help and Support window by clicking the Windows Help and Support button on the Taskbar.

8. Follow the instructions in the *Pin an app to the taskbar* section of the Windows Help and Support window to pin the Snipping Tool to the Taskbar.

   When you pin an application to the Taskbar, the button for the application will be added to the Taskbar and remain there until it is unpinned (even when you restart the computer). Pinning applications you use often to the Taskbar reduces the steps required to open them.

9 Read information in the *Pin an app to the taskbar* section of the Windows Help and Support Window on how to remove a pinned application from the Taskbar and then unpin the Snipping Tool.

> Note that if the Snipping Tool is open when you unpin the button from the Taskbar, the button will be unpinned, but it will still display on the Taskbar until the Snipping Tool is closed.

10 Close the Windows Help and Support window and the Snipping Tool application by clicking the Close button in the upper right corner of each window.

> North Shore Medical Clinic requires that employees work with the display of file extensions turned on. This practice helps employees to identify the source application associated with a file and often prevents employees from accidentally opening file attachments that may contain harmful data. In the next steps, you will turn on the display of file extensions.

11 Click the File Explorer button on the Taskbar.

> When you first open File Explorer, the This PC window displays by default. The This PC window contains icons you can double-click to navigate to common file locations.

12 Click the View tab on the ribbon.

> In Windows 8.1, File Explorer windows contain a ribbon that displays various tabs, depending on which file location is currently active in the File Explorer window. With the This PC window open, three tabs display: File, Computer, and View. These tabs contain options and buttons to change File Explorer settings.

13 Click the *File name extensions* check box in the Show/hide group to insert a check mark. ***Note: If the check box appears with a check mark in it, file extensions are already displayed and you can skip this step.***

> Inserting a check mark in a check box makes that option active.

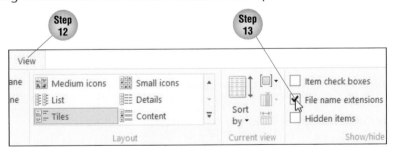

14 Close the File Explorer window by clicking the Close button at the right side of the Title bar.

In Brief
Display Help and Support Window
1. Display Start screen.
2. Click down-pointing arrow in lower left corner of Start screen.
3. Click Help and Support tile.

In Addition

Browsing the Windows Help and Support Window by Topic Lists

You can also locate help information by browsing the contents list in the Windows Help and Support window. To do this, click the <u>Browse help</u> link (located below the search text box) in the Windows Help and Support window. This displays the Windows Help topics list. Click a category in the topics list and then read the associated information. Continue clicking topic hyperlinks until you find the information you need.

Features Summary

Feature	Button	Action
close window	✕	Click Close button on Title bar.
Date and Time dialog box		Click time on Taskbar and then click <u>Change date and time settings</u>.
maximize window	▢	Drag window to top of screen or click Maximize button on Title bar.
minimize window	▬	Click Minimize button on Title bar.
move window on desktop		Click in Title bar and then drag to new location.
restore window	▥	Drag maximized window down or click Restore Down button on Title bar.
shut down computer		Click Settings button on Charm bar, click Power tile, and then click *Shut down*.
Speakers slider bar	🔊	Click Speakers button on Taskbar.
Start button	⊞	Click Start button on Taskbar.
Taskbar and Start Menu Properties dialog box		Right-click unused section of Taskbar and then click *Properties* at shortcut menu.
Taskbar shortcut menu		Right-click unused section of Taskbar.
Windows Help and Support window		Display Start screen, display all apps, and then click Help and Support tile.

Knowledge Check

Completion: In the space provided at the right, indicate the correct term, command, or option.

1. This term refers to tapping the left mouse button twice in quick succession.
2. Click this button in a window's Title bar to reduce the window to a button on the Taskbar.
3. Click this button in a window's Title bar to expand the window so it fills the entire screen.
4. Click the time located in the Notification area of the Taskbar and then click this option to open the Date and Time dialog box.
5. Display this bar on the desktop for quick access to a variety of Windows 8.1 features.
6. Press this key to open a Windows Help and Support window from the desktop.

Skills Review

Review 1 Opening and Manipulating Windows

1. At the Windows 8.1 desktop, click the File Explorer button on the Taskbar. *Hint: If the This PC window fills the desktop, drag the window down from the top of the screen or click the Restore Down button in the upper right corner of the window.*
2. Double-click the Recycle Bin icon on the desktop. *Hint: If the Recycle Bin window fills the desktop, drag the window down from the top of the screen or click the Restore Down button.*
3. Position the mouse pointer on the Title bar in the Recycle Bin window, hold down the left mouse button, and then drag the Recycle Bin window so the Title bar of the This PC window is visible.
4. Click the Title bar in the This PC window to make it the active window.
5. Right-click a blank, unused section of the Taskbar and then click *Cascade windows* at the shortcut menu.
6. Click the Minimize button in the Title bar of the This PC window to reduce the window to a task button behind the File Explorer button on the Taskbar.
7. Click the Minimize button in the Title bar of the Recycle Bin window to reduce the window to a task button behind the File Explorer button on the Taskbar.
8. Point to the File Explorer button on the Taskbar and then click the thumbnail preview for the Recycle Bin window to restore the Recycle Bin window on the desktop.
9. Point to the File Explorer button on the Taskbar and then click the thumbnail preview for the This PC window to restore the This PC window on the desktop.
10. Drag the This PC window to the top of the screen and then release the mouse button. (The window expands to fill the entire screen.)
11. Drag the This PC window down from the top of the screen and then release the mouse button to restore the window to its previous size.
12. Drag the This PC window off the right edge of the screen until a transparent box displays on the right half of the screen and then release the mouse button.
13. Drag the Recycle Bin window off the left edge of the screen until a transparent box displays on the left half of the screen and then release the mouse button.
14. Close the This PC window.
15. Close the Recycle Bin window.

Review 2 Exploring the Taskbar

1. At the Windows 8.1 desktop, click the time that displays in the Notification area at the right side of the Taskbar and then click <u>Change date and time settings</u>.
2. At the Date and Time dialog box, click the Change date and time button.
3. At the Date and Time Settings dialog box with the current month displayed in the calendar, click the right arrow in the calendar to display the next month.
4. Click OK twice.
5. Click the Start button, display all apps by clicking the All Apps button in the lower left corner of the screen, and then click the Notepad tile in the *Windows Accessories* category.
6. Close the Notepad window by clicking the Close button at the right side of the Title bar.

Skills Assessment

Assessment 1 Manipulating Windows

1. Click the File Explorer button on the Taskbar and then double-click the Pictures icon.
2. Position the mouse pointer on the File Explorer button on the Taskbar, click the mouse wheel, and then double-click the Music icon. *Note: If you do not have a wheel on your mouse, right-click the File Explorer button on the Taskbar and then click* **File Explorer** *at the shortcut menu.*
3. Stack the two windows.
4. Make the Pictures window the active window and then reduce it to a task button on the Taskbar.
5. Reduce the Music window to a task button on the Taskbar.
6. Restore the Pictures window.
7. Restore the Music window.
8. Arrange the two windows side-by-side on the desktop with each window filling one-half the width of the screen.
9. Close the Music window and then close the Pictures window.

Assessment 2 Customizing the Taskbar and Using the Charm Bar

1. At the Windows 8.1 desktop, display the Date and Time Settings dialog box.
2. Change the current time to one hour ahead and then close the dialog box.
3. Display the Speakers slider bar, drag the slider button to increase the volume, and then click the desktop outside the slider bar to close it.
4. Display the Taskbar Properties dialog box, use the *Taskbar location on screen* option box to change the Taskbar location on the screen to *Top*, and then close the dialog box. (Notice that the Taskbar is now positioned along the top edge of the screen.)
5. Display the Charm bar and then click the Search button.
6. At the Search panel, type **Calculator** in the text box and then press Enter.
7. Close the Calculator application.

Assessment 3 Restoring the Default Settings and the Taskbar

1. At the Windows 8.1 desktop, display the Date and Time Settings dialog box and then change the date and time to the current date and time.
2. Display the Speakers slider bar and then drag the slider button back to the original position.
3. Display the Taskbar Properties dialog box and then change the location of the Taskbar back to the bottom of the screen.

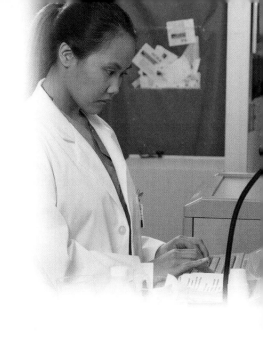

Windows 8.1 SECTION 2

Maintaining Files and Customizing Windows

Skills

- Browse the contents of storage devices
- Change folder and view options
- Create a folder
- Rename a file and folder
- Select, move, copy, and paste folders and files
- Delete files and folders to and restore files and folders from the Recycle Bin
- Explore the Control Panel
- Use search tools to find applications, folders, and/or files
- Customize the appearance of the desktop
- Change the screen resolution

Student Resources

Before beginning the activities in Windows Section 2, copy to your storage medium the WindowsMedS2 folder from the Student Resources CD. This folder contains the data files you need to complete the projects in this Windows section.

Projects Overview

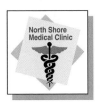
North Shore Medical Clinic

Organize files and folders by creating and renaming folders and moving, copying, renaming, deleting, and restoring files. Search for specific files and customize your desktop to the clinic's computer standard.

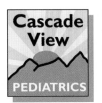
Cascade View PEDIATRICS

Organize files for Cascade View Pediatrics by creating folders and copying, moving, renaming, and deleting files.

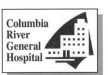
Columbia River General Hospital

Organize files by creating folders and copying, moving, renaming, and deleting files. Assist your supervisor by searching for information on setting up a computer for multiple users and working with libraries.

Activity 2.1

Browsing Storage Devices and Files in the This PC Window

The This PC window displays by default when you click the File Explorer button on the Taskbar. Use the This PC window to view the various storage devices connected to your computer. The Content pane of the This PC window displays an icon for each hard disk drive and each removable storage medium such as a CD, DVD, or USB device. Next to each storage device icon, Windows provides the amount of storage space available as well as a bar with the amount of used space shaded with color. With this visual cue, you can see at a glance the amount of space available relative to the capacity of the device. Double-click a device icon in the Content pane to display a list of the files stored on the device. You can access another device or folder by using the Navigation pane or the Address bar of the This PC window.

Project

As a medical office assistant at North Shore Medical Clinic, you are getting ready to organize the filing system. You decide to start by exploring the contents of the various storage devices on the computer you are using.

Note: To complete the projects in this section, you will need to use a USB flash drive or computer hard drive (do not use OneDrive). Before beginning the projects in this section, make sure you have copied the WindowsMedS2 folder from the Student Resources CD to your storage medium.

1. If you have not already done so, insert into an empty USB port the storage medium that you are using for the files in this course.

2. Click the File Explorer button [ ] on the Taskbar to display the This PC window, as shown in Figure WIN2.1. Your window will look slightly different from the one shown in the figure.

FIGURE WIN2.1 This PC Window

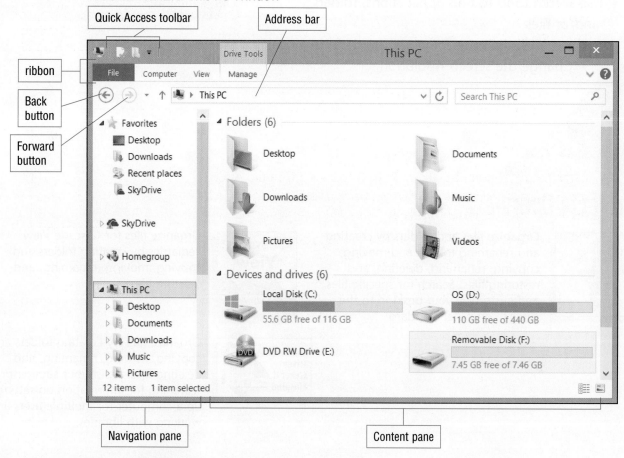

(3) Double-click the icon for the hard disk drive named *Local Disk (C:)*.

In Brief
Display This PC Window
Click File Explorer button on Taskbar.

The Content pane of the This PC window displays the files and folders stored on the local hard disk drive with the drive letter *C:*. The Address bar in the This PC window also updates to show the location where you are viewing Local Disk (C:) within your PC. You can navigate back to the This PC window by clicking either the Back button or *This PC* in the Address bar.

(4) Click the Back button 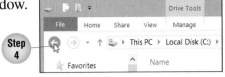 to return to the This PC window.

(5) Double-click the icon for the storage medium onto which you copied the WindowsMedS2 folder.
Note: The screen captures in this section show **Removable Disk (F:)** *as the storage medium in the* **This PC window. Your icon label and drive letter may vary.**

USB flash drives are shown in the *Devices and drives* section of the Content pane. Each device is assigned an alphabetic drive letter, usually starting at C and continuing through the alphabet, depending on the number of drives and removable devices that are currently in use. Next to the drive letter, a label displays. The content of this label depends on the drive or drive manufacturer. If no manufacturer label is present for a USB flash drive, Windows displays *Removable Disk*.

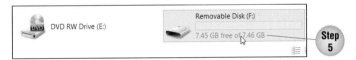

(6) Double-click the *WindowsMedS2* folder to view its contents in the Content pane.

(7) Look at the Address bar and notice how it displays the path to the current content: *This PC* ▶ *Removable Disk (F:)* ▶ *WindowsMedS2*.

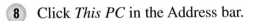

You can use the Address bar to navigate to any other device or folder by clicking the drive or folder name in the Address bar, or by clicking one of the right-pointing arrows to view a drop-down list of folders or other devices.

(8) Click *This PC* in the Address bar.

(9) Click the right-pointing arrow ▶ next to *This PC* in the Address bar (the arrow becomes a down-pointing arrow) and then click the drive letter representing your removable storage device.

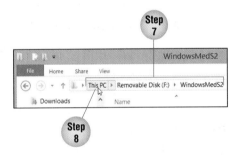

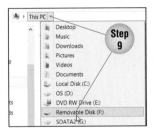

(10) Click *Desktop* in the *Favorites* section of the Navigation pane.

You can also change what displays in the Content pane by clicking the device or folder name in the Navigation pane. Click the right-pointing arrow next to a device or folder name in the Content pane to view what is stored within the item.

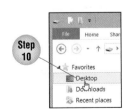

(11) Close the This PC window.

Activity 2.2

Changing Folder and View Options

When working with File Explorer, you can change the view to display items as icons, as a list, as tiles, or with thumbnail images of their contents. With the Content pane in Details view, you can click a column heading to sort the list alphabetically in ascending or descending order. In Activity 1.5, you displayed file extensions by inserting a check mark in the *File name extensions* check box on the View tab. File extensions are helpful for identifying the application in which the file was created. You can also use other buttons on the View tab to customize the File Explorer environment. You can change how panes are displayed, the layout of the Content pane, how content is sorted, and which features are shown or hidden.

Project

You decide to experiment with various view options as you continue to become acquainted with the Windows 8.1 environment and prepare to organize your filing system.

1. Click the File Explorer button on the Taskbar.

2. Click the drive letter representing your storage medium in the *This PC* section of the Navigation pane.

3. Double-click the *WindowsMedS2* folder in the Content pane.

4. Click the View tab located below the Title bar in the WindowsMedS2 window.

5. Click the *Large icons* option in the Layout group on the View tab.

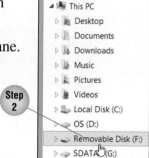

After you click an option on the View tab, the View tab collapses to provide more space in the File Explorer window.

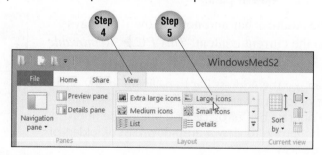

6. Click the View tab.

7. Click the *Details* option in the Layout group on the View tab.

8. With folders now displayed in Details view, click the *Name* column heading to sort the list in descending order by name.

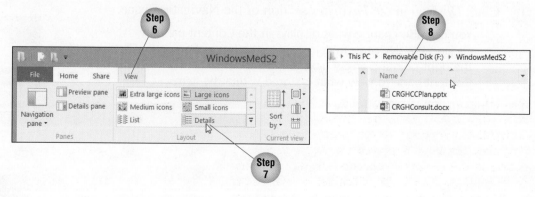

9 Click the *Name* column heading again to sort the list in ascending order by name.

10 Click the View tab and then click the Options button 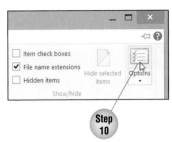 to open the Folder Options dialog box.

In Brief
Change Current View
1. Click View tab.
2. Click desired option in Layout group.

Change Folder and View Options
1. Click View tab.
2. Click Options button.
3. Click desired option(s).
4. Click OK.

Step 10

11 Click the *Open each folder in its own window* option in the *Browse folders* section of the General tab and then click OK.

12 Close the WindowsMedS2 window.

13 Click the File Explorer button on the Taskbar and then click the drive representing your storage medium in the *This PC* section of the Navigation pane.

14 Double-click the *WindowsMedS2* folder.

> Notice that a new window with the WindowsMedS2 content opens on top of the original File Explorer window.

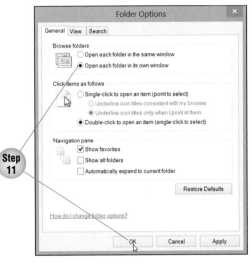

Step 11

15 Close the WindowsMedS2 window.

16 Click the View tab, click the Options button, click the Restore Defaults button located near the bottom of the General tab, and then click OK.

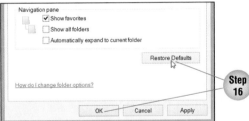

Step 16

17 Close the Removable Disk (F:) window.

In Addition

Changing the Default View for All Folders

You can set a certain view as the default for all folders of a similar type (such as all disk drive folders or all documents folders). To do this, open a File Explorer window, navigate to a type of folder for which you want to change the default view, and then change the current view to the desired view. Next, click the View tab and then click the Options button at the right side of the ribbon. At the Folder Options dialog box, click the View tab, click the Apply to Folders button in the *Folder views* section (as shown at the right), and then click OK. Click Yes at the Folder Views message box asking if you want all folders of this type to match this folder's view settings.

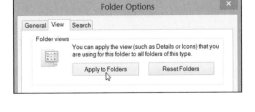

Activity 2.3

Creating a Folder; Renaming a Folder or File

As you begin working with programs, you will create files in which data (information) is saved. A file might be a Word document, an Excel workbook, a PowerPoint presentation, or pictures and videos that you transfer from your digital camera. As you begin creating and working with files, it is important to develop a system of organization so that you can easily retrieve a document or image when you need it. The first step in organizing your files is to create folders, which act as containers in which you can place similar types of files. File management tasks such as creating a folder, renaming a folder or file, and copying and moving files and folders can be completed at a variety of locations, including within File Explorer windows.

Project

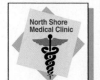

To begin organizing files for the North Shore Medical Clinic, you will create some new folders.

1 Click the File Explorer button on the Taskbar.

2 Double-click the icon representing the storage medium onto which you copied the WindowsMedS2 folder.

3 Click the New folder button ▊ on the Quick Access toolbar.

> A new folder icon appears in the Content pane with the text *New folder* already selected.

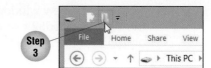

4 With the text *New folder* selected next to the folder icon, type **PatientInfo** and then press Enter. (As soon as you type the *P* in *PatientInfo*, the existing text *New Folder* is immediately deleted.)

> This changes the folder name from *New Folder* to *PatientInfo*.

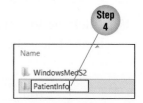

5 You can also create a new folder by using a shortcut menu. Right-click a blank, unused area of the Content pane, point to *New*, and then click *Folder*.

6 With the text *New folder* already selected next to the folder icon, type **Procedures** and then press Enter.

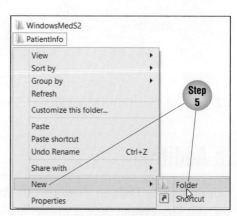

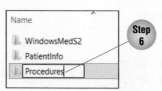

7 Click the *PatientInfo* folder to select it.

8 Click the Home tab and then click the Rename button in the Organize group.

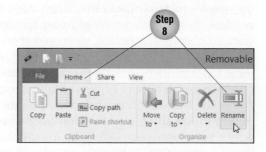

9 With the text *PatientInfo* selected, type Education and then press Enter.

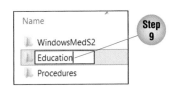

> You can also use the shortcut menu to rename a file or folder.

10 Right-click the *Procedures* folder and then click *Rename* at the shortcut menu.

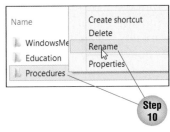

11 With the text *Procedures* selected, type Administration and then press Enter.

12 Double-click the *WindowsMedS2* folder.

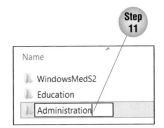

13 Right-click ***NSMCNotice.docx*** and then click *Rename* at the shortcut menu.

14 Type NSMCDiabetesHWANotice and then press Enter.

> When you rename a file, notice that Windows does not select the file extension. Programs such as Microsoft Word and Microsoft Excel automatically assign a file extension to each document or workbook you create. These file extensions should remain intact so that Windows will know which program is needed to open each file. If you rename or remove a file extension by accident, Windows prompts you with a message that the file may no longer be usable and asks you if you are sure.

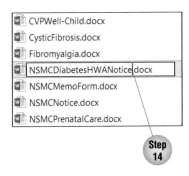

15 Close the WindowsMedS2 window.

In Brief

Create New Folder
1. Display This PC window.
2. Double-click device on which to create folder.
3. Click New folder button on Quick Access toolbar.
4. Type folder name and then press Enter.

Rename Folder or File
1. Display This PC window.
2. Navigate to desired location.
3. Right-click file to be renamed.
4. At shortcut menu, click *Rename*.
5. Type new file name and then press Enter.

In Addition

Learning More about Organizing Files into Folders

Think of a folder on the computer the same way you think of a file folder in which you would store paper documents in a filing cabinet. Generally, you put similar types of documents into the same folder. For example, all of your rent receipts might be placed inside a file folder on which you have written the label *Rent*. Similarly, on the computer, you could create a folder named *Rent* in which you store the electronic copies of all of your rental documents. On the computer, folders can be placed within other folders for added organization. A folder within a folder is referred to as a ***subfolder***. For example, you may have thousands of pictures stored on your computer. Saving all of the pictures in one folder named *Pictures* would be too cumbersome—you would have to search a long time to locate a particular picture. Instead, you might create subfolders labeled by month or event within the Pictures folder to keep related pictures together in one place.

Activity 2.4

Selecting, Copying, and Pasting Folders and Files

In addition to creating and renaming files and folders, file management activities include selecting, moving, copying, and deleting files or folders. Open a File Explorer window to perform file management tasks. You can use options on the Home tab or at the shortcut menus. More than one file or folder can be moved, copied, or deleted at one time. Select adjacent files and folders using the Shift key and select nonadjacent files and folders using the Ctrl key. When selecting multiple files or folders, you may want to change the view in the File Explorer window so that you can see all the files or folders you want to select.

Project As you continue to organize files for the North Shore Medical Clinic, you will copy files to the Education folder you created.

1. At the Windows desktop, click the File Explorer button to open the This PC window.

2. Double-click the icon representing your storage medium.

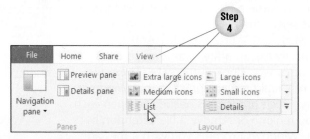

3. Double-click the *WindowsMedS2* folder in the Content pane.

4. Click the View tab and then click the *List* option in the Layout group.

5. Click *Fibromyalgia.xlsx* in the Content pane.

   Click once to select a file. Windows displays file properties for the selected file in the bottom left corner of the window.

6. Hold down the Shift key, click *NSMCTable02.docx*, and then release the Shift key.

   Clicking *NSMCTable02.docx* while holding down the Shift key causes all files from *Fibromyalgia.xlsx* through *NSMCTable02.docx* to be selected.

7. Position the mouse pointer within the selected group of files, right-click, and then click *Copy* at the shortcut menu.

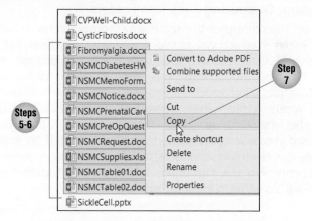

8 Click the Back button at the left side of the Address bar.

9 Double-click the *Education* folder.

10 Right-click in the Content pane and then click *Paste* at the shortcut menu.

> When a large file or group of files is copied and pasted, Windows displays a message box with a progress bar to indicate the approximate time required to copy the files from one location to another. The message box closes when the process is complete.

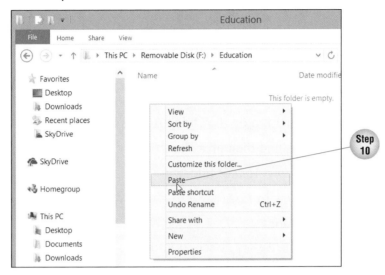

In Brief
Copy and Paste
Folders and Files
1. Select folders or files.
2. Click Home tab.
3. Click Copy button.
4. Navigate to destination.
5. Click Paste button.

OR

1. Select files or folders.
2. Right-click files or folders.
3. Click *Copy*.
4. Navigate to destination.
5. Right-click blank area of Content pane.
6. Click *Paste*.

11 Click in a blank area of the Content pane to deselect the file names.

12 Close the Education window.

In Addition

Copying and Pasting by Dragging and Dropping

You can copy a file or folder to another location using a drag-and-drop technique. To do this, open a File Explorer window and display the desired file or folder in the Content pane. Position the mouse pointer on the file or folder to be copied, hold down the left mouse button, drag to the destination drive or folder name in the *Favorites, OneDrive,* or *This PC* sections of the Navigation pane (as shown at the right), and then release the mouse button. By default, when you drag a file from one disk drive to another, Windows uses a Copy command. When you drag from one folder to another on the same disk drive, you must hold down the Ctrl key as you drag to create a copy. If you do not hold down the Ctrl key, the file will simply be moved. Alternatively, you can open two windows and arrange them side-by-side on the desktop. In one window, display the files that you want to copy. In the other window, display the destination folder. Select the files to be copied and then hold down the Ctrl key (if necessary) while dragging the selected files to the destination window.

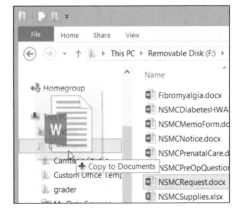

Activity 2.5

Moving Folders and Files

Move files in a File Explorer window in a manner similar to how you would copy and paste them. Select the file(s) and/or folder(s) that you want to move, position the mouse pointer over them, right-click, and then click *Cut* at the shortcut menu. Navigate to the desired destination location, right-click a blank area of the Content pane, and then click *Paste* at the shortcut menu. You can also use the Copy, Cut and Paste buttons in the Clipboard group on the Home tab of a File Explorer window.

Project

As you continue to develop the file organization system for North Shore Medical Clinic, you decide to create another folder and move some files into the new folder.

1. At the Windows desktop, display the This PC window.

2. Double-click the icon representing your storage medium.

3. Click the New folder button on the Quick Access toolbar.

4. Type **OtherProviders** and then press Enter.

5. Double-click the *WindowsMedS2* folder.

6. Change the current view to *List*.

7. Click **CRGHConsult.docx**.

   Clicking once on the file simply selects it; double-clicking the file would instruct Windows to open Word and then open the document.

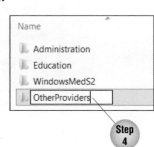

8. Hold down the Ctrl key, click **CRGHRadiologyReq.xlsx**, click **CVPMemoForm.docx**, and then release the Ctrl key.

   Use the Ctrl key to select multiple nonadjacent files.

9. Click the Home tab and then click the Cut button in the Clipboard group.

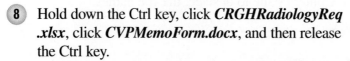

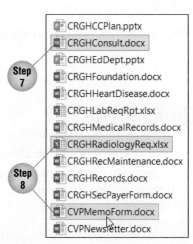

10. Click the Back button at the left side of the Address bar.

11. Double-click the *OtherProviders* folder.

12 Click the Home tab and then click the Paste button in the Clipboard group.

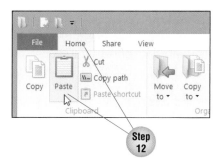

Step
12

In Brief
Move Nonadjacent Files to New Folder
1. Click first file name.
2. Hold down Ctrl key, click additional file names, and then release Ctrl key.
3. Click Cut button in Clipboard group on Home tab.
4. Navigate to desired destination drive and/or folder.
5. Click Paste button in Clipboard group on Home tab.

13 Click in a blank area of the Content pane to deselect the file names.

14 Click the Back button at the left side of the Address bar.

15 Double-click the *WindowsMedS2* folder.

> Notice the three files *CRGHConsult.docx*, *CRGHRadiologyReq.xlsx*, and *CVPMemoForm.docx* no longer reside in the WindowsMedS2 folder.

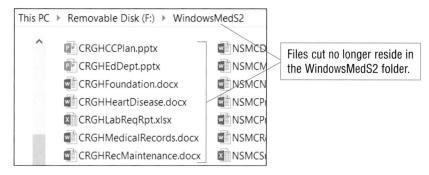

Files cut no longer reside in the WindowsMedS2 folder.

16 Close the WindowsMedS2 window.

In Addition

Displaying Disk or Drive Properties

Information such as the amount of used space and free space on a disk or drive and the disk or drive hardware is available at the Properties dialog box. To display the Local Disk (C:) Properties dialog box, similar to the one shown at the right, display the This PC window. At the This PC window, right-click *Local Disk (C:)* and then click *Properties* at the shortcut menu. With the General tab selected, information displays about used and free space on the drive. Click the Tools tab to display error-checking, backup, and defragmentation options. The Hardware tab displays the name and type of all disk drives as well as the device properties. The Sharing tab displays options for sharing folders and changing user permissions. To enable quota management, where you can set space limits for each user, click the Quota tab.

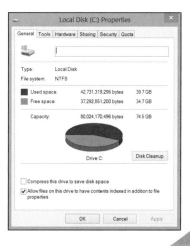

Activity 2.6

Deleting Folders and Files to the Recycle Bin

To delete a file or folder, display a File Explorer window and then display in the Content pane the file(s) and/or folder(s) you want to delete. Select the file(s) and/or folder(s) and then press the Delete key on the keyboard, or right-click the selected files and then click *Delete* at the shortcut menu. At the message asking you to confirm the deletion, click Yes.

Deleting the wrong file can be a nuisance, but the Recycle Bin in Windows helps protect your work so that an accidental deletion doesn't become a disaster. The Recycle Bin acts just like an office wastepaper basket: you can "throw away" (delete) unwanted files, but you can "reach in" to the Recycle Bin and take out (restore) a file if you threw it away by accident. Files or folders deleted from a hard disk drive are automatically sent to the Recycle Bin, but files or folders deleted from a removable disk, such as your USB flash drive, are deleted permanently.

Project As you continue organizing files, you will copy a file and a folder from your storage medium to the Documents folder on the hard drive and then delete a file and folder to the Recycle Bin.

1. At the Windows desktop, display the This PC window.

2. Double-click the icon representing your storage medium.

3. Click the *OtherProviders* folder to select it.

4. Position the mouse pointer over the selected folder name, hold down the left mouse button, drag the folder to the Documents folder in the *This PC* section of the Navigation pane, and then release the mouse button.

   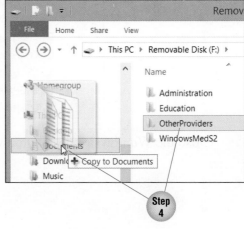

   As you point to the Documents folder in the Navigation pane, Windows displays the ScreenTip *Copy to Documents*.

5. Double-click the *Education* folder.

6. Click *Fibromyalgia.docx* to select it.

7. Position the mouse pointer over the selected file name, hold down the left mouse button, drag the file to the Documents folder in the *This PC* section of the Navigation pane, and then release the mouse button.

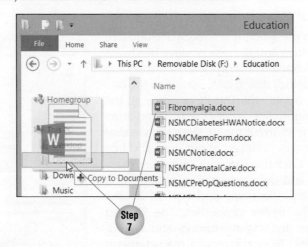

8 Click the *Documents* folder in the *This PC* section of the Navigation pane to display its contents in the Content pane.

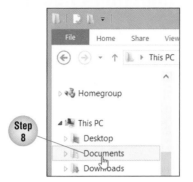

In Brief
Delete File or Folder
1. Click file or folder to select it.
2. Press Delete key.
3. At confirmation message, click Yes.

9 Click the *OtherProviders* folder to select it.

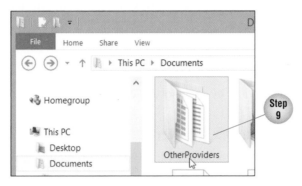

10 Press the Delete key on the keyboard.

11 Right-click ***Fibromyalgia.docx*** in the Content pane and then click *Delete* at the shortcut menu.

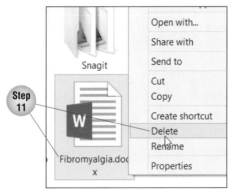

12 Close the Documents window.

In Addition

Deleting by Dragging and Dropping

Another method for deleting a file or folder is to drag the file or folder to the Recycle Bin icon on the desktop and then release the mouse button. This moves the file from its current location into the Recycle Bin. You can also select multiple files or folders and then drag and drop them into the Recycle Bin.

Activity 2.7

Restoring Folders and Files; Emptying Files from the Recycle Bin

A file or folder deleted to the Recycle Bin can be restored using options at the Recycle Bin window. Display this window by double-clicking the Recycle Bin icon on the Windows desktop. When you restore a file or folder, it is removed from the Recycle Bin and returned to its original location. Just like a wastepaper basket can overflow, the Recycle Bin can become overfilled with too many files and folders, so it is important to empty it regularly. Emptying the Recycle Bin permanently deletes all files and folders. You can also delete a single file or folder from the Recycle Bin (rather than all files and folders).

Project You decide to learn more about the Recycle Bin by experimenting with restoring a file and deleting items from the Recycle Bin.

North Shore
Medical Clinic

1 At the Windows desktop, double-click the Recycle Bin icon.

The Recycle Bin window displays similar to the one shown in Figure WIN2.2.

2 At the Recycle Bin window, change the current view to *List*.

Change to List view by clicking the View tab and then clicking the *List* option in the Layout gallery.

3 Click **Fibromyalgia.docx** to select it.

Depending on the contents of the Recycle Bin, you may need to scroll down to display this document.

FIGURE WIN2.2 Recycle Bin Window

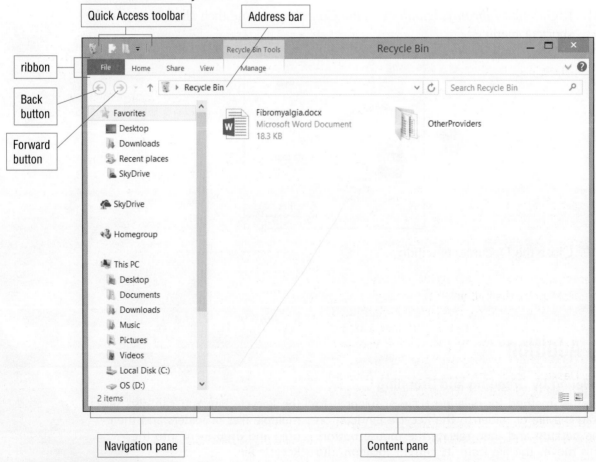

4 Click the Recycle Bin Tools Manager tab and then click the Restore the selected items button in the Restore group.

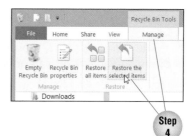

Step 4

> The file is removed from the Recycle Bin and returned to the location from which it was deleted.

5 Click the *OtherProviders* folder to select it.

6 Click the Restore the selected items button in the Restore group.

7 Close the Recycle Bin window.

8 At the Windows desktop, open the This PC window.

9 Double-click the *Documents* folder in the Content pane.

> Notice that the file and folder that you deleted have been restored from the Recycle Bin.

10 Delete the file and folder you restored. To do this, click the *OtherProviders* folder, hold down the Ctrl key, click ***Fibromyalgia.docx***, release the Ctrl key, and then press the Delete key.

11 Close the Documents window.

12 At the Windows desktop, double-click the Recycle Bin icon.

13 Click the *OtherProviders* folder, hold down the Ctrl key, click ***Fibromyalgia.docx***, and then release the Ctrl key.

Step 14

14 Click the Home tab and then click the Delete button in the Organize group.

15 At the Delete Multiple Items message box asking if you are sure you want to permanently delete the 2 items, click Yes.

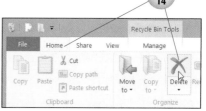

> To empty the entire contents of the Recycle Bin, click the Empty the Recycle Bin button in the Manage group on the Recycle Bin Tools Manage tab.

16 Close the Recycle Bin window.

In Brief

Restore File or Folder from Recycle Bin
1. At Windows desktop, double-click Recycle Bin icon.
2. At Recycle Bin window, click file or folder to select it.
3. Click Restore the selected items button on Recycle Bin Tools Manage tab.

Delete File or Folder from Recycle Bin
1. At Windows desktop, double-click Recycle Bin icon.
2. At Recycle Bin window, click file or folder to select it.
3. Press Delete key.
4. At confirmation message, click Yes.

In Addition

Showing or Hiding the Recycle Bin Icon on the Desktop

Even though the Recycle Bin icon displays on the desktop by default, you can choose to hide it if you wish. To do so, right-click a blank area of the desktop and then click *Personalize* at the shortcut menu. At the Personalization window, click *Change desktop icons* in the left pane. At the Desktop Icon Settings dialog box (shown at the right), click the *Recycle Bin* check box to remove the check mark and then click OK. Note the other desktop icons you can also choose to show or hide at this dialog box.

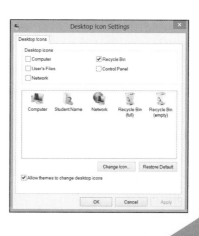

Activity 2.8

Exploring the Control Panel

The Windows 8.1 Control Panel offers a variety of categories, each containing icons you can use to customize the appearance and functionality of your computer. Display the Control Panel window by right-clicking the Start button and then clicking *Control Panel* at the shortcut menu. At the Control Panel window, available categories display in the Content pane. (By default, the Control Panel window opens in Category view. If your window opens in Large icons view or Small icons view, click the down-pointing arrow next to *View by*, located near the top right of the Control Panel window, and then click *Category* at the drop-down list.) Click a category or hyperlinked option and a list of tasks, a list of icons, or a separate window displays.

Project

You want to know how to customize your computer for your own needs, so you decide to explore the Control Panel window.

1. At the Windows desktop, right-click the Start button and then click *Control Panel* at the shortcut menu.

   The Control Panel window displays similar to the one shown in Figure WIN2.3.

2. At the Control Panel window, click the <u>Appearance and Personalization</u> hyperlink.

3. After viewing the tasks and icons available in the Appearance and Personalization category, click the Back button.

4. Click the <u>Hardware and Sound</u> hyperlink.

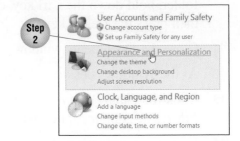

FIGURE WIN2.3 Control Panel Window

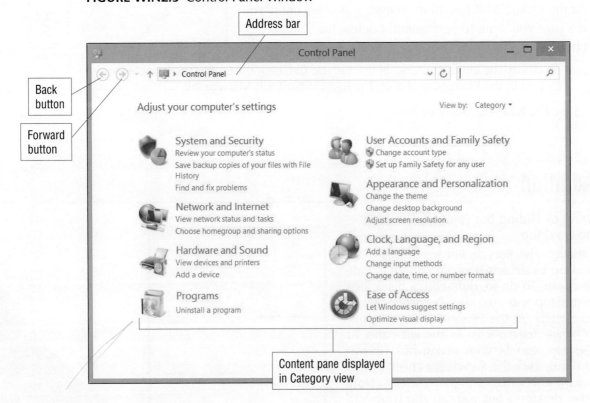

5 Click the <u>Mouse</u> hyperlink in the Devices and Printers category.

This displays the Mouse Properties dialog box.

In Brief

Display Control Panel
1. Right-click Start button.
2. Click *Control Panel*.

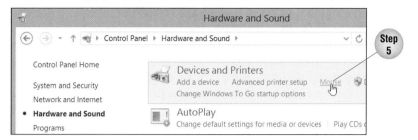

6 At the Mouse Properties dialog box, click each tab and review the available options.

7 Click the Cancel button to close the Mouse Properties dialog box.

8 Click the Back button.

9 Click the <u>Programs</u> hyperlink in the Content pane.

10 At the Programs window, click the <u>Programs and Features</u> hyperlink.

This is where you would uninstall a program on your computer.

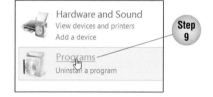

11 Click the Back button twice.

12 Click the <u>System and Security</u> hyperlink.

13 Click the <u>System</u> hyperlink.

14 Maximize the window.

15 Close the Control Panel window.

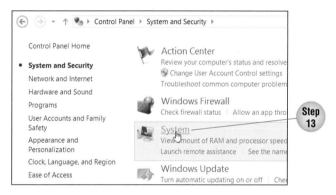

In Addition

Changing the Control Panel View

By default, the Control Panel window displays categories of tasks in what is called Category view. This view can be changed to *Large icons* or *Small icons*. In the Large icons view (shown at the right), options in the Control Panel are shown alphabetically by icon name. To change from Category view to Large icons view or Small icons view, click the down-pointing arrow next to *View by*, located near the top right of the Control Panel window, and then click the desired option at the drop-down list.

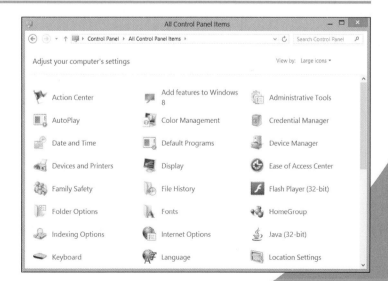

Activity 2.9

Using Windows Search Tools

Windows includes a Search feature that is accessed through the Charm bar. You can quickly find an application, setting, or file by typing the first few letters of the name. If your computer has many applications and files stored on the hard disk, using the search tool allows you to locate what you need in a few seconds and with minimal mouse clicks.

You can also search for items using the search text box located in the upper right corner of each File Explorer window. Type in this text box the first few letters of a file you need to locate. The Content pane is filtered instantly to display items that match the text you entered.

Windows can return search results very quickly because the operating system maintains an index in the background in which all of the keywords associated with the applications, settings, and files on your computer are referenced. This index is constantly updated as you work. When you type an entry in a search text box, Windows consults the index rather than conducting a search of the entire hard drive.

Project

You decide to experiment with the search capabilities of Windows to see how you can locate programs and documents more quickly in the future.

1. At the Windows desktop, display the Charm bar and then click the Search button.

2. With the insertion point positioned in the search text box at the top of the Search panel, type **calc**.

    As soon as you begin typing in the search text box, Windows begins to display relevant results. Notice that two Calculator programs display below the search text box.

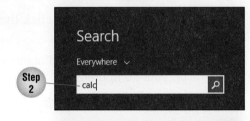

3. Click the second Calculator tile in the list.

4. Close the Calculator window.

5. Display the Charm bar and then click the Search button.

6. Type **note** in the search text box.

    Windows lists all applications stored on the computer you are using that are associated with the text *note*. This includes the Notepad application, which you can use to create, edit, and save simple text-based documents.

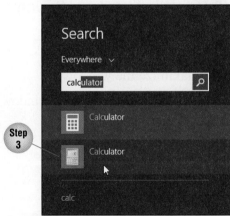

7. Press the Esc key.

    Pressing the Esc key clears the search text box and the search results list.

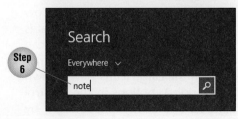

8. Display the This PC window.

9. Double-click the icon representing your storage medium.

10. Double-click the *WindowsMedS2* folder and then change the current view to *Large icons*.

11. Click in the *Search WindowsMedS2* text box at the right side of the Address bar.

12 Type **nsmc**.

As soon as you begin typing, Windows filters the list of files in the Content pane based on the letters you have typed. Notice that the Address bar displays *Search Results in WindowsMedS2* to indicate that the search results displayed are only from the current folder. If you want to search other locations or using other file properties, click one of the options on the Search Tools Search tab.

In Brief

Search from Charm bar
1. Click Search button on Charm bar.
2. Type search criteria in search text box.

Search from File Explorer Window
1. Open This PC or Documents window.
2. Type search criteria in search text box.

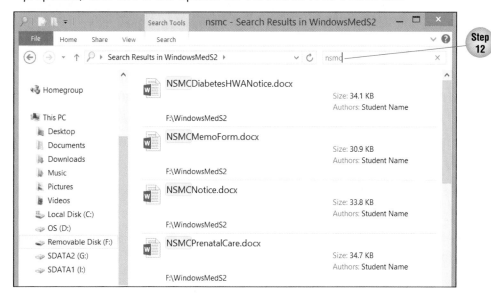

13 With the insertion point still positioned in the search text box, press the Backspace key to remove *nsmc* and then type **cvp**.

The list of files in the Content pane changes to display those files that begin with *CVP*.

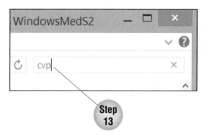

14 Double-click ***CVPWell-Child.docx***.

The file opens in Microsoft Word.

15 Close Microsoft Word by clicking the Close button in the upper right corner of the window.

16 Close the WindowsMedS2 window.

In Addition

Using a Wildcard Character in a Search

When conducting a search, you can type an asterisk (*) in place of any number of letters, numbers, or symbols within a file name. For example, typing ***pre*** into the *Search WindowsMedS2* text box would return **NSMCPrenatalCare.docx** and **NSMCPreOpQuestions.docx** as search results. Notice that both of the files have *pre* in the middle of the file name but any number of other characters before and after *pre*.

Activity 2.10

Customizing the Desktop

The Windows 8.1 operating environment is customizable. You can change background patterns and colors; specify a screen saver to display when the screen sits idle for a specific period of time; or change the color scheme for windows, Title bars, and system fonts. Make these types of changes at the Personalization window. Be careful when customizing your desktop at work, however — many companies adopt a corporate standard for computer display properties.

Project

North Shore Medical Clinic

You decide to look at the customization options available for the desktop and set the screen resolution to the corporate standard for computers at the North Shore Medical Clinic. *Note: Before completing this activity, check with your instructor to determine if you can customize the desktop. If necessary, practice these steps on your home computer.*

1. At the Windows desktop, right-click a blank area and then click *Personalize* at the shortcut menu.

2. At the Personalization window, click the <u>Desktop Background</u> hyperlink at the bottom of the window.

   Make a note of the current desktop background name.

3. Scroll up and down through the available images, click an image that you like, and then click the Save changes button.

4. Click the <u>Screen Saver</u> hyperlink.

   Make a note of the current screen saver name.

5. At the Screen Saver Settings dialog box, click the option box below *Screen saver* and then click *Ribbons* at the drop-down list.

   A preview of the screen saver displays toward the top of the dialog box.

6. Click the up- or down-pointing arrows next to the *Wait* measurement box until *1* displays.

7. Click OK.

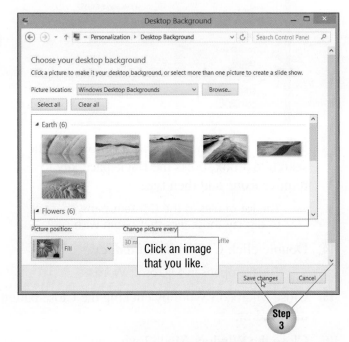

Click an image that you like.

Step 3

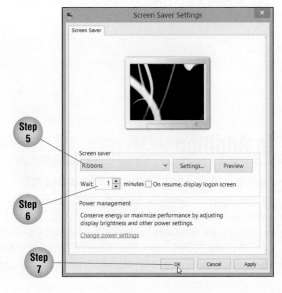

Step 5

Step 6

Step 7

8 Click the <u>Color</u> hyperlink.

> Make a note of the color that displays next to *Current color* below the color boxes.

9 Click the *Color 9* box (second column in the bottom row) and then click the Save changes button.

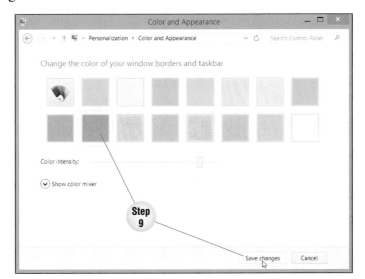

10 Close the Personalization window. Let the screen remain idle for one minute until the screen saver displays.

11 Move the mouse to deactivate the screen saver and then double-click the Recycle Bin icon.

> Notice that the Color 9 color scheme has been applied to the Taskbar and the window borders.

12 Close the Recycle Bin window.

13 Reinstate the original desktop settings by right-clicking a blank area of the desktop, clicking *Personalize* at the shortcut menu, and then returning the desktop background, screen saver, and window color to the original settings you noted before you began making changes.

14 Right-click a blank area of the desktop and then click *Screen resolution* at the shortcut menu.

> In the next steps, you will set the screen resolution to *1600 × 900 pixels*, which is the corporate standard for all desktops at North Shore Medical Clinic. Standardizing display properties is considered a best practice in organizations that support many computer users.

15 At the Screen Resolution window, look at the current setting displayed in the *Resolution* option box; for example, *1920 × 1080*. If your screen is already set to *1600 × 900*, click OK to close the window and complete this activity.

> Screen resolution is measured in pixels. The term ***pixel*** is an abbreviation of *picture element* and refers to a single dot or point on the display monitor. Changing the screen resolution to a higher number of pixels means that more information can be seen on the screen as items are scaled to a smaller size.

continues

In Brief
Change Screen Resolution
1. Right-click blank area of desktop.
2. Click *Screen resolution*.
3. Click Resolution option box.
4. Click desired resolution.
5. Click OK.
6. Click Keep changes button.

16 Click the *Resolution* option box and then drag the slider bar up or down until the screen resolution is set to *1600 × 900*. If necessary, check with your instructor for alternate instructions.

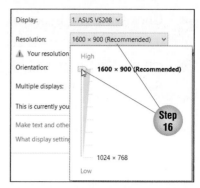

17 Click in the window outside the drop-down list, click OK, and then click the Keep changes button at the Display Settings message box asking if you want to keep the display settings.

18 At the Screen Resolution window, click the Make text and other items larger or smaller hyperlink located toward the lower left corner of the window.

19 At the Display window, make sure the *Let me choose one scaling level for all my displays* check box contains a check mark and then click the *Medium - 125%* option.

20 Click the Apply button.

21 At the message indicating that you must sign out of your computer, click the Sign out now button.

22 Log back into your account.

> The screen captures in this textbook use 1600 × 900 screen resolution and the display of text and items is set to Medium - 125%. If the computer you are using has a different screen resolution, your screen may not match the textbook illustrations. For additional information, refer to the In Addition below.

In Addition

Understanding Screen Resolution and the Display of the Microsoft Office Ribbon

Before you begin learning the applications in the Microsoft Office 2013 suite, take a moment to check the display settings on the computer you are using. The ribbon in the Microsoft Office suite adjusts to the screen resolution setting of your computer monitor. Computer monitors set at a high resolution will have the ability to show more buttons on the ribbon than will monitors set to low resolution. The screen captures in this textbook were taken at a screen resolution of 1600 x 900 pixels. Below, the Word ribbon is shown three ways: at a lower screen resolution (1366 x 768 pixels), at the screen resolution featured throughout this textbook, and at a higher screen resolution (1920 x 1080 pixels). Note the differences in the appearance of the ribbon in all three examples. If possible, set your display to 1600 x 900 pixels to match the illustrations you will see in this textbook.

1366 x 768 pixels

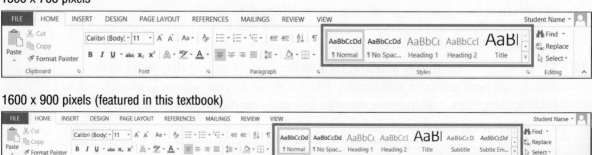

1600 x 900 pixels (featured in this textbook)

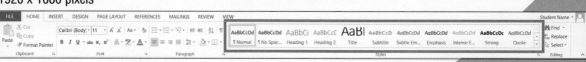

1920 x 1080 pixels

Features Summary

Feature	Button/Icon	Action
Control Panel window		Right-click Start button and then click *Control Panel.*
copy files/folders		At File Explorer window, select files/folders to be copied, right-click in selected group, click *Copy*, navigate to destination folder, right-click in Content pane, and then click *Paste.*
create new folder		At File Explorer window, click New Folder button on Quick Access toolbar.
delete files/folders		At File Explorer window, select files to be deleted, press Delete key, and then click Yes.
folder options		Click View tab and then click Options button.
move files/folders		At File Explorer window, select files/folders to be moved, right-click in selected group, click *Cut*, navigate to destination folder, right-click in Content pane, and then click *Paste.*
Recycle Bin		Double-click Recycle Bin icon.
rename file/folder		At File Explorer window, right-click file/folder, click *Rename,* type new name, and then press Enter.
restore files/folders from Recycle Bin		At Recycle Bin window, select desired files/folders, click Recycle Bin Tools Manage tab, and then click *Restore the selected items* button.
search for programs or documents		Display Charm bar, click Search button, and then type search criteria in search text box; or, open This PC window and then type search criteria in search text box.
select adjacent files/folders		Click first file/folder, hold down Shift key, and then click last file/folder.
select nonadjacent files/folders		Click first file/folder, hold down Ctrl key, and then click any other files/folders.
This PC window		Click File Explorer button on Taskbar.

Knowledge Check

Completion: In the space provided at the right, indicate the correct term, command, or option.

1. Navigate to any other device or folder from the current device or folder using the Navigation pane or this bar in a File Explorer window. _____

2. Click this button to display in the Content pane the contents of the location previously viewed. _____

3. Change the display of files and folders in a File Explorer window to *List* or *Details* using this group on the View tab. _____

4. Tell File Explorer to open each folder in its own window at this dialog box. _____

5. Click this button on the Quick Access toolbar to create a new folder in a File Explorer window. _____

6. To select adjacent files, click the first file, hold down this key, and then click the last file. _____

7. To select nonadjacent files, click the first file, hold down this key, and then click any other desired files. _____

8. Click this button in the Clipboard group on the Home tab to move selected files. _____

9. Files deleted from the hard drive are sent here. _____

10. Open this window to display a list of categories or icons you can use to customize the appearance and functionality of your computer. _____

11. Access the Windows Search feature using this bar at the desktop. _____

12. Access options for changing the background, screen saver, and color scheme of the desktop at this window. _____

Skills Review

Review 1 Browsing Devices and Changing the View

1. Open the This PC window.
2. Change to Large Icons view.
3. Turn on the option to open each folder in its own window.
4. Display the contents of your storage medium.
5. Display the contents of the WindowsMedS2 folder.
6. Change to Details view.
7. Close the WindowsMedS2 window.
8. Close the window for your storage medium.
9. Display the Folder Options dialog box and then select the option to open each folder in the same window.
10. Change to Tiles view and then close the This PC window.

Review 2 Creating a Folder

1. Open the This PC window.
2. Display the contents of your storage medium.
3. Right-click a blank area of the Content pane, point to *New*, and then click *Folder*.
4. Type Worksheets and then press Enter.
5. Close the File Explorer window.

Review 3 Selecting, Copying, Moving, and Deleting Files

1. Open the This PC window.
2. Display the contents of your storage medium.
3. Display the contents of the WindowsMedS2 folder.
4. Change the current view to *List* if it is not already set to that option.
5. Click *CRGHLabReqRpt.xlsx* to select it, hold down the Ctrl key, and then click *CVPTravelExpenses.xlsx*.
6. Right-click either of the selected files and then click *Copy* at the shortcut menu.
7. Click the Back button.
8. Double-click the *Worksheets* folder.
9. Right-click in the Content pane, click *Paste*, and then click in a blank area to deselect the files.
10. Click the Back button and then double-click the *WindowsMedS2* folder.
11. Click *NSMCSupplies.xlsx* in the Content pane.
12. Click the Home tab, click the Organize button, and then click *Cut* at the drop-down list.
13. Click the Back button and then double-click the *Worksheets* folder.
14. Click the Home tab, click the Organize button, and then click *Paste* at the drop-down list.
15. Click the right-pointing arrow next to your storage medium in the Address bar and then click *WindowsMedS2* at the drop-down list.
16. Click *NSMCRequest.docx* in the Content pane, hold down the Shift key, and then click *NSMCTable02.docx*.
17. Press the Delete key and then click Yes at the Delete Multiple Items confirmation message.
18. Close the WindowsMedS2 window.

Review 4 Renaming Files

1. Open the This PC window.
2. Display the contents of your storage medium.
3. Display the contents of the WindowsMedS2 folder.
4. Right-click *CRGHCCPlan.pptx* and then click *Rename*.
5. Type CRGHReorgPlan and then press Enter.
6. Right-click *SickleCell.pptx* and then click *Rename*.
7. Type CCMASickleCellPres and then press Enter.
8. Close the WindowsMedS2 window.

Review 5 Searching for Files

1. Open the This PC window.
2. Display the contents of the WindowsMedS2 folder on your storage medium.
3. Type *dia* in the *Search WindowsMedS2* text box and view the search results.
4. Press the Esc key until the search text is cleared and all files are redisplayed.
5. Close the WindowsMedS2 window.
6. Click the Search button on the Charm bar.
7. Type *word* in the search text box. Notice the applications displayed.
8. Press the Esc key and then click outside the Search panel to close it.

Skills Assessment

Assessment 1 Managing Folders and Files

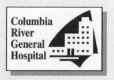

1. Create a new folder on your storage medium and name it *ColumbiaRiverGenHosp*.
2. Display the contents of the WindowsMedS2 folder.
3. If necessary, change the view to *List*.
4. Copy and paste all files beginning with *CRGH* into the ColumbiaRiverGenHosp folder.
5. If they are not already displayed, display the contents of the ColumbiaRiverGenHosp folder and then change the view to *List*.
6. Create a new folder within the ColumbiaRiverGenHosp folder and name it *Records*.
7. Move **CRGHMedicalRecords.docx** and **CRGHRecords.docx** from the ColumbiaRiverGenHosp folder into the Records subfolder.
8. Delete **CRGHReorgPlan.pptx** from the ColumbiaRiverGenHosp folder.
9. Rename **CRGHEdDept.pptx**, located in the ColumbiaRiverGenHosp folder, to **EducationPlan.pptx**.

Assessment 2 Managing Folders and Files

1. Display the contents of your storage medium.
2. Create a new folder named *CascadeViewPed*.
3. Display the contents of the WindowsMedS2 folder.
4. Copy all files beginning with *CVP* to the CascadeViewPed folder.
5. If necessary, display the contents of the CascadeViewPed folder and change the view to *List*.
6. Create a new folder within the CascadeViewPed folder and name it *Forms*.
7. Create a new folder within the Forms folder and name it *Travel*.
8. Move **CVPRules.docx** from the CascadeViewPed folder into the Forms subfolder.
9. Move **CVPTravelExpenses.xlsx** from the CascadeViewPed folder into the Travel subfolder.
10. Delete **CVPVancouver.pptx** from the CascadeViewPed folder.
11. Rename **CVPWell-Child.docx**, located in the CascadeViewPed folder, to **ChildAppointment.docx**.

Assessment 3 Deleting Folders and Files

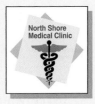

Note: Check with your instructor before completing this assessment. You may need to show him or her that you completed the activities within this section before you begin deleting the folders.

1. Display the contents of your storage medium.
2. Delete the Administration folder.
3. Delete the Education folder.
4. Delete the OtherProviders folder.

Assessment 4 Copying Folders from the Student CD

1. Display the contents of the student CD that accompanies this textbook in a File Explorer window.
2. Display the contents of the Unit3Word folder in the Content pane.
3. Select all of the subfolders in the Unit3Word folder and then copy them to your storage medium.
4. Display the contents of the Unit4Excel folder in the Content pane and then copy all of the subfolders in the Unit4Excel folder to your storage medium.
5. Display the contents of the Unit5PowerPoint folder in the Content pane and then copy all of the subfolders in the Unit5PowerPoint folder to your storage medium.
6. Display the contents of the IntegratingPrograms folder and then copy all of the subfolders to your storage medium.

Assessment 5 Searching for Information on User Accounts

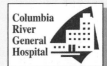

1. You have been asked by your supervisor at Columbia River General Hospital to learn about sharing your computer with other users. Your supervisor is considering adding an evening shift in your department and wants to find out how existing computer equipment can be set up for other users. Using the Windows Help and Support feature, search for information on user accounts. ***Hint: Type*** *user accounts* ***in the search text box and then press Enter. Consider reading the topic*** **Standard accounts versus administrator accounts** ***as your first step***.
2. Locate topics with information about the two types of user accounts: Standard and Administrator. Also determine the pros and cons of a Microsoft account versus a local account. Specifically, your supervisor would like to know which type of account is best suited for day-to-day work, and why.
3. Create a new folder on your storage medium and name it *WindowsEOS*.
4. Compose a memo to your instructor that describes the differences between the two types of user accounts and then provide your recommendation for which type of account should be used for individual users on each shift. Make sure to support your response with details from your research.
5. Save the memo in the WindowsEOS folder and name it **WinMedS2-UserAccounts**.
6. Print the memo.

Assessment 6 Searching for Information on Windows Touchscreen Features

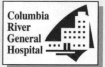

1. Your supervisor at Columbia River General Hospital is interested in upgrading the office computers to include a touchscreen, and she has asked you to research the touchscreen features in Windows 8.1. She wants you to find out how a touchscreen can be useful to her, as well as how to complete various tasks using a touchscreen. Using the Windows Help and Support feature, search for information on touchscreen interactions. *Hint: Type* touch *in the search text box and then press Enter. Consider reading the topic* **Touch: Swipe, tap, and beyond** *as your first step*.
2. Locate topics with information about using touchscreens in Windows 8.1.
3. Using Notepad or Word 2013, compose a list for your instructor that provides four common touch interactions (such as Tap or Slide) and what they accomplish.
4. Save the list in the WindowsEOS folder and name it **WinMedS2-TouchList**.
5. Print the memo.

Using INTERNET EXPLORER 11 *in the* Medical Office

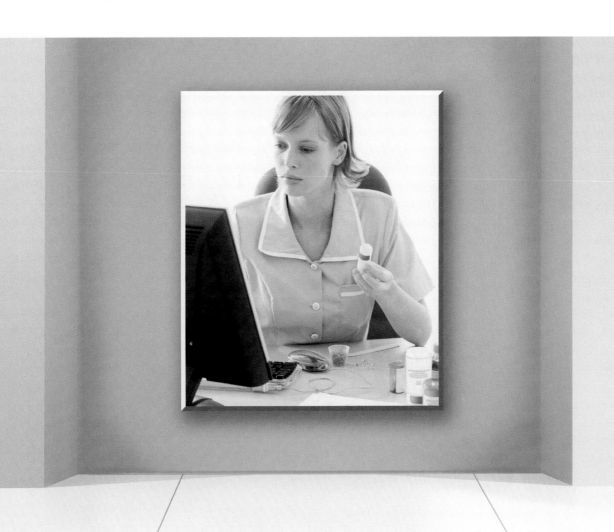

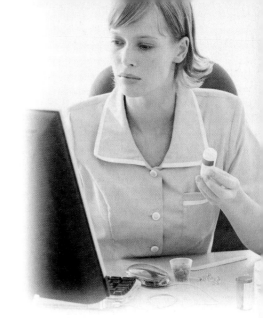

Internet Explorer

Browsing the Internet Using Internet Explorer 11

Skills

- Navigate to a site by typing a web address
- Use hyperlinks to navigate among web pages
- Search for information using search tools
- Use advanced search options to narrow a search
- Download content from a web page
- Evaluate content found on a web page

Projects Overview

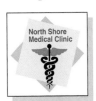

Visit websites for the Department of Health and Human Services and the Centers for Disease Control and Prevention. Search for websites that sell office forms, equipment, and supplies. Use advanced search options to locate information on the symptoms of and treatments for Hodgkin's disease. Locate images related to diabetes management and download the images to the desktop. Read newspaper home pages for current articles.

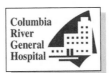

Search for two websites for medical schools in your state or province, browse each site, and compare navigation systems.

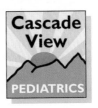

Search for websites about healthy living and download an online image to your computer.

51

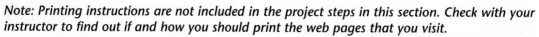

Activity 1.1

Navigating the Internet Using Web Addresses

In today's world, the Internet is used for a variety of tasks including locating information about any topic one can imagine, communicating with others through email and social networking sites, and buying and selling goods and services. In this section, you will use the Microsoft Internet Explorer web browser to locate information on the Internet. A *web browser* is software that allows you to view the text, images, and other content stored on web pages on the Internet. *Uniform Resource Locators*, referred to as *URLs*, identify web servers that have content on the Internet. A URL is often referred to as a *web address*. Just as you need a specific mailing address in order to identify your location to the post office, a server has a unique web address that identifies its location to the Internet.

Project

Dr. St. Claire is preparing a presentation on current health issues and has asked you to display and print the web pages of the Department of Health and Human Services and the Centers for Disease Control and Prevention.

Note: Printing instructions are not included in the project steps in this section. Check with your instructor to find out if and how you should print the web pages that you visit.

1. Display the Windows desktop and make sure you are connected to the Internet.

   Check with your instructor to determine if you need to complete additional steps to access the Internet.

2. Open Microsoft Internet Explorer by clicking the Internet Explorer button *e* on the Windows Taskbar.

   Figure IE1.1 identifies the elements of the Internet Explorer, version 11, window. The web page that displays in your Internet Explorer window may vary from what you see in Figure IE1.1. Refer to Figure IE1.2 on the next page for descriptions of the tools available in Internet Explorer.

3. At the Internet Explorer window, click in the Address bar (refer to Figure IE1.1), type **www.hhs.gov**, and then press Enter.

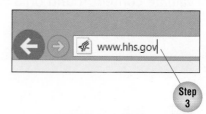

Step 3

FIGURE IE1.1 Internet Explorer Window

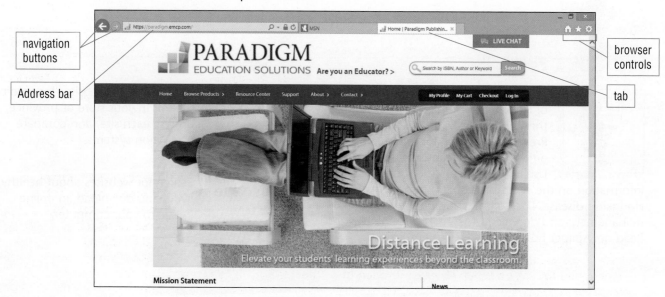

navigation buttons

Address bar

browser controls

tab

④ Scroll down the home page of the United States Department of Health and Human Services website by pressing the Down Arrow key on the keyboard or by clicking the down-pointing arrow on the vertical scroll bar at the right side of the Internet Explorer window.

> The first web page that appears for a website is called the *home page*.

⑤ Display the home page for the Centers for Disease Control and Prevention by clicking in the Address bar, typing **www.cdc.gov**, and then pressing Enter.

> As you begin to type the first few characters in the Address bar, a drop-down list appears below the Address bar with the names of websites that you have already visited that are spelled the same. Matched characters are displayed in blue for quick reference. If the web address you want displays in the drop-down list, you do not need to continue typing the address—simply click the desired URL at the drop-down list.

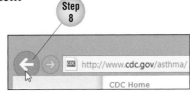

⑥ Click the <u>Diseases & Conditions</u> hyperlink located in the *HEALTH & SAFETY TOPICS* section in the middle of the page.

> Most web pages contain hyperlinks that you can click to connect to another page within the website or to another site on the Internet. Hyperlinks can display in a web page in a variety of ways. They can appear as underlined text, buttons, images, or icons, among others. To use a hyperlink, position the mouse pointer over it until the mouse pointer turns into a hand and then click the left mouse button.

⑦ Click the <u>Asthma</u> hyperlink and then view the content on the Asthma web page.

⑧ Click the Back button in the upper left corner of the screen (see Figure IE1.2) to return to the Diseases & Conditions web page.

⑨ Click the Forward button to return to the Asthma web page.

In Brief
Display Specific Website
1. At Windows desktop, click Internet Explorer button on Taskbar.
2. Click in Address bar and type web address.
3. Press Enter.

FIGURE IE1.2 Browsing and Navigating in Internet Explorer

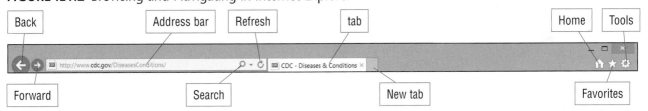

In Addition

Using Internet Explorer in the Modern UI

Windows 8.1 contains a new user interface (UI) that has been optimized for touch devices. If you access Internet Explorer through the Windows 8.1 Start screen, the Modern UI version of Internet Explorer displays. This version displays differently than the desktop version of Internet Explorer and is designed for use on touch devices. To open the Modern UI version of Internet Explorer, display the Windows 8.1 Start screen and then click the Internet Explorer tile. When the application opens, the Address bar and buttons appear at the bottom of the screen and are increased in size. All of the activities in this section use the desktop version of Internet Explorer. If the Internet Explorer button does not appear on the Taskbar, ask your instructor for help with accessing the desktop version of Internet Explorer.

Activity 1.2

Finding Information Using Search Tools

If you do not know the web address for a specific site or you want to find information on the Internet but do not know what site to visit, use a search engine to find what you need. A variety of search engines are available on the Internet. You can visit one of these websites to conduct a search, or you can search directly from the Internet Explorer window. To do this, simply click in the Address bar, type a keyword or phrase related to your search, and then press Enter. Within a few seconds, Internet Explorer's built-in search engine, Bing, will display your results in the Internet Explorer window.

Project

You work at North Shore Medical Clinic. Lee Elliott, the office manager, has asked you to locate sites on the Internet that sell medical office forms, equipment, and supplies. The clinic will be purchasing these items in the near future.

1 With the Internet Explorer window active, click in the Address bar.

2 Type **medical office forms** and then press Enter.

When you press the Enter key, a Bing page with a list of the search results displays. Bing is Microsoft's online search portal and is the default search engine used by Internet Explorer. Bing organizes search results by topic and provides related search suggestions.

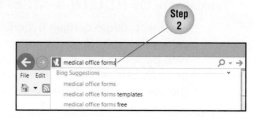

Step 2

3 Scroll down the search list, position the mouse pointer over a hyperlink that interests you until the pointer turns into a hand, and then click the left mouse button.

4 Browse the content at the page you selected.

5 Use the Yahoo! search engine to find sites that sell medical office equipment by clicking in the Address bar, typing **www.yahoo.com**, and then pressing Enter.

6 At the Yahoo! website, type **medical office equipment** in the search text box and then press Enter.

As you begin to type, the Yahoo! search assist feature displays search suggestions in a list below the search text box. Characters in each suggested search phrase that match the ones you typed are displayed in another font style for quick reference. You can click a suggested phrase in the list to select it. Because each search engine has its own way of cataloguing and indexing search terms, you may notice that different search engines provide different suggested search phrases, even when you enter the same characters.

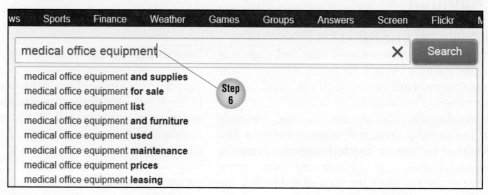

Step 6

7 Click a hyperlink to a site that interests you.

> Hyperlinks clicked from a Yahoo! search results page will open in a new tab within Internet Explorer.

8 Use the Google search engine to find sites that sell medical office supplies by clicking in the Address bar, typing **www.google.com**, and then pressing Enter.

9 At the Google website, type **medical office supplies** in the search text box and then press Enter.

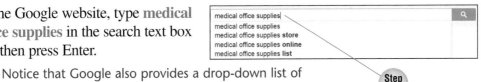

> Notice that Google also provides a drop-down list of suggested search phrases based on the characters you typed.

Step 9

10 Click a hyperlink that interests you.

11 Use the Dogpile search engine to find sites that sell medical office forms by clicking in the Address bar, typing **www.dogpile.com**, and then pressing Enter.

> Dogpile is a *metasearch* search engine, which means it sends your search phrase to other search engines and then compiles the results into one list. This allows you to view results from multiple search engines at the same time, even though you only typed your search criteria once. Dogpile compiles search results from Google, Yahoo!, and Yandex.

12 At the Dogpile website, type **medical office forms** in the search text box and then press Enter.

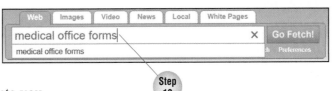

Step 12

13 Click a hyperlink that interests you.

> Hyperlinks clicked from a Dogpile search results page will open in a new tab within Internet Explorer.

In Brief
Conduct Internet Search
1. At Internet Explorer window, type search text in Address bar.
2. Press Enter.

In Addition

Customizing Internet Explorer

Internet Explorer 11 has been streamlined to provide users with more browsing space and reduced clutter. By default, Microsoft has turned off many features in Internet Explorer 11, including the Menu bar, Command bar, and Status bar. You can turn on these features by right-clicking the empty space above the Address bar (see Figure IE1.1 on page 52) and then clicking the desired option at the shortcut menu that displays. For example, to display the Menu bar (the bar that contains File, Edit, and so on), right-click the empty space above the Address bar and then click *Menu bar* at the shortcut menu. (This inserts a check mark next to *Menu bar*.)

Adding Web Pages to Favorites

If you visit a web page on a regular basis, you may want to add the page to the Favorites Center or create a button for the web page on the Favorites bar. To display the Favorites bar, right-click the empty space above the Address bar and then click *Favorites bar*

at the shortcut menu. To add a web page to the Favorites bar, display the web page and then click the Favorites button (the white star in the upper right corner of the window). When the Favorites Center displays, click the Add to favorites button arrow and then click *Add to favorites bar* at the drop-down list. If you prefer, you can add the website to the Favorites Center list. To do this, click the Favorites button and then click the Add to favorites button at the Favorites Center. At the Add a Favorite dialog box that displays, make sure the information in the *Name* text box is the title by which you want to refer to the website (if not, type your own name for the page) and then click the Add button. The new website is added to the Favorites Center drop-down list, making it possible for you to access the site simply by clicking the Favorites button and then clicking the site name at the drop-down list.

Activity
1.3

The Internet contains an extraordinary amount of information. Depending on what you are searching for on the Internet and the search engine you use, some searches can result in several thousand "hits" (sites). Wading through a long list of results can be very time consuming. You can achieve a more targeted list of search results by using the advanced search options offered by many search engines. Look for an advanced search options link at your favorite search engine site the next time you need to locate information, and experiment with various methods to limit the search results. Effective searching is a skill best obtained through practice.

Project

Lee Elliott has asked you to locate sites on the Internet that contain information on the symptoms of and treatments for Hodgkin's disease.

1. With the Internet Explorer window active, click in the Address bar, type **www.google.com**, and then press Enter.

2. At the Google home page, click the <u>Settings</u> hyperlink in the bottom right corner of the window.

3. Click *Advanced search* at the pop-up list.

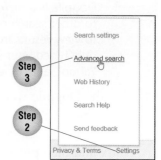

4. At the Advanced Search page, click in the *this exact word or phrase* text box and then type **symptoms of Hodgkin's disease**.

   This limits the search to websites that contain the exact phrase "symptoms of Hodgkin's disease."

5. Click in the *site or domain* text box and then type **.com**.

   This tells Google to only display websites with a .com extension in the search results.

6. Click the Advanced Search button.

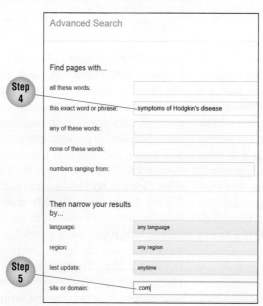

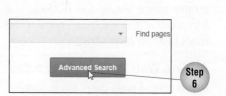

7 When the list of websites displays, click a hyperlink that interests you.

8 Click the Back button until the Google Advanced Search page displays.

9 Select and then delete the text *symptoms of Hodgkin's disease* in the *this exact word or phrase* text box.

10 Click in the *all these words* text box and then type **treatment Hodgkin's disease lymphoma**.

> This helps focus your search on websites that offer information on the treatment of Hodgkin's disease lymphoma.

11 Select and then delete the text *.com* in the *site or domain* text box.

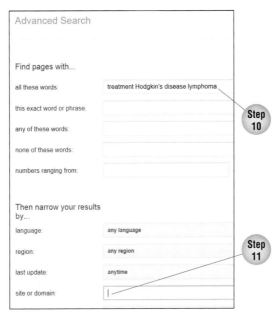

12 Click the Advanced Search button.

13 When the list of websites displays, click a hyperlink that interests you.

In Brief

Complete Advanced Search Using Google

1. At Internet Explorer window, click in Address bar, type www.google.com, and then press Enter.
2. Click Settings hyperlink and then click *Advanced search*.
3. Click in desired search text box and then type search criteria text.
4. Select search method and search options.
5. Click Advanced Search button.

In Addition

Displaying a List of Sites Visited

As you view various web pages, Internet Explorer keeps a list of the websites you have visited in the History pane. Display the History pane by clicking the Favorites button and then clicking the History tab in the Favorites Center. Click a timeframe to expand the list and display the sites visited. For example, click *Last Week* to view the pages that you visited within the past week. Click a hyperlink to revisit the page. At the top of the History pane, click the View option box (currently displays *View By Date*) to change the order in which the history list is displayed. You can choose from *View By Date*, *View By Site*, *View By Most Visited*, or *View By Order Visited Today*. Click *Search History* at the View button drop-down list to search the websites in the History pane by keyword or phrase.

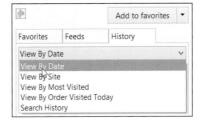

Activity 1.4

Downloading Content from a Web Page

Downloading content from a web page involves saving to your hard disk or other storage medium images, text, video, audio, or even an entire web page. Copyright laws protect much of the information on the Internet. Before using information or other media files you have downloaded from the Internet, check the source site for usage restrictions. When in doubt, contact the website administrator or other contact person identified on the site and request permission to use the content. Finally, make sure to credit the source of any content you use that was obtained from a web page. Generally, you are allowed to use content from a website that is considered public domain, such as a site for a government agency.

Project

Dr. St. Claire has asked you to use the Internet to locate two images related to diabetes to be used in a presentation she is giving to support staff next month.

1. With the Internet Explorer window active, click in the Address bar, type **www.google.com**, and then press Enter.

2. At the Google home page, type **glucose test** in the search text box and then press Enter.

3. At the search results page, click the <u>Images</u> hyperlink that displays below the search text box.

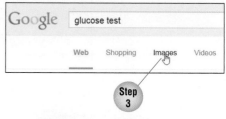

Step 3

4. Browse the images that display in the search results.

5. Position the mouse pointer over an image you want to download, right-click, and then click *Save picture as* at the shortcut menu.

   The image that you choose may vary from the one shown here.

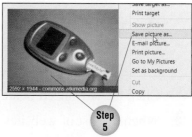

Step 5

6. At the Save Picture dialog box, click *Desktop* in the *Favorites* section of the Navigation pane, select the current text in the *File name* text box, type **glucosetest1** and then click Save or press Enter.

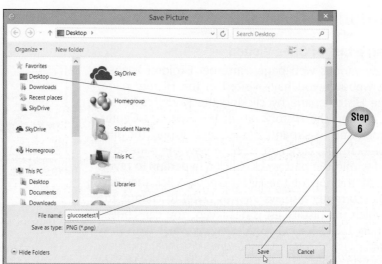

Step 6

7 Click in the Address bar, type **www.dogpile.com**, and then press Enter.

8 Click the Images tab at the Dogpile home page.

9 Click in the search text box, type **blood sugar testing**, and then press Enter or click the Go Fetch! button.

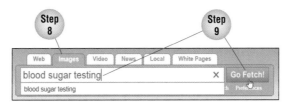

Step 8 · Step 9

10 Browse the images that display in the search results, right-click an image you want to download, and then click *Save picture as* at the shortcut menu.

11 At the Save Picture dialog box, with *Desktop* already selected in the Address bar and with the current file name already selected in the *File name* text box, type **bloodsugartest1** and then click Save or press Enter.

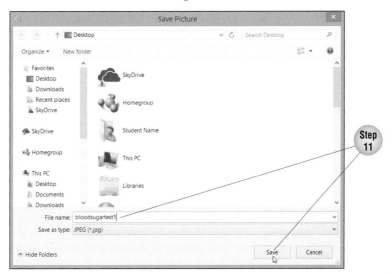

Step 11

In Brief

Download Image from Web Page
1. Display desired web page in Internet Explorer window.
2. Right-click desired image.
3. Click *Save picture as*.
4. Navigate to desired drive and/or folder.
5. Type file name in *File name* text box.
6. Click Save.

In Addition

Downloading an Application

Using Internet Explorer, you can download applications and programs to install onto your computer. When an application is downloaded, Internet Explorer displays the download bar toward the bottom of the screen (as shown below) asking if you want to run or save the application. If you want to install the application, click the Run button. Click the Save button if you want Internet Explorer to save the application in a temporary folder. If you want to save the application in a specific location on your computer, click the Save button arrow and then click *Save As* at the drop-down list. This displays the Save As dialog box, where you can specify the drive or file in which you want to save the file. Applications downloaded from the Internet could potentially contain a virus, so make sure the website and file are from a trusted source.

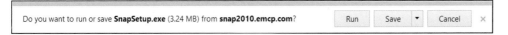

Do you want to run or save **SnapSetup.exe** (3.24 MB) from **snap2010.emcp.com**?   Run   Save ▾   Cancel   ×

Activity 1.5

Evaluating Content on the Web

The Internet is a vast repository of information that is easily accessible and constantly changing. Although a wealth of accurate and timely information is available at your fingertips, some information may be outdated, inaccurate, or of poor quality and should not be relied upon. Since anyone with an Internet connection and the right software can publish information on the Web, knowing how to recognize accurate, up-to-date content is a worthwhile skill.

To evaluate online content, first look for an author, publisher, or website owner name and consider if the source is credible. For example, is the author associated with a recognizable company, government, or news organization? Second, look for the date the information was published. Is the content outdated? If yes, consider the impact that more current information might have on the information you are evaluating. Third, look for indications that a bias may exist in the content. For example, is there a sponsor on the site that might indicate the information is one-sided? Can the information be validated by another source?

Project

Dr. St. Claire asks you to find information on the Internet about diabetes management. You want to make sure that the information you provide for the project is credible.

1. With the Internet Explorer window active, click in the Address bar, type **www.google.com**, and then press Enter.

2. At the Google home page, type **diabetes management** in the search text box and then click the Search button or press Enter.

3. Click a hyperlink that interests you.

4. At the web page, try to locate the author or publisher name, the date the article was published, and/or the date the page was last updated. If the web page contains any advertisements or sponsors, consider if these elements have an impact on the content.

   Some pages put this type of information at the bottom of the page, while other pages place the author and date at the beginning of the article. If you cannot find an author or date, look for a Contacts link to see if you can determine the name of the company that published the information. Also, look over the web address to see if it provides a clue to the authorship. For example, a web address with a *.edu* domain indicates the source is from a page affiliated with a university.

5. Click the New Tab button to open a new tab in the browsing window.

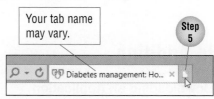

6. Click in the Address bar, type **www.nlm.nih .gov/medlineplus/diabeticdiet.html**, and then press Enter.

7. Scroll to the bottom of the page to read the publisher name and address, the date the page was last updated, and the date the topic was last reviewed.

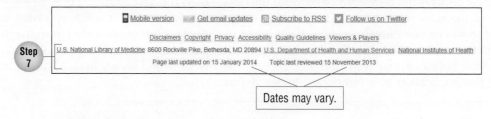

8 Click the tab for the first web page that you visited about diabetes management and then click the Back button to return to the search results list.

9 Click another hyperlink that interests you and try to locate information about the date and publisher of the content.

10 Examine the page shown in Figure IE1.3. Notice that the page provides a date and author and that the publisher is a trusted government website.

> A page that does provide information about the author, publisher, and date may not necessarily contain inaccurate data or be a poor source of information; however, the absence of an author or date of revision means that you would have difficulty citing the source for a research paper or other academic assignment.

11 Close Internet Explorer. At the dialog box that displays, click the Close all tabs button.

FIGURE IE1.3 Web Page with Author, Date, and Publisher Notations

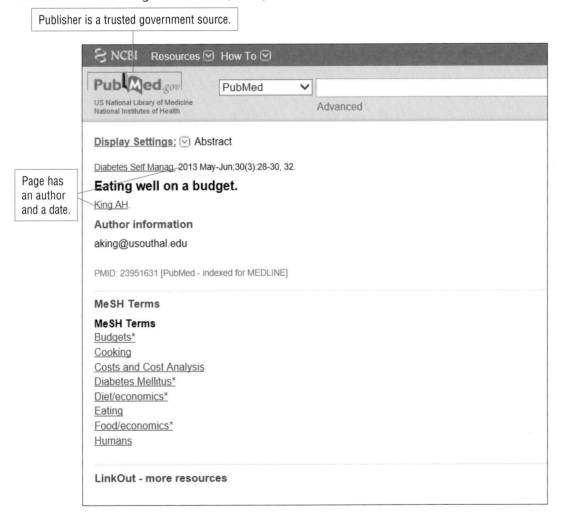

Features Summary

Feature	Button	Keyboard Shortcut
display Favorites Center	⭐	Alt + C
display Tools drop-down list	⚙	Alt + X
go back to previous web page	←	Alt + Left Arrow OR Backspace
go forward to next web page	→	Alt + Right Arrow
go to home page	🏠	Alt + Home
select Address bar contents	https://paradigm.emcp.com/	Alt + D

Knowledge Check

Completion: In the space provided at the right, indicate the correct term, command, or option.

1. Type a URL in this bar at the Internet Explorer window. _____
2. The letters *URL* stand for this. _____
3. Click this button on the Internet Explorer toolbar to display the previous web page. _____
4. Bing is the default search engine in Internet Explorer; list two other search engines. _____
5. Refine your search results by using these options at a search engine's website. _____
6. Download an image from a website to your computer by right-clicking the image and then clicking this option at the shortcut menu. _____

Skills Review

Note: Check with your instructor before completing the Skills Review activities to find out if you should print the pages that you visit.

Review 1 Browsing the Internet and Navigating with Hyperlinks

1. Open Internet Explorer.
2. Click in the Address bar, type **www.medicare.gov**, and then press Enter to visit the home page for Medicare.
3. Click a link to a topic that interests you and read the page.
4. Click another link and read the page.
5. Click the Back button until the Medicare home page displays.

Review 2 Searching for Specific Sites

1. At the Internet Explorer window, use the Address bar to search for websites on good nutrition habits.
2. In the search results, click a hyperlink that interests you.
3. Display the Google website and then use advanced options to search for websites on good nutrition that have a *.org* domain.
4. Visit at least two sites in the search results that interest you.

Review 3 Downloading Content from a Web Page

1. Using your favorite search engine, search for websites on holistic medicine. Find a site that contains an image that you like.
2. Download the image to the desktop, saving it with the name **holisticmed1**.
3. Close Internet Explorer.

Skills Assessment

Note: Check with your instructor before completing the Skills Assessment activities to find out if you should print the pages that you visit.

Assessment 1 Visiting Web Pages for Current News Articles

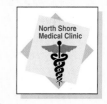

1. Lee Elliott, office manager at North Shore Medical Clinic, likes to keep up-to-date with current events by reading the daily headlines for various newspapers. Lee has asked you to scan the home pages for two online newspapers—the *New York Times* and *USA Today*—for articles of interest. To begin, open Internet Explorer.
2. Go to the website of the *New York Times* at www.nytimes.com. Scan the headlines for today's publication, click the link to an article that interests you, and then read the article.
3. Visit the website of *USA Today* at www.usatoday.com, click the link to an article that interests you, and then read the article.

Assessment 2 Navigating Websites for Medical Schools

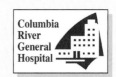

1. Laura Latterell, education director at Columbia River General Hospital, has asked you to visit the web pages for medical schools at two universities to compare programs.
2. Using your favorite search engine, find the web pages for two medical schools in your state or province.
3. At each website, click a link to an article or page that interests you.
4. Write a memo to your instructor with the URLs of each medical school website, the page that you read, and your perception of which medical school's site was easier to navigate and why.

Assessment 3 Downloading Content on Healthy Living

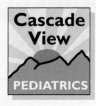

1. You work as a medical assistant at Cascade View Pediatrics and are preparing a brochure on healthy living. You need some information and images for the brochure. Search the Internet for information on healthy living.
2. Visit a website that interests you and locate an appropriate image.
3. Download an image from the web page to the desktop, saving it with the name **healthyliving1**.
4. Close Internet Explorer.

Assessment 4 Deleting Downloaded Content on the Desktop

1. At the Windows 8.1 desktop, right-click the *healthyliving1* file and then click *Delete* at the shortcut menu.
2. Delete all of the other downloaded files you saved to the desktop during this section.

Using WORD in the Medical Office

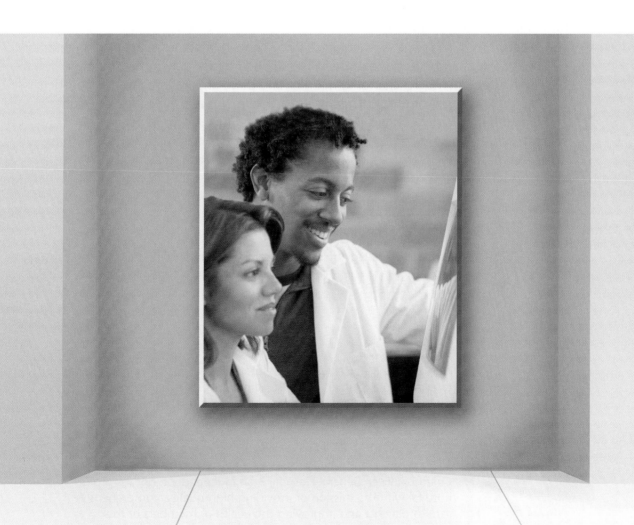

Introducing

WORD 2013

Microsoft Word 2013 is a word processing program used to create documents such as memos, letters, medical reports, medical research papers, brochures, announcements, newsletters, envelopes, labels, and much more. Word provides a wide variety of editing and formatting features as well as sophisticated visual elements.

This unit on Microsoft Word 2013 in the medical office contains four sections that guide you in learning and applying the features of Word 2013. In Section 1, you will create and edit medical documents by inserting, replacing, and deleting text; checking the spelling and grammar in documents; using the AutoCorrect feature and Thesaurus; changing document views; creating documents using a template; and managing documents. Section 2 focuses on formatting characters and paragraphs and includes applying fonts, aligning text in paragraphs, indenting text, changing line and paragraph spacing, inserting bullets and numbers, inserting symbols, setting tabs, adding borders and shading, and applying styles and style sets. In Section 3, you will learn how to format and enhance documents by finding and replacing text; cutting, copying, and pasting text; using the Clipboard task pane; inserting page breaks and page numbers; changing margins and page orientation; inserting headers and footers, images, WordArt, and shapes in a document; and preparing envelopes and labels. In Section 4, you will learn how to merge main documents with data sources, sort and filter records, create and modify tables, and prepare and edit forms.

In each of the four Word sections, you will prepare medical documents for two clinics and a hospital as described below.

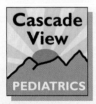

Cascade View Pediatrics is a full-service pediatric clinic that provides comprehensive primary pediatric care to infants, children, and adolescents.

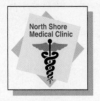

North Shore Medical Clinic is an internal medicine clinic dedicated to providing exceptional care to all patients. The physicians in the clinic specialize in a number of fields including internal medicine, family practice, cardiology, and dermatology.

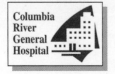

Columbia River General Hospital is an independent, not-for-profit hospital with the mission of providing high-quality, comprehensive care to patients and improving the health of members of the community.

Word SECTION 1

Creating and Editing a Document

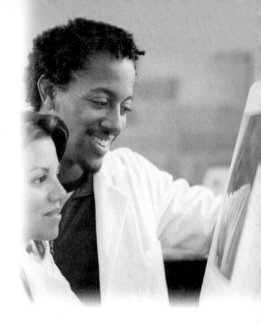

Skills

- Complete the word processing cycle
- Move the insertion point
- Insert and delete text
- Scroll and navigate in a document
- Select and delete text
- Use Undo and Redo
- Check the spelling and grammar in a document
- Use AutoCorrect
- Use the Thesaurus
- Change document views
- Use the Help feature
- Preview and print a document
- Insert the date and time in a document
- Insert quick parts in a document
- Close a document
- Create a document using a template
- Create and rename a folder
- Save a document in a different format

Student Resources

Before beginning the activities in Word Section 1, copy to your storage medium the WordMedS1 folder from the Student Resources CD. This folder contains the data files you need to complete the projects in this Word section.

Projects Overview

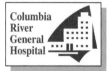

Edit and format a history and physical examination document, manage files, and edit and format a consultation report document.

Prepare an x-ray report document, prepare a letter requesting interpreting services, edit and format a notice to employees regarding a diabetes presentation, research a medical spell checking dictionary, prepare a letter to a doctor, and prepare a chart note.

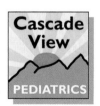

Prepare a memo regarding well-child checkups and edit and format a document containing information on scheduling appointments.

Activity 1.1

Completing the Word Processing Cycle

The process of creating a document in Microsoft Word generally follows a word processing cycle. The steps in the cycle vary but typically include the following: opening Word; creating and editing a document; saving, printing, and closing the document; and then closing Word.

Project

As the medical office assistant for North Shore Medical Clinic, you are responsible for preparing and updating medical records. You need to type the results of a portable chest x-ray for a patient at the clinic.

1 At the Windows 8.1 Start screen, click the Word 2013 tile.

Depending on your system configuration, these steps may vary.

2 At the Word 2013 opening screen, click the *Blank document* template.

3 At the blank Word document, identify the various features by comparing your screen with the one shown in Figure W1.1.

Refer to Table W1.1 for a description of the screen features.

4 Type **Name: Joseph Ingram** as shown in Figure W1.2. When you have finished typing, hold down the Shift key, press the Enter key, and then release the Shift key.

Shift + Enter is the New Line command. Use this command to start a new line without starting a new paragraph. Starting a new line creates less space between the lines than starting a new paragraph.

5 Type **Procedure: Portable chest x-ray** and then press Shift + Enter.

6 Type **Date of Procedure: 05/18/2016** and then press Enter.

Pressing the Enter key begins a new paragraph in the document.

FIGURE W1.1 Word Document Screen

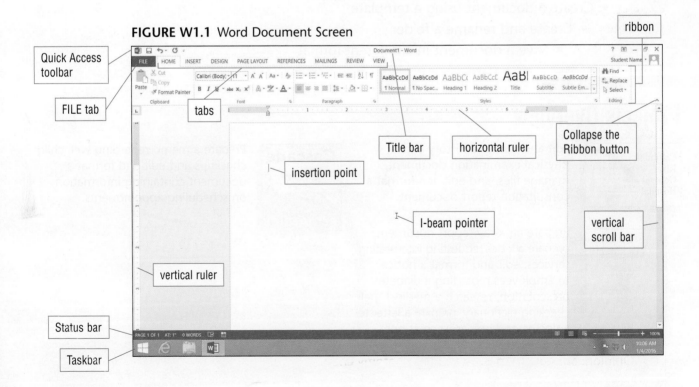

Enter twice while writing a business letter

TABLE W1.1 Word Screen Features and Descriptions

Feature	Description
Collapse the Ribbon button	when clicked, removes the ribbon from the screen; when double-clicked, redisplays the ribbon
FILE tab	when clicked, displays backstage area that contains options for working with and managing documents
horizontal ruler	used to set margins, indents, and tabs
I-beam pointer	used to move the insertion point or to select text
insertion point	indicates location of next character entered at the keyboard
Quick Access toolbar	contains buttons for commonly used commands, making it possible to execute them with a single mouse click
ribbon	area containing the tabs with options and buttons divided into groups
Status bar	displays number of pages and words, view buttons, and Zoom slider bar
tabs	contain commands and buttons organized into groups
Taskbar	divided into three sections—the Start button, the task buttons area, and the Notification area
Title bar	displays document name followed by program name
vertical ruler	used to set top and bottom margins
vertical scroll bar	used to view parts of the document beyond the current screen

7 Type the remainder of the text shown in Figure W1.2.

Type the text as shown. When you type *adn* and then press the spacebar, the AutoCorrect feature will automatically change it to *and*. When you type *teh* and then press the spacebar, AutoCorrect changes it to *the*. Do not press the Enter key at the end of each line of text. Word will automatically wrap text to the next line.

8 Save the document by clicking the Save button on the Quick Access toolbar.

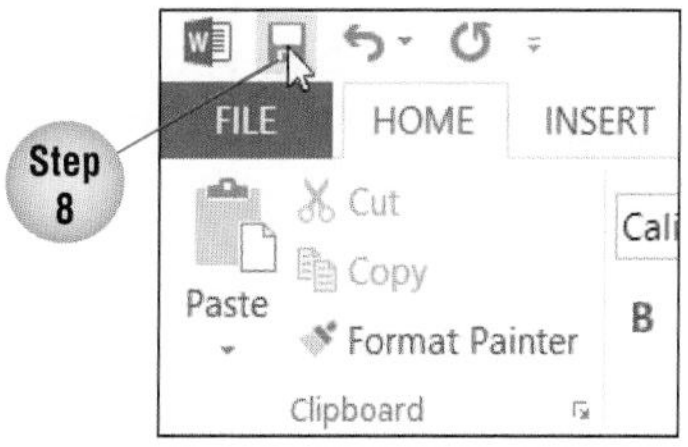

FIGURE W1.2 Steps 4–7

Name: Joseph Ingram
Procedure: Portable chest x-ray
Date of Procedure: 05/18/2016

Comparison: A single portable view of teh chest is provided and comparison is made with earlier study of the same date.

Findings: Endotracheal tube adn right chest tubes are in place. Heart appears to be generous in size and right border is somewhat indistinct of perihilar vascular structure. No sign of pneumothorax was observed.

Opinion: Satisfactory post median sternotomy chest.

Word → Design → Drop down → select design → Layout → Merge → center

Print Scn → screenshot

Mailings ↓ Mail Merge ↓ step by step mail merge wizard ↓ Letters ↓ create → OK ↓ Save
write letter ↓ Address block ↓ Greeting Line ↓ Type Letter ↓ More items ↓ company name ↓ sincerely ↓ name ↓ initial (lowercase)

Home → Paragraph (expend) ↓ Tabs (put measurement) select set → OK put cursor before (hit tab) ↓ Next ↓ Edit individual letters ↓ All → OK

continues

9 At the Save As backstage area, click the desired location in the middle panel (contains the four location options). For example, click the *OneDrive* option preceded by your name if you are saving to your OneDrive or click the *Computer* option if you are saving to a USB flash drive.

10 Click the Browse button.

11 At the Save As dialog box, navigate to your storage medium and then double-click the *WordMedS1* folder.

> Press the F12 function key to display the Save As dialog box without displaying the Save As backstage area.

12 Click in the *File name* text box, type **WMedS1-Results**, and then press Enter or click the Save button.

> Word automatically adds the file extension *.docx* to the end of a document name. The Address bar at the Save As dialog box displays the active folder. To make the WordMedS1 folder active (if it is not already), click the drive in the Navigation pane that contains your storage medium and then double-click the *WordMedS1* folder in the Content pane.

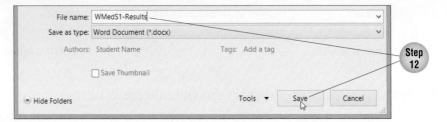

13 Print the document by clicking the FILE tab, clicking the *Print* option, and then clicking the Print button at the backstage area.

> The FILE tab is located in the upper left corner of the screen at the left side of the HOME tab. When you click the FILE tab, the backstage area displays with options for working with and managing documents. Refer to Table W1.2 for descriptions of these options and the information you will find at each backstage area.

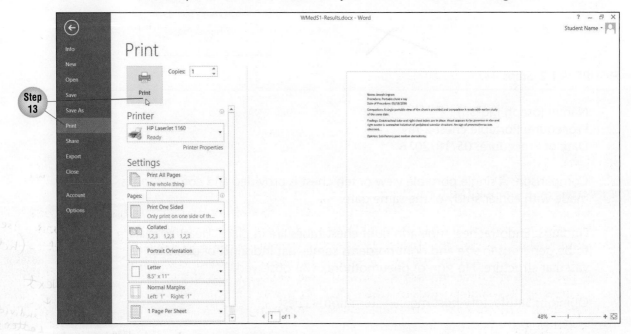

TABLE W1.2 Backstage Area Options

Tab	Options and Information
Info	permissions, possible issues with sharing the document, document versions, properties (for example, number of pages, number of words), date created, date last modified, date last printed, author
New	available templates such as Blank document as well as templates from Office.com
Open	options for opening documents; list of recently opened documents
Save	saves previously saved document or displays Save As backstage area with options for saving a document, current folder, and recent folders
Save As	options for saving a document, current folder, and recent folders
Print	number of copies, printer, settings (for example, one-sided pages, letter size, normal margins, one page per sheet)
Share	share document with specific people; share document using email, present document online, and share as a blog post
Export	export document as PDF or XPS document; change file type
Close	close currently open document
Account	user information, connected services, product information
Options	Word Options dialog box with options for customizing Word

14 Close the document by clicking the FILE tab and then clicking the *Close* option.

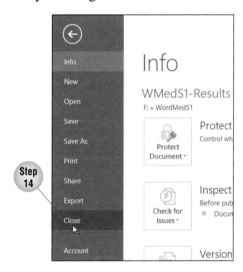

In Addition

Understanding Default Document Formatting

A Word document is based on a template that applies default formatting. Default formatting refers to formatting automatically applied by Word. Some of the default settings include 11-point Calibri font, 1.08 line spacing, and 8 points of spacing after each paragraph (added when you press the Enter key). You will learn more about fonts and paragraph spacing in Section 2.

Correcting Errors

Word contains a spelling feature that inserts a wavy red line below words that are not found in the built-in spelling dictionary. You can edit the word or leave it as written. The wavy red line does not print. You will learn more about checking for and correcting spelling errors in Activity 1.4.

Activity 1.2

Moving the Insertion Point; Inserting and Deleting Text

After you create a document, you will often want to make changes to it. These changes may include adding text, called *inserting*, or removing text, called *deleting*. To insert text, position the insertion point in the desired location and then type the text. Delete text in a document by positioning the insertion point in the desired location and then pressing the Backspace key to delete text to the left of the insertion point or the Delete key to delete text to the right of the insertion point.

Project

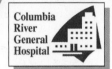

Columbia River General Hospital

As a medical office assistant for Columbia River General Hospital, you are responsible for typing history and physical examination documents for patients admitted to the hospital.

1. At a blank Word document, click the FILE tab.

   This displays the Open backstage area. When you click the FILE tab from an existing document that contains text or objects, you have to click the *Open* option to display the Open backstage area.

2. At the Open backstage area, click the desired location in the middle panel.

   For example, click the *OneDrive* option preceded by your name if you are opening a document from your OneDrive or click the *Computer* option if you are opening a document from your USB flash drive.

3. Click the Browse button.

4. At the Open dialog box, navigate to your storage medium and then double-click the *WordMedS1* folder.

   Press Ctrl + F12 to display the Open dialog box without displaying the Open backstage area.

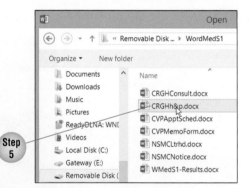

Step 5

5. Double-click ***CRGHh&p.docx*** in the Content pane of the Open dialog box.

6. At the document, click the FILE tab and then click the *Save As* option.

7. At the Save As backstage area, click the *WordMedS1* folder name that displays below the *Current Folder* heading in the *Computer* section.

8. At the Save As dialog box, press the Home key to move the insertion point to the beginning of the file name, type **WMedS1-** in the *File Name* text box, and then press the Enter key. (The file name in the *File Name* text box should display as **WMedS1-CRGHh&p.docx**.)

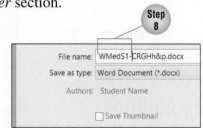

Step 8

File name: WMedS1-CRGHh&p.docx
Save as type: Word Document (*.docx)
Authors: Student Name
☐ Save Thumbnail

   Pressing the Home key saves you from having to type the entire document name. If you open an existing document, make changes to it, and then want to save it with the same name, click the Save button on the Quick Access toolbar. If you want to keep the original document and save the updated document with a new name, click the FILE tab and then click the *Save As* option.

9. Position the mouse pointer at the beginning of the *HISTORY OF PRESENT ILLNESS* paragraph and then click the left mouse button.

   This moves the insertion point to the location of the mouse pointer.

10 Press the Up Arrow, Down Arrow, Left Arrow, and Right Arrow keys located toward the right side of the keyboard.

> Pressing the arrow keys is one way to move the insertion point in a document. Use the information shown in Table W1.3 to practice using other methods for moving the insertion point.

11 Move the insertion point to the beginning of the name *Shawn Lipinski, MD*, located toward the beginning of the document, and then type **Physician:**. Press the spacebar once after typing the colon.

> By default, text you type in a document is inserted in the document and existing text is moved to the right.

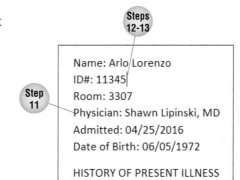

Steps 12-13

Step 11

Name: Arlo Lorenzo
ID#: 11345
Room: 3307
Physician: Shawn Lipinski, MD
Admitted: 04/25/2016
Date of Birth: 06/05/1972

HISTORY OF PRESENT ILLNESS

12 Click immediately to the right of the last number in the ID number *10572* and then press the Backspace key until all of the numbers are deleted.

> Press the Backspace key to delete any character located immediately to the left of the insertion point.

13 Type **11345**.

14 Click any character in the last sentence in the *HISTORY OF PRESENT ILLNESS* section (the sentence that begins *He notes that he usually*).

15 Press the Backspace key until the insertion point is positioned immediately to the right of the period that ends the previous sentence. Press the Delete key until you have deleted the remainder of the sentence.

> Press the Delete key to delete any character located immediately to the right of the insertion point.

16 Click the Save button on the Quick Access toolbar.

> Clicking the Save button saves the document with the same name (**WMedS1-CRGHh&p.docx**).

In Brief

Open Document
1. Click FILE tab.
2. At Open backstage area, click desired location.
3. Click Browse button.
4. At Open dialog box, navigate to desired folder.
5. Double-click document name.

Save Document with Save As
1. Click Save button on Quick Access toolbar.
2. At Save As backstage area, click desired location.
3. Click Browse button.
4. At Save As dialog box, navigate to desired folder.
5. Type document name.
6. Click Save or press Enter.

TABLE W1.3 Insertion Point Movement Keys

Press	To move insertion point
End	to end of line
Home	to beginning of line
Page Up	up one screen
Page Down	down one screen
Ctrl + Home	to beginning of document
Ctrl + End	to end of document

In Addition

Adding Buttons to the Quick Access Toolbar

You can add buttons to the Quick Access toolbar that represent commonly used features. For example, you might want to add the Open button to make it easier to open a document or the Quick Print button to save steps when printing a document. To add a button to the Quick Access toolbar, click the Customize Quick Access Toolbar button that displays at the right side of the toolbar and then click the desired button name at the drop-down list or click *More Commands* to access more button options.

Activity 1.3

Scrolling; Selecting and Replacing or Deleting Text; Using Undo and Redo

In addition to moving the insertion point, you can use the mouse to change the display of text in the document screen. The vertical scroll bar displays toward the right side of the screen. Click the arrows located at the top or bottom of the vertical scroll bar, click the scroll bar itself, or click and drag the scroll box to scroll through text in a document. Scrolling in a document changes the text displayed but does not move the insertion point. Previously, you learned to delete text by positioning the insertion point and then pressing the Backspace key or the Delete key. You can also select the text and then delete it or replace it with other text. If you make a change to text, such as deleting it, and then change your mind, use the Undo button on the Quick Access toolbar to restore it. If you change your mind again, click the Redo button to delete the text once more.

Project

To minimize the need for additional editing, you have decided to review carefully the History and Physical Examination document you have open on your screen.

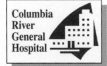

1 With **WMedS1-CRGHh&p.docx** open, press Ctrl + Home to move the insertion point to the beginning of the document.

2 Position the mouse pointer on the down-pointing arrow at the bottom of the vertical scroll bar and then click the left mouse button to scroll down the document.

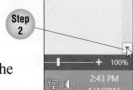

3 Position the mouse pointer on the vertical scroll bar below the scroll box and then click the left mouse button two times.

> The scroll box on the vertical scroll bar indicates the location of the text in the document screen in relation to the remainder of the document. Clicking below the scroll box on the vertical scroll bar scrolls down one screen of text at a time.

4 Position the mouse pointer on the scroll box on the vertical scroll bar, hold down the left mouse button, drag the scroll box to the top of the vertical scroll bar, and then release the mouse button.

5 Position the mouse pointer on the word *leg* (the last word in the first sentence in the *HISTORY OF PRESENT ILLNESS* section) and then double-click the left mouse button. (This selects the word *leg*.)

> **HISTORY OF PRESENT ILLNESS**
> Mr. Lorenzo is a 43-year-old male admitted to thrombophlebitis in his left lower leg. He was healthy, never been hospitalized, and has had

> Selected text displays with a gray background. You can also click and drag through text with the mouse to select the text. When you select text, the Mini toolbar displays. You will learn more about the Mini toolbar in Activity 2.1.

6 Type **extremity**.

> When you type *extremity*, it takes the place of *leg*.

7 Move the insertion point immediately to the left of the comma after the word *healthy* (located in the third sentence in the *HISTORY OF PRESENT ILLNESS* section) and then press the F8 function key on the keyboard. Press the Right Arrow key until the words *never been hospitalized* and the comma that follows *hospitalized* are selected.

> **HISTORY OF PRESENT ILLNESS**
> Mr. Lorenzo is a 43-year-old male admitted to thrombophlebitis in his left lower extremity. He been healthy, never been hospitalized, and has ago, when he developed a superficial thrombo

> Pressing the F8 function key turns on Extend mode. Use the insertion point movement keys to select text in Extend mode.

8 Press the Delete key.

> Pressing the Delete key deletes the selected text. If you change your mind about deleting text after you have selected it, press the Esc key and then press any arrow key.

9 Position the mouse pointer on any character in the second sentence in the *HISTORY OF PRESENT ILLNESS* section (the sentence that begins *He was brought to the hospital*), hold down the Ctrl key, click the mouse button, and then release the Ctrl key.

> Holding down the Ctrl key while clicking the mouse button selects the entire sentence.

10 Press the Delete key to delete the selected sentence.

11 Click the Undo button ⤺ ▾ on the Quick Access toolbar.

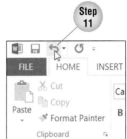

> When you click the Undo button, the deleted sentence reappears. Clicking the Undo button reverses the last command or deletes the last entry you typed. Click the down-pointing arrow at the right side of the Undo button and a drop-down list displays with the changes made to the document since it was opened. Click an action and the action, along with any actions listed above it, is undone.

12 Click the Redo button ⤻ on the Quick Access toolbar.

> Clicking the Redo button deletes the selected sentence once more. If you click the Undo button and then decide you do not want to reverse the original action, click the Redo button to carry out the original command.

13 Position the mouse pointer between the left edge of the page and the heading *CONSULTATION* until the pointer turns into an arrow pointing up and to the right (instead of the left) and then click the left mouse button.

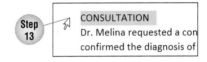

> The space between the left edge of the page and the text is referred to as the *selection bar*. Use the selection bar to select specific sections of text. Refer to Table W1.4 for more information on selecting text.

14 Deselect the text by clicking in the document.

> Deselecting cancels the selection of text.

15 Save the document by clicking the Save button on the Quick Access toolbar.

TABLE W1.4 Selecting Text with the Mouse

To select	Complete these steps using the mouse
a word	Double-click the word.
a line of text	Click in the selection bar to the left of the line.
multiple lines of text	Drag in the selection bar to the left of the lines.
a sentence	Hold down the Ctrl key and then click anywhere in the sentence.
a paragraph	Double-click in the selection bar next to the paragraph or triple-click anywhere in the paragraph.
multiple paragraphs	Drag in the selection bar.
an entire document	Triple-click in the selection bar.

In Addition

Resuming Reading or Editing in a Document

When you work in a multiple-page document and then close the document, Word remembers the page where the insertion point was last positioned. When you reopen the document, Word displays a Welcome Back message at the right side of the screen near the vertical scroll bar. The message tells you that you can pick up where you left off and identifies the page where your insertion point was last located. Click the message and the insertion point is positioned at the top of that page.

Activity 1.4

Checking the Spelling and Grammar in a Document

Use Word's spelling checker to find and correct misspelled and duplicated words (such as *and and*). The spelling checker compares words in your document with words in its dictionary. If a match is found, the word is passed over. If no match is found for the word, the spelling checker stops, selects the word, and offers replacements. The grammar checker will search a document for errors in grammar, punctuation, and word usage. The spelling checker and the grammar checker can help you create a well-written document but do not replace the need for proofreading.

Project

Continuing with the editing process, you are ready to check the spelling and grammar in the History and Physical Examination document.

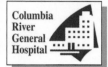

1. With **WMedS1-CRGHh&p.docx** open, press Ctrl + Home to move the insertion point to the beginning of the document.

2. Click the REVIEW tab and then click the Spelling & Grammar button in the Proofing group.

   When you click the Spelling & Grammar button, Word selects the first misspelled word or grammar error and displays the Spelling task pane at the right side of the screen with options for correcting the error, ignoring the error, or adding the word to the spelling dictionary. It also displays a brief definition of the selected word in the list box.

3. When the word *traetment* is selected in the document and *treatment* is selected in the list box in the Spelling task pane, click the Change button in the task pane.

   Refer to Table W1.5 for an explanation of the buttons in the Spelling and Grammar task panes.

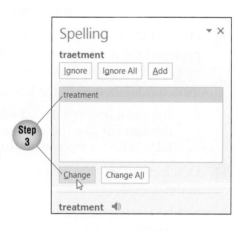

4. When the word *pyelogram* is selected in the document, click the Ignore All button in the Spelling task pane.

   This medical term is spelled correctly.

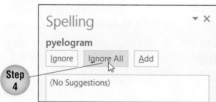

5. When the word *swolen* is selected in the document and *swollen* is selected in the list box in the Spelling task pane, click the Change button.

6. When the word *juandice* is selected in the document and *jaundice* is selected in the Spelling task pane, click the Change button.

7. When the word *Their* is selected in the document and *There* is selected in the list box in the Grammar task pane, click the Change button.

8. When the *HENT* heading and first sentence of the section are selected in the document, click the Ignore button in the Grammar task pane.

TABLE W1.5 Spelling and Grammar Task Pane Buttons

Button	Function
Ignore	during spell checking, skips that occurrence of the word; in grammar checking, leaves currently selected text as written
Ignore All	during spell checking, skips that occurrence and all other occurrences of the word in the document
Add	adds selected word to the main spelling check dictionary
Delete	deletes the currently selected word(s)
Change	replaces selected word in sentence with selected word in list box
Change All	replaces selected word in sentence with selected word in list box and all other occurrences of the word

In Brief

Check Spelling and Grammar
1. Click REVIEW tab.
2. Click Spelling & Grammar button in Proofing group.
3. Ignore or change as needed.
4. Click OK.

9 When the word *thyromegaly* is selected in the document, click the Ignore All button in the Spelling task pane.

This medical term is spelled correctly.

10 If the word *hepatosplenomegaly* is selected in the document, click the Ignore All button in the Spelling task pane.

This medical term is spelled correctly.

11 When the word *were* is selected (this word occurs twice), click the Delete button in the Spelling task pane.

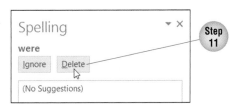

12 If the text *SL:SN* is selected in the document, click the Ignore button in the Spelling task pane.

13 Click OK at the message box telling you the spelling and grammar check is complete.

14 Click the Save button on the Quick Access toolbar to save the changes made to the document.

In Addition

Changing Spelling Options

Control spelling and grammar checking options at the Word Options dialog box with the *Proofing* option selected. Display this dialog box by clicking the FILE tab and then clicking *Options*. At the Word Options dialog box, click *Proofing* in the left panel. With options in the dialog box, you can tell the spelling checker to ignore certain types of text, create custom dictionaries, show readability statistics, and hide spelling and/or grammar errors in the document.

Editing While Checking Spelling and Grammar

When checking the spelling and grammar in a document, you can temporarily leave the Spelling or Grammar task pane by clicking in the document. To resume the spelling and grammar check, click the Resume button in the Spelling or Grammar task pane.

Activity 1.5

Using AutoCorrect and the Thesaurus

The AutoCorrect feature automatically detects and corrects some typographical errors, misspelled words, and incorrect capitalization. In addition to correcting errors, you can use the AutoCorrect feature to insert frequently used text. Use the Thesaurus to find synonyms, antonyms, and other related terms for a particular word.

Project

Columbia River General Hospital

You need to insert additional text in the History and Physical Examination document. To speed up the process, you will create a new AutoCorrect entry. You will also use the Thesaurus to find synonyms for specific words in the document.

1. With **WMedS1-CRGHh&p.docx** open, click the FILE tab and then click *Options*.

2. At the Word Options dialog box, click *Proofing* in the left panel and then click the AutoCorrect Options button in the *AutoCorrect options* section.

3. At the AutoCorrect dialog box with the AutoCorrect tab selected, type **tc** in the *Replace* text box and then press the Tab key.

4. Type **tachycardia** in the *With* text box and then click the Add button.

5. With the *tc* selected in the *Replace* text box, type **pl** and then press the Tab key.

6. With *tachycardia* selected in the *With* text box, type **pulmonary**, click the Add button, and then click OK to close the dialog box.

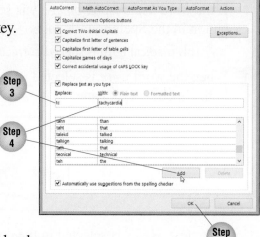

7. Click OK to close the Word Options dialog box.

8. Press Ctrl + End to move the insertion point to the end of the document. Move the insertion point so it is positioned immediately to the right of the period after the sentence *The neurologic assessment was normal* (below the *NEUROLOGIC* heading) and then press the Enter key.

9. Type **DIAGNOSIS** and then press Shift + Enter.

   Shift + Enter is the New Line command.

10. Type the remaining text shown in Figure W1.3. *Note: Type the text exactly as shown. AutoCorrect will change* **tc** *to* **tachycardia** *and* **pl** *to* **pulmonary**. *Do not press Enter at the end of each line in the figure. Word will automatically wrap text to the next line.*

FIGURE W1.3 Steps 9–10

DIAGNOSIS
Patient is diagnosed with deep vein thrombophlebitis in the left lower extremity and tc. This patient will be admitted. A pl ventilation perfusion scan is mandated by the presence of tc. A baseline study needs to be done to exclude the presence of plembolization. He will be treated with bed rest and anticoagulation. Further notation will be made as the case progresses. Appropriate studies for coagulopathy were performed.

11 Click anywhere in the word *done* (located in the fourth sentence of the paragraph you just typed), click the REVIEW tab, and then click the Thesaurus button 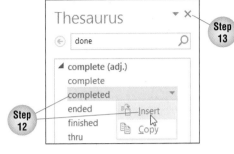 in the Proofing group.

12 At the Thesaurus task pane, right-click the word *completed* in the list box and then click *Insert* at the drop-down list.

13 Close the Thesaurus task pane by clicking the Close button ☒ in the upper right corner.

14 Position the mouse pointer on the word *exclude* (located in the fourth sentence of the paragraph you just typed) and then click the right mouse button.

15 At the shortcut menu that displays, point to *Synonyms* and then click *eliminate* at the side menu.

16 Click the Save button to save the document with the same name.

17 Click the FILE tab and then click *Options*. Click *Proofing* in the left panel of the dialog box and then click the AutoCorrect Options button.

18 At the AutoCorrect dialog box, type **pl** in the *Replace* text box.

> This selects the *pulmonary* entry in the list box.

19 Click the Delete button.

20 Type **tc** in the *Replace* text box and then click the Delete button.

21 Click OK to close the AutoCorrect dialog box and then click OK to close the Word Options dialog box.

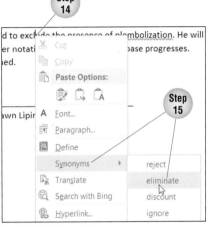

In Brief

Add AutoCorrect Entry
1. Click FILE tab.
2. Click *Options*.
3. Click *Proofing*.
4. Click AutoCorrect Options button.
5. Type text in *Replace* text box.
6. Type text in *With* text box.
7. Click Add button.
8. Click OK.
9. Click OK.

Use Thesaurus
1. Click in desired word.
2. Click REVIEW tab.
3. Click Thesaurus button.
4. Right-click desired word.
5. Click *Insert*.

In Addition

Using the Thesaurus Task Pane

Depending on the word you are looking up, the words in the Thesaurus task pane list box may display followed by *(n.)* for *noun*, *(v.)* for *verb*, *(adj.)* for *adjective*, or *(adv.)* for *adverb*. Click a word in the list box and a definition of the word displays below the list box. You may need to install a dictionary before you can see a definition. To install a dictionary, click the Get a dictionary hyperlink. At the Dictionaries pane, click the desired dictionary and then click the Download button.

Activity 1.6

Changing Document Views

By default, a document generally displays in Print Layout view. In this view, you have the capability to show or hide the white space at the top and bottom of each page. You can change the view to Read Mode, Web Layout, Outline, or Draft. You can also change the zoom percentage for viewing a document by using the Zoom button on the VIEW tab and/or the Zoom slider bar on the Status bar. Use the Navigation pane to browse in a document, search for specific text or items in the document, and rearrange the content of the document.

Project Your supervisor, as well as Dr. Lipinski, will be reviewing the History and Physical Examination document electronically, so you decide to experiment with various views to determine the best one to use for on-screen reviewing.

Columbia River General Hospital

1. With **WMedS1-CRGHh&p.docx** open, press Ctrl + Home to move the insertion point to the beginning of the document. Change to Draft view by clicking the VIEW tab and then clicking the Draft button in the Views group.

2. Click the Print Layout button in the Views group.

3. Change the zoom by clicking the Zoom button in the Zoom group on the VIEW tab. At the Zoom dialog box, click the *75%* option in the *Zoom to* section and then click OK.

   You can also display the Zoom dialog box by clicking the percentage that displays at the right side of the Zoom slider bar, located toward the bottom of the screen at the right side of the Status bar.

   Step 3

   Step 4

4. Return the zoom percentage to 100% by positioning the mouse pointer on the button on the Zoom slider bar and then dragging the button to the right until *100%* displays at the right side of the bar.

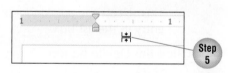

5. Hide the white and light gray space that displays at the top and bottom of each page by positioning the mouse pointer on the light gray space at the top of the page until the pointer turns into the hide white space icon and then double-clicking the left mouse button.

   Step 5

6. Redisplay the white and light gray space at the top and bottom of each page by positioning the mouse pointer on the gray line at the top of the page until the pointer turns into the show white space icon and then double-clicking the left mouse button.

7. Click the Read Mode button in the Views group and then navigate in the document using the commands shown in Table W1.6.

   Read Mode displays a document for easy reading. You can also display the document in Read Mode by clicking the Read Mode button in the view area on the Status bar.

TABLE W1.6 Navigating in Read Mode

Press this key	To complete this action
Page Down or spacebar	Move to next page or section.
Page Up or Backspace key	Move to previous page or section.
Right Arrow	Move to next page.
Left Arrow	Move to previous page.
Home	Move to first page in document.
End	Move to last page in document.
Esc	Return to previous view.

8 Return to Print Layout view by pressing the Esc key on the keyboard.

> You can also return to Print Layout view by clicking the VIEW tab and then clicking *Edit Document* at the drop-down list.

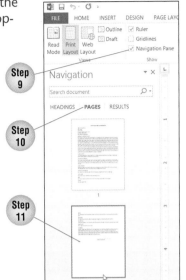

In Brief

Display Draft View
1. Click VIEW tab.
2. Click Draft button in Views group.

Display Read Mode View
1. Click VIEW tab.
2. Click Read Mode button in Views group.

OR

Click Read Mode button in view area on Status bar.

Display Navigation Pane
1. Click VIEW tab.
2. Click *Navigation Pane* check box.

9 Click the *Navigation Pane* check box in the Show group on the VIEW tab.

> The Navigation pane displays at the left side of the screen and includes a search text box and three tabs. Click the HEADINGS tab to browse headings in a document (heading styles must be applied to the text for headings to display in this pane), click the PAGES tab to browse pages in the document, and click the RESULTS tab to browse search results.

10 Click the PAGES tab in the Navigation pane.

> Clicking the PAGES tab displays thumbnails of each document page in the Navigation pane.

11 Click the page 2 thumbnail in the Navigation pane.

> This moves the insertion point to the beginning of page 2.

12 Click in the search text box in the Navigation pane (contains the text *Search document*) and then type **LUNGS**.

> When you type *LUNGS*, each occurrence of the text is highlighted in the document.

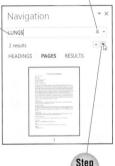

13 Click the Next Search Result button in the Navigation pane (displays as a down-pointing arrow) to select the next occurrence of *LUNGS*. Click the button again to select the next occurrence.

> You can click the Previous Search Result button to display the previous occurrence of the search text.

14 Click the button containing an X that displays at the right side of the search text box.

> Clicking this button ends the current search, removes the search text in the Navigation pane, and selects the current search result in the document.

15 Close the Navigation pane by clicking the Close button that displays in the upper right corner of the pane or by clicking the *Navigation Pane* check box in the Show group on the VIEW tab.

16 Click the Multiple Pages button in the Zoom group to display two pages on the screen and then click the One Page button.

17 Click the Page Width button in the Zoom group to display the document so that the width of the page matches the width of the window.

18 Drag the button on the Zoom slider bar or click the Zoom Out button or the Zoom In button until *100%* displays at the left side of the slider bar.

In Addition

Displaying Ribbon Options

Control how much of the ribbon displays on screen with the Ribbon Display Options button, located in the upper right corner of the screen. Click this button and a drop-down list displays with options for hiding the ribbon, showing only the tabs, or showing tabs and commands. You can also hide the ribbon by clicking the Collapse the Ribbon button above the vertical scroll bar or with the keyboard shortcut Ctrl + F1. Redisplay the ribbon by double-clicking any tab or by pressing Ctrl + F1.

Activity 1.7

Using the Help Feature and Printing a Document

Microsoft Word includes a Help feature that contains information on Word features and commands. To access Help, click the Microsoft Word Help button in the upper right corner of the screen to display the Word Help window. You can also get help from within a dialog box by clicking the Help button that displays in the upper right corner of the dialog box. When you do so, the Word Help window displays with specific information about the dialog box and its features.

To print a document, click the FILE tab and then click the *Print* option. The Print backstage area displays with various buttons and options. At the Print backstage area, you can preview your document, specify the number of copies to print, and choose specific pages for printing. To close the Print backstage area, click the Back button located in the upper left corner of the screen or press the Esc key.

Project

You are ready to print certain sections of the History and Physical Examination document. But first you want to learn more about printing a document from the Print backstage area. You decide to use the Help feature to do so.

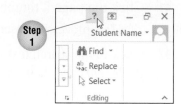

1. With **WMedS1-CRGHh&p.docx** open, press Ctrl + Home to move the insertion point to the beginning of the document and then click the Microsoft Word Help button ? in the upper right corner of the screen.

   You can also press the F1 function key to display the Word Help window.

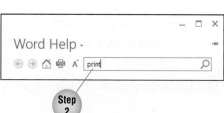

2. At the Word Help window, type **print** and then press Enter.

3. At the Word Help window, click a hyperlink that pertains to printing a document.

4. Read the information and then close the Word Help window by clicking the Close button in the upper right corner of the window.

5. Click the FILE tab to display the backstage area and then click the Microsoft Word Help button in the upper right corner of the screen.

6. Click a hyperlink in the Word Help window that interests you, read the information, and then close the window.

7. Click the *Print* option to display the Print backstage area.

   At the Print backstage area, your document displays at the right side of the screen and looks as it will when printed. The left side of the Print backstage area displays three categories—*Print*, *Printer*, and *Settings*. Click the Print button in the *Print* category to send the document to the printer. Specify the number of copies you want printed with the *Copies* option in the *Print* category. Use the gallery in the *Printer* category to specify the desired printer. The *Settings* category contains a number of galleries, each with options for specifying how you want your document printed, such as whether or not you want the pages collated when printed; the orientation, page size, and margins of your document; and how many pages of your document you want to print on each sheet of paper.

8 Click the Next Page button located below and to the left of the preview page to display the next page in the document.

9 Click twice on the Zoom In button (contains a plus symbol) that displays at the right side of the Zoom slider bar.

> Click the Zoom In button to increase the size of the page or click the Zoom Out button (contains a minus symbol) to decrease the size of the page.

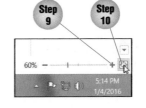

10 Click the Zoom to Page button located at the right side of the Zoom slider bar.

> Click the Zoom to Page button to increase or decrease the page size so an entire page displays in the preview area.

11 Print only page 2 of the document by clicking in the *Pages* text box in the *Settings* category, typing 2, and then clicking the Print button.

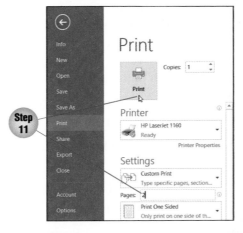

12 Position the insertion point anywhere in page 1, click the FILE tab, and then click the *Print* option.

13 Click the top gallery in the *Settings* category and then click *Print Current Page* at the drop-down list.

14 Click the Print button.

15 Save **WMedS1-CRGHh&p.docx**.

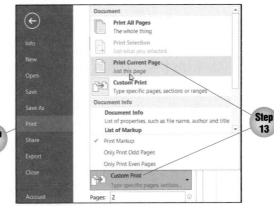

In Addition

Printing a Range of Pages

Identify a specific page, multiple pages, and/or a range of pages for printing at the Print backstage area. To print specific pages, click in the *Pages* text box and then type the page numbers of the pages you want to print. If you want to print multiple pages, use a comma to indicate *and* and a hyphen to indicate *through*. For example, to print pages 2 and 5, you would type *2,5* in the *Pages* text box. To print pages 6 through 10, you would type *6-10*. You can enter both commas and hyphens when specifying page numbers.

Getting Help on a Button

When you hover your mouse over certain buttons, the ScreenTip that displays may include a Help icon and the text *Tell me more*. Click this hyperlinked text and the Word Help window opens with information about the button feature. You can also hover the mouse pointer over a button and then press F1 to display the Word Help window with information about the button feature.

Activity 1.8

Inserting the Date, Time, and Quick Parts; Closing a Document

Insert the current date and/or time into a document with options at the Date and Time dialog box. The Date and Time dialog box contains a list of date and time options in the *Available formats* list box. If the *Update automatically* check box at the Date and Time dialog box does not contain a check mark, the date and/or time are inserted in the document as text that can be edited in the normal manner. You can also insert the date and/or time as a field in a document. The advantage to inserting the date or time as a field is that you can automatically update the field by pressing the Update Field key, F9. Insert the date and/or time as a field by inserting a check mark in the *Update automatically* check box before you select an option from the *Available formats* list box. Word also contains a Quick Parts button with options for inserting predesigned building blocks to help you build a document. Building blocks include cover pages, headers and footers, page numbers, tables, text boxes, and watermarks, which are all located at the Building Blocks Organizer dialog box.

Project

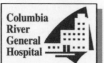

You are satisfied with the recent revisions to the History and Physical Examination document. The final steps are to identify the document as confidential, insert the date and time, and then close the document.

1. With **WMedS1-CRGHh&p.docx** open, press Ctrl + End to move the insertion point to the end of the document.

2. Type Date: and then press the spacebar once.

3. Click the INSERT tab and then click the Date & Time button 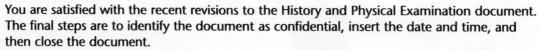 in the Text group.

4. At the Date and Time dialog box, click the third option from the top in the *Available formats* list box. (Your date will vary from what you see below.)

5. Click the *Update automatically* check box to insert a check mark and then click OK to close the dialog box.

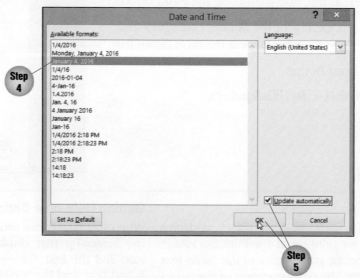

6. Press Shift + Enter, type Time:, and then press the spacebar once.

7. Click the Date & Time button.

8 At the Date and Time dialog box, click the option that will insert the time in numbers with the hour, minutes, and seconds (for example, *2:19:30 PM*). Make sure the *Update automatically* check box contains a check mark and then click OK to close the dialog box.

> This option may be the fourteenth or fifteenth from the top in the *Available formats* list box.

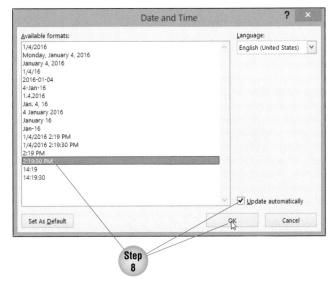

9 Print only page 2 of the document.

10 To identify the document as confidential, insert a building block that displays the word *CONFIDENTIAL* as a watermark (a lightened image that displays behind text). To begin, click the Quick Parts button in the Text group on the INSERT tab and then click *Building Blocks Organizer* at the drop-down list.

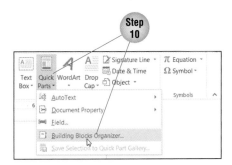

11 At the Building Blocks Organizer dialog box, click the *Gallery* column heading.

> This sorts the building blocks alphabetically by gallery.

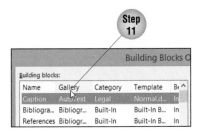

continues

⑫ Scroll to the end of the list box, click *CONFIDENTIAL 1*, and then click the Insert button.

You will not see the entire name of the quick part in the list box, but if you click the first part of the name, the full name of the quick part will display in the lower right corner of the dialog box below the preview section.

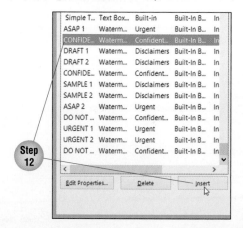

Step 12

⑬ To begin inserting a predesigned cover page quick part, press Ctrl + Home to move the insertion point to the beginning of the document, click the Quick Parts button in the Text group on the INSERT tab, and then click *Building Blocks Organizer* at the drop-down list.

⑭ At the Building Blocks Organizer dialog box, click *Semaphore* in the list box and then click the Insert button.

After you click *Semaphore*, check the Gallery column to make sure it contains the text *Cover Page*.

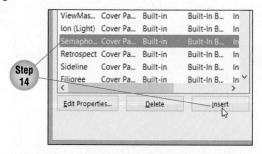

Step 14

⑮ Click anywhere in the placeholder text *[DATE]* to select it, click the down-pointing arrow at the right of the placeholder, and then click the Today button at the drop-down list.

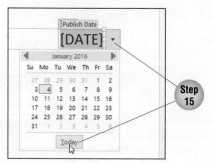

Step 15

16 Click anywhere in the placeholder text *[DOCUMENT TITLE]* and then type History and Physical Examination.

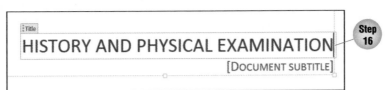

Step 16

17 Click anywhere in the placeholder text *[DOCUMENT SUBTITLE]*, click the placeholder tab, and then press the Delete key.

Clicking a placeholder's tab selects that object.

Step 17

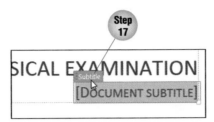

18 Click the text that displays below the title (might be a personal name or a school name), click the placeholder tab, and then type your first and last names.

19 Click anywhere in the placeholder text *[COMPANY NAME]* and then type Columbia River General Hospital.

20 Click anywhere in the placeholder text *[Company address]*, click the placeholder tab, and then press the Delete key.

21 Press Ctrl + End to move the insertion point to the end of the document, click anywhere in the time text, and then press F9 to update the time.

Pressing F9, the Update Field key, updates the time. You can also update the time by clicking the Update tab that displays above the selected time.

22 Click the Save button on the Quick Access toolbar.

23 Print the document by clicking the FILE tab, clicking the *Print* option, and then clicking the Print button.

24 Close the document by clicking the FILE tab and then clicking the *Close* option at the backstage area.

In Brief

Display Date and Time Dialog Box
1. Click INSERT tab.
2. Click Date & Time button.

Display Building Blocks Organizer Dialog Box
1. Click INSERT tab.
2. Click Quick Parts button.
3. Click *Building Blocks Organizer*.

In Addition

Sorting Data in the Building Blocks Organizer

The Building Blocks Organizer dialog box provides a single location where you can view all of the predesigned building blocks available in Word. You can sort the building blocks in the dialog box alphabetically by clicking the column headings. For example, to sort building blocks alphabetically by name, click the *Name* column heading.

Activity 1.9

Creating a Document Using a Template

Word includes a number of template documents formatted for specific uses. Each Word document is based on a template, with the Normal template the default. With Word templates, you can easily create a variety of documents with specialized formatting, such as letters, faxes, and awards. Display available templates by clicking the FILE tab and then clicking the *New* option. Search for Microsoft online templates with the *Search for online templates* option. Type a category in the search text box and then press Enter to display relevant templates. Click the desired template and then click the Create button. You must be connected to the Internet to download online templates.

Project

Your supervisor at North Shore Medical Clinic has asked you to send a letter requesting information on interpreting services.

1. Click the FILE tab and then click the *New* option.

2. At the New backstage area, click in the search text box (contains the text *Search for online templates*), type **business letter**, and then press Enter.

3. Scroll down the list of templates and then click the *Letter (Equity theme)* template.

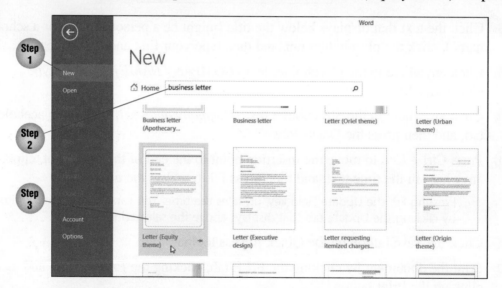

4. Click the Create button.

5. At the letter document, click the placeholder text *[Pick the date]* and then type the current date. (Your date will automatically change to numbers when you click outside the placeholder.)

6. Select the name that automatically displays below the date and then type your first and last names.

7. Click the placeholder text *[Type the sender company name]* and then type North Shore Medical Clinic.

8. Click the placeholder text *[Type the sender company address]*, type 7450 Meridian Street, Suite 150, press the Enter key, and then type Portland, OR 97202.

9. Click the placeholder text *[Type the recipient name]* and then type Community Interpreting Services.

10. Click the placeholder text *[Type the recipient address]*, type 4525 Lawrence Street, press the Enter key, and then type Portland, OR 97216.

11. Click the placeholder text *[Type the salutation]* and then type Ladies and Gentlemen:.

12. Click any character in the three paragraphs of text in the body of the letter and then type the text shown in Figure W1.4.

13. Click the placeholder text *[Type the closing]* and then type Sincerely,.

14. Make sure your name displays below *Sincerely*. If not, select the name that displays and then type your first and last names.

15. Click the placeholder text *[Type the sender title]* and then type Medical Office Assistant.

16. Click the Save button on the Quick Access toolbar.

17. At the Save As backstage area, click the *WordMedS1* folder that displays below the *Recent Folders* heading. (Alternatively, click your OneDrive or the *Computer* option, click the Browse button, and then navigate to the WordMedS1 folder.)

18. At the Save As dialog box with the WordMedS1 folder active (either on your OneDrive or USB flash drive), type WMedS1-RequestLtr in the *File name* text box and then press Enter or click the Save button.

   > If a dialog box displays telling you that your document will be upgraded to the newest file format, click OK.

19. Print the letter by clicking the FILE tab, clicking the *Print* option, and then clicking the Print button.

20. Close the document by clicking the FILE tab and then clicking the *Close* option.

FIGURE W1.4 Step 12

At North Shore Medical Clinic, our goal is to provide the best possible medical care for our patients. Since some of our patients are non-English speakers, we occasionally need interpreting services. Up to this point, we have been hiring interpreters from various agencies. We recently determined that we would like to contract with one agency to provide all interpreting services at our clinic.

We are interested in learning about all interpreting services available at your agency and would like a representative to contact us to schedule a face-to-face meeting. Please call our clinic at (503) 555-2330 and ask for the clinic director. We look forward to working with your agency.

In Addition

Specifying a Category

When you search for online templates, a *Category* list box displays at the right side of the screen. The list box displays the category name and the number of templates in the category. Click the desired category in the list box to display templates matching that category in the New backstage area.

Activity 1.10

Creating and Renaming Folders; Saving a Document in a Different Format

As you continue creating documents, you will need to consider document management tasks such as creating folders and copying, moving, and deleting documents. You can complete many document management tasks at the Open dialog box.

By default, Word saves a file as a Word document and adds the extension *.docx* to the name. Using the *Save as type* option box at the Save As dialog box, you can save a document in a different format, such as an earlier version of Word, rich text format, a template, or a PDF or XPS file.

Project

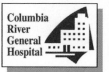

To begin managing your documents, you decide to create a folder named H&P in which you will save all history and physical examination documents. You also need to send a document to a colleague who uses an earlier version of Word, so you will use the Save As dialog box to save the document in that format.

1. Click the FILE tab. At the Open backstage area, click your OneDrive or click *Computer* in the middle panel.

2. Click the *WordMedS1* folder that displays below the *Recent Folders* heading. (If the WordMedS1 folder does not display below the *Recent Folders* heading, click the Browse button.)

3. At the Open dialog box with WordMedS1 the active folder, click the New folder button.

4. Type **H&P** and then press Enter.

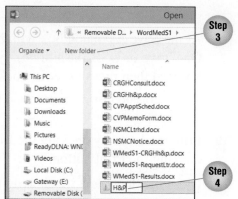

5. Click **CRGHh&p.docx** in the Content pane of the Open dialog box, hold down the Ctrl key, click **WMedS1-CRGHh&p.docx**, click **WMedS1-Results.docx**, and then release the Ctrl key.

   Use the Ctrl key to select multiple nonadjacent documents. Use the Shift key to select multiple adjacent documents.

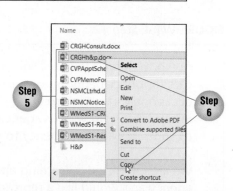

6. Right-click any of the selected documents and then click *Copy* at the shortcut menu.

7. Double-click the *H&P* folder.

   Folders display before documents in the Content pane of the Open dialog box. Folders display preceded by a folder icon 📁 and documents display preceded by a document icon 📄.

8. Position the mouse pointer over a blank portion of the Content pane in the Open dialog box, right-click, and then click *Paste* at the shortcut menu.

   The copied documents are inserted in the H&P folder.

9. You need to send **WMedS1-CRGHh&p.docx** to a colleague who uses Word 2003, so you need to save the document in that format. At the Open dialog box with the H&P folder active, double-click **WMedS1-CRGHh&p.docx**.

10 Click the FILE tab and then click the *Save As* option.

11 At the Save As backstage area, click the *WordMedS1* folder that displays below the *Recent Folders* heading.

12 At the Save As dialog box, type **WMedS1-CRGHh&pW2003** in the *File name* text box.

13 Click the *Save as type* option box and then click *Word 97-2003 Document (*.doc)* at the drop-down list.

14 Click the Save button in the lower right corner of the dialog box and then close the document.

> If a compatibility checker message displays, click the Continue button.

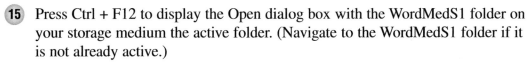

Step 12

Step 13

In Brief

Create Folder
1. Display Open dialog box.
2. Click New folder button.
3. Type folder name.
4. Press Enter.

Save Document in Different Format
1. Display Save As dialog box.
2. Type document name in *File name* text box.
3. Click *Save as type* option box.
4. Click desired format.
5. Click Save button.

15 Press Ctrl + F12 to display the Open dialog box with the WordMedS1 folder on your storage medium the active folder. (Navigate to the WordMedS1 folder if it is not already active.)

16 At the Open dialog box, rename the H&P folder. To do this, right-click the folder name and then click *Rename* at the shortcut menu. Type **H&PEDocs** and then press Enter.

> The new folder name replaces the original folder name. You can also rename a folder by selecting the folder, clicking the Organize button, clicking *Rename* at the drop-down list, and then typing the new folder name.

17 Delete the H&PEDocs folder. To do this, click once on the folder to select it, click the Organize button on the toolbar, and then click *Delete* at the drop-down list. At the message asking if you are sure you want to delete the folder and all of its contents, click the Yes button.

> You can also delete a folder by clicking the folder and then pressing the Delete key or by right-clicking the folder and then clicking *Delete* at the shortcut menu.

Step 17

18 Close the Open dialog box.

19 Close Word by clicking the Close button in the upper right corner of the screen.

In Addition

Editing a PDF File in Word

New to Word 2013 is the ability to open a PDF file in Word and make edits to it. PDF, which stands for Portable Document Format, is a common format for sharing files. When you open a PDF file, Word converts it to a .docx file so that you can edit it. The data in the file may not display in the exact format as in the PDF file. Converting a PDF file to a Word document works best with text-based documents.

Features Summary

Feature	Ribbon Tab, Group	Button	Quick Access Toolbar	FILE Tab Option	Keyboard Shortcut
AutoCorrect dialog box				*Options, Proofing, AutoCorrect Options*	
close				*Close*	Ctrl + F4
close Word		⊠			Alt + F4
date	INSERT, Text				Shift + Alt + D
Draft view	VIEW, Views				
Help		?			F1
Navigation pane	VIEW, Show				Ctrl + F
New backstage area				*New*	
Open backstage area				*Open*	Ctrl + O
Open dialog box					Ctrl + F12
Print backstage area				*Print*	Ctrl + P
Print Layout view	VIEW, Views				
quick parts	INSERT, Text				
Read Mode	VIEW, Views				
redo			↷		Ctrl + Y
Save As backstage area				*Save* OR *Save As*	
Save As dialog box					F12
save document					Ctrl + S
Spelling & Grammar	REVIEW, Proofing	ABC✓			F7
Thesaurus	REVIEW, Proofing				Shift + F7
time	INSERT, Text				Shift + Alt + T
undo			↶▾		Ctrl + Z
Word Options dialog box				*Options*	

Knowledge Check

Completion: In the space provided at the right, indicate the correct term, command, or option.

1. This area on the screen contains tabs and commands divided into groups. _____
2. Click this tab to display the backstage area. _____
3. Use this keyboard command to move the insertion point to the beginning of the document. _____
4. To select a sentence, hold down this key and then click anywhere in the sentence. _____
5. This toolbar contains the Undo and Redo buttons. _____
6. To begin checking the spelling and grammar in a document, click this tab and then click the Spelling & Grammar button in the Proofing group. _____
7. This feature automatically detects and corrects some typographical errors. _____
8. Use this feature to find synonyms for a word. _____
9. Display a document in this view for easy reading. _____
10. The *Navigation Pane* check box is located in this group on the VIEW tab. _____
11. Click the Date & Time button located in the Text group on this tab to display the Date and Time dialog box. _____
12. Click this button on the Open dialog box toolbar to create a new folder. _____
13. Select nonadjacent documents at the Open dialog box by holding down this key while clicking each document name. _____

Skills Review

Review 1 Moving the Insertion Point, Scrolling, and Inserting Text

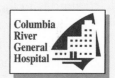

1. Open **CRGHConsult.docx**.
2. Save the document with the name **WMedS1-R-CRGHConsult**.
3. Using the mouse pointer and/or keyboard, practice moving the insertion point by completing the following steps:
   a. Move the insertion point to the end of the document.
   b. Move the insertion point back to the beginning of the document.
   c. Scroll to the end of the document.
   d. Scroll back to the beginning of the document.
   e. Move the insertion point to the beginning of the second page.
   f. Move the insertion point to the beginning of the document.
4. Move the insertion point to the beginning of the date *04/25/2016* located toward the beginning of the document, type Date of Admission:, and then press the spacebar once.
5. Move the insertion point to the beginning of the date *06/05/1939*, type Date of Birth:, and then press the spacebar once.
6. Save **WMedS1-R-CRGHConsult.docx**.

Review 2 Selecting and Deleting Text

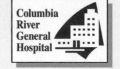

1. With **WMedS1-R-CRGHConsult.docx** open, select and then delete the words *as well* located at the end of the second sentence in the HISTORY section. (Make sure the period that ends the sentence is positioned immediately right of the word *area*.)
2. Select and then delete the words *was brought to the Emergency Room by her husband and* located in the fourth sentence in the *HISTORY* section.
3. Use the selection bar to select the line containing the sentence *Review of systems is unremarkable* in the second paragraph in the *HISTORY* section and then delete the line. *Note: Make sure no extra space displays above the EXAMINATION heading.*
4. Undo the deletion.
5. Redo the deletion.
6. Select and then delete the last sentence in the *HISTORY* section (*The rest of her social and family history is noted on the admission report.*).
7. Undo the deletion.
8. Deselect the text.
9. Save **WMedS1-R-CRGHConsult.docx**.

Review 3 Checking the Spelling and Grammar in a Document

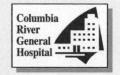

1. With **WMedS1-R-CRGHConsult.docx** open, move the insertion point to the beginning of the document.
2. Complete a spelling and grammar check on the document. *Note: The medical term **nontender** is spelled correctly.*
3. Save **WMedS1-R-CRGHConsult.docx**.

Review 4 Creating an AutoCorrect Entry; Using the Thesaurus; Inserting the Date and Time and a Cover Page

1. With **WMedS1-R-CRGHConsult.docx** open, add the following entries to the AutoCorrect dialog box:
   a. Insert *ic* in the *Replace* text box and *intertrochanteric* in the *With* text box.
   b. Insert *tr* in the *Replace* text box and *trochanter* in the *With* text box.
2. Move the insertion point to the blank line above the RECOMMENDATIONS heading (below the *EXAMINATION* section) and then type the text shown in Figure W1.5. *Hint: Press Shift + Enter after typing* **X-RAY** *and after typing* **IMPRESSION.**

FIGURE W1.5 Review 4, Step 2

X-RAY
Review of x-rays demonstrates a comminuted right ic hip fracture with comminution of the greater tr, as well as lesser tr.

IMPRESSION
Right comminuted ic hip fracture, noninsulin dependent diabetes mellitus, and hypercholesterolemia.

3. Use the Thesaurus to make the following changes:
   a. Change *aware* in the first sentence of the *EXAMINATION* section to *alert*.
   b. Change *unidentified*, located toward the end of the *HISTORY* section, to *unknown*.
4. Move the insertion point to the end of the document, insert the current date (you choose the format), press Shift + Enter, and then insert the current time (you choose the format).
5. Delete the AutoCorrect entries for *ic* and *tr*.
6. Insert the Retrospect cover page. **Hint: Choose the Retrospect cover page at the Building Blocks Organizer dialog box.**
7. Click in the placeholder text *[Document title]* and then type Consultation Report.
8. Click in the placeholder text *[DOCUMENT SUBTITLE]* and then type ID# 09232.
9. Select the name that displays toward the bottom of the cover page (in the orange section) and then type your first and last names.
10. Delete the *[COMPANY NAME]* and *[COMPANY ADDRESS]* placeholders and then delete the vertical bar that displays between the two placeholders and the blank line on which the bar was previously located.
11. Save, print, and then close **WMedS1-R-CRGHConsult.docx**.

Review 5 Creating a Fax Using a Template

1. Click the FILE tab and then click the *New* option.
2. At the New backstage area, click in the search text box, type equity fax, and then press the Enter key.
3. Click the *Fax (Equity theme)* template and then click the Create button.
4. Insert the following information in the specified locations:
   a. *[Type the recipient name]*   = Andres Diaz
   b. Select the text that displays after the *From:* heading and then type your first and last names.
   c. *[Type the recipient fax number]*   = (503) 555-0988
   d. *[Type number of pages]*   = Cover page plus 1 page
   e. *[Type the recipient phone number]*   = (503) 555-0900
   f. *[Pick the date]*   = 5.30.2016
   g. *[Type text]* (located after *Re:*)   = Interpreting Services and Fees
   h. Click the *[Type text]* placeholder that displays after *CC:*, click the placeholder tab, and then delete the placeholder.
   i. Click in the square that displays immediately to the left of *Please Comment* and then type the letter X.
   j. *[Type comments]*   = Interpreting services and fees are shown on the following document.
5. Save the completed fax and name it **WMedS1-R-Fax**.
6. Print and then close **WMedS1-R-Fax.docx**.

Skills Assessment

Assessment 1 Inserting Text in a Document

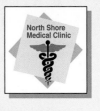

1. Open **NSMCNotice.docx**.
2. Save the document with the name **WMedS1-A1-NSMCNotice**.
3. In the first paragraph of text, make the following changes:
   a. Change the day from *Thursday* to *Wednesday*.
   b. Change the date from *20* to *19*.
   c. Change the time from *7:30 to 9:00* to *7:00 to 8:30*.
4. Press Ctrl + End to move the insertion point to the end of the document and then type the information shown in Figure W1.6.
5. Save, print, and then close **WMedS1-A1-NSMCNotice.docx**.

FIGURE W1.6 Assessment 1, Step 4

The presentation will include information on the prevalence of diabetes among people of different age and ethnic groups, health complications related to diabetes, and treatment and prevention of diabetes. For more information on the presentation, please contact Lee Elliott.

Assessment 2 Preparing a Memo

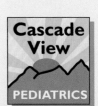

1. Open **CVPMemoForm.docx**.
2. Save the document with the name **WMedS1-A2-CVPMemoForm**.
3. Insert the following information after the specified heading:

To:	**All Front Office Staff**
From:	**Sydney Larsen, Office Manager**
Date:	(Insert current date)
Re:	**Well-child Checkup Appointments**

4. Move the insertion point below the *Re:* heading and then write the body of the memo using the following information (write the information in paragraph form—do not use bullets):
   - With the recent hiring of Dr. Joseph Yarborough, pediatric specialist, we will be scheduling additional well-child checkup appointments.
   - Schedule appointments at the ages of 2 weeks and 2, 4, 6, 12, 18, and 24 months.
   - Appointment length is generally 20 minutes.
   - Schedule well-child checkup appointments for Dr. Yarborough on Tuesdays and Thursdays.
   - Evening hours for appointments with Dr. Yarborough will be added next month.
5. Complete a spelling and grammar check on the memo.
6. Save, print, and then close **WMedS1-A2-CVPMemoForm.docx**.

Assessment 3 Adding Text to a Scheduling Information Document

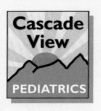

1. Open **CVPApptSched.docx**.
2. Save the document with the name **WMedS1-A3-CVPApptSched**.
3. Create an AutoCorrect entry that inserts *Appointments* when you type *Aps*.
4. Insert the following text in the document:
   a. Move the insertion point to the beginning of the second paragraph (begins with *These are short visits*), type Acute Illness Aps (20 minutes), and then press Shift + Enter. (The AutoCorrect feature will insert *Appointments* when you press the spacebar after typing *Aps*.)
   b. Move the insertion point to the beginning of the paragraph that begins *These appointments, available within one week*, type Routine Aps (20 minutes), and then press Shift + Enter.
   c. Move the insertion point to the beginning of the paragraph that begins *Physical examination appointments are usually*, type Physical Examination Aps (30 minutes), and then press Shift + Enter.
   d. Move the insertion point to the beginning of the paragraph that begins *All children should be seen*, type Well-child Checkup Aps (20 minutes), and then press Shift + Enter.
5. Complete a spelling and grammar check on the document.
6. Move the insertion point to the end of the document and then insert the current date and time.
7. Delete the AutoCorrect entry *Aps*.
8. Insert the DRAFT 1 watermark
9. Save, print, and then close **WMedS1-A3-CVPApptSched.docx**.

Assessment 4 Locating Information about Word 2013 Features

1. At a blank document, display the Word Help window and then click the <u>See what's new</u> hyperlink in the *Getting started* section.
2. Read about the new features in Word 2013.
3. Using the information you learn, prepare a memo to your instructor describing at least three new Word 2013 features.
4. Save the memo and name it **WMedS1-A4-NewFeatures**.
5. Print and then close **WMedS1-A4-NewFeatures.docx**.

Assessment 5 Researching a Medical Spell Checking Dictionary

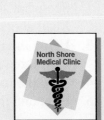

1. As you learned in Activity 1.4, the standard spell checking dictionary in Word does not contain many medical terms. Most offices, clinics, and hospitals that prepare medical documents and forms add a supplemental medical spell checking dictionary to their Word software. One of the most popular is *Stedman's Medical Dictionary*. As the medical office assistant at North Shore Medical Clinic, your supervisor has asked you to locate information about the Stedman's medical spell checking dictionary. Using the Internet, go to the Stedman's home page at www.stedmans.com. (If this website is not available, search for another company that sells a medical spell checking dictionary and visit their home page.)
2. After looking at the information at the Stedman's website, prepare a memo to your supervisor, Lee Elliott, Office Manager. Include information on the medical dictionary, including its web address, price, features, and how to order it.
3. Save the completed memo and name it **WMedS1-A5-Dictionary**.
4. Print and then close **WMedS1-A5-Dictionary.docx**.

Marquee Challenge

Challenge 1 Preparing a Presurgery Letter to a Doctor

1. Open **NSMCLtrhd.docx** and then save it with the name **WMedS1-C1-NSMCInfoLtr**.
2. Type the letter as shown in Figure W1.7.
3. Remove the hyperlink from the email address (displays in underlined blue font) by right-clicking the email address and then clicking *Remove Hyperlink* at the shortcut menu.
4. Save, print, and then close **WMedS1-C1-NSMCInfoLtr.docx**.

Challenge 2 Preparing Patient Chart Notes

1. Open **NSMCLtrhd.docx** and then save it with the name **WMedS1-C2-NSMCNote**.
2. Type the chart notes as shown in Figure W1.8 on page 100.
3. Save, print, and then close **WMedS1-C2-NSMCNote.docx**.

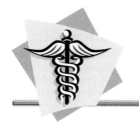

North Shore Medical Clinic
7450 Meridian Street, Suite 150
Portland, OR 97202
(503) 555-2330
www.emcp.net/nsmc

Date: _____

Dear Doctor _____:

Our mutual patient _____, D.O.B. _____, is scheduled for
surgery on _____. Please assist us by providing the following information:

      Pathology report
      Copy of most recent EKG
      New lab work (Basic Metabolic Panel, HCT/Hemoglobin, Protime/INR, K+)
      Clearance for surgery

The surgeon would like the patient to stop taking Coumadin as soon as possible prior to surgery. Please
let us know if instructing the patient to do so is safe and how long the patient can be off the medication.

Please email or fax requested information to us as soon as possible. Our email address is
www.emcp.net/nsmc and our fax number is (503) 555-2335. If you have any questions, please call the
clinic at (503) 555-2330.

Sincerely,

Darrin Lancaster, CMA
Medical Assistant

WMedS1-C1-NSMCInfoLtr.docx

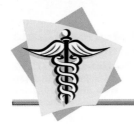

North Shore Medical Clinic
7450 Meridian Street, Suite 150
Portland, OR 97202
(503) 555-2330
www.emcp.net/nsmc

PATIENT: Grace Montgomery
DATE OF VISIT: 04/18/2016

SUBJECTIVE
Patient is complaining of itching and a rash that began about three weeks ago, starting on the hands and arms and spreading to the chest and back. She is currently taking Benadryl at bedtime with little relief. She stated that she tried a new perfume after her shower three or four days before the rash appeared.

OBJECTIVE
GENERAL APPEARANCE: Normal.
VITAL SIGNS: Temperature 98.6 degrees, blood pressure 140/74, weight 145, height 5 feet 6 inches, heart rate 74, respirations 22.
SKIN: Patient has a smooth, erythematous rash over her neck extending over her trunk and back. She has a confluent, erythematous rash extending to fingertips on her upper extremities. Wheals with patechiae are noted in the antecubital fossae bilaterally.

ASSESSMENT
Contact dermatitis, secondary to allergy to perfume.

PLAN
Avoid use of any perfume or perfumed soap.
Wash or dry-clean all clothing and linens exposed to suspected perfume.
Take diphenhydramine (Benadryl) 25 mg q6 h x 3 days.

_____

Jonathon Melina, MD

JM:SN
Date: (Insert current date)
Time: (Insert current time)

Word SECTION 2

Formatting Characters and Paragraphs

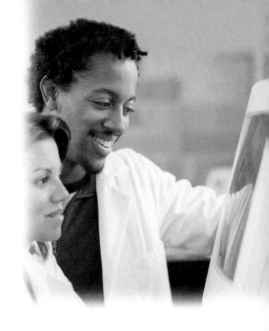

Skills

- Apply fonts and font effects
- Use Format Painter
- Repeat a command
- Align text in paragraphs
- Indent text
- Change line and paragraph spacing
- Insert bullets and numbering
- Insert symbols and special characters
- Set tabs and apply leaders
- Add borders and shading to text
- Insert a page border
- Apply styles and style sets
- Apply themes

Student Resources

Before beginning the activities in Word Section 2, copy to your storage medium the WordMedS2 folder from the Student Resources CD. This folder contains the data files you need to complete the projects in this Word section.

Projects Overview

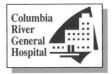

Edit and format an informational document on heart disease and format a legal document on records storage and maintenance.

Edit and format a document on well-child checkup appointment recommendations and suggestions and prepare a document containing information on clinic hours.

Edit and format a document on diabetes, format a document on cystic fibrosis, edit and format a document on how to request medical records, prepare a letter to the local community college indicating the availability of an internship, prepare a memo describing Word features, prepare a memo describing aspects of the medical assisting field, prepare a job announcement, and prepare a flyer advertising a free diabetes presentation.

Activity 2.1

Applying Formatting with the Font Group and the Mini Toolbar

The appearance of a document in the document screen and how it looks when printed is called the *format*. Use buttons in the Font group on the HOME tab to apply character formatting to text. The top row of the group contains buttons for changing the font and font size as well as changing the text case and clearing formatting. The bottom row contains buttons for applying formatting such as bold, italics, underlining, strikethrough, superscript, subscript, text effects, highlighting, and font color. Microsoft Word has taken some commonly used commands and placed them on the Mini toolbar. When you select text, the Mini toolbar displays above the selected text. The Mini toolbar disappears when you move the mouse pointer away from it.

Project Your supervisor at Columbia River General Hospital has asked you to format and edit an informational document on heart disease. You decide to improve the appearance of the document by applying different types of fonts and effects to the text.

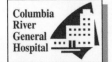

1 Open **CRGHHeartDisease.docx** and then save it with the name **WMedS2-CRGHHeartDisease**.

2 Select the text *Heart Disease* and then click the Bold button **B** in the Font group on the HOME tab.

3 With *Heart Disease* still selected, click the Change Case button **Aa ▾** in the Font group and then click *UPPERCASE* at the drop-down list.

> Use options at the Change Case drop-down list to specify the case of selected text.

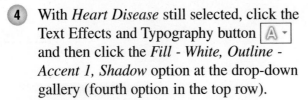

4 With *Heart Disease* still selected, click the Text Effects and Typography button **A ▾** and then click the *Fill - White, Outline - Accent 1, Shadow* option at the drop-down gallery (fourth option in the top row).

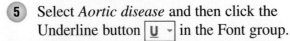

5 Select *Aortic disease* and then click the Underline button **U ▾** in the Font group.

6 Select and then underline the remaining headings: *Arrhythmia (abnormal heart rhythm), Cardiomyopathy (heart muscle disease), Congenital heart disease, Coronary artery disease, Heart failure, Heart valve disease, Pericardial disease*, and *Vascular disease*.

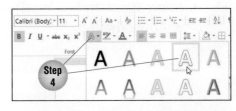

7 Select the words *abnormal heart rhythm* in the parentheses after the word *Arrhythmia* in the second underlined heading and then click the Italic button **I** on the Mini toolbar that displays above the selected text.

> The Mini toolbar displays above selected text. The toolbar disappears when you move the mouse pointer away from it.

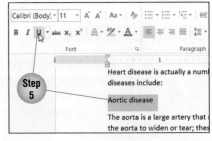

8 Select the words *heart muscle disease* in the parentheses after the word *Cardiomyopathy* and then click the Italic button on the Mini toolbar.

9 Select the heading *HEART DISEASE* and then click the Clear All Formatting button in the Font group.

10 Select the entire document by clicking the Select button in the Editing group on the HOME tab and then clicking *Select All* at the drop-down list.

11 Click the Font button arrow in the Font group. Hover the mouse pointer over various typefaces in the Font drop-down gallery and notice how the text in the document reflects the selected font.

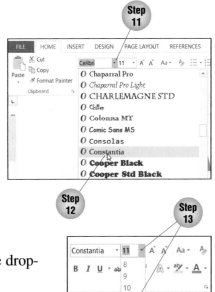

> This feature is referred to as *live preview*. It provides you with an opportunity to see how the document will appear with formatting before you make a final choice.

12 Scroll down the gallery and then click *Constantia*.

13 Click the Font Size button arrow and then click *12* at the drop-down gallery.

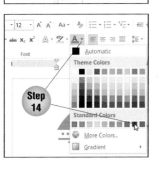

14 Click the Font Color button arrow and then click the *Dark Blue* option at the drop-down gallery (second color from the right in the *Standard Colors* row).

15 Deselect the text by clicking anywhere in the document.

16 You decide to highlight specific text to identify it for review by colleagues. To do this, click the Text Highlight Color button in the Font group and then select the first sentence under the heading *Aortic disease* (the sentence that begins *The aorta is a large artery that*).

> When you click the Text Highlight Color button, the mouse pointer displays with a highlighter pen attached. To turn off highlighting, click the Text Highlight Color button again.

17 Select the sentence under the *Arrhythmia* heading to highlight it and then click the Text Highlight Color button to turn off highlighting.

18 Remove the text highlighting by pressing Ctrl + A, clicking the Text Highlight Color button arrow, and then clicking *No Color* at the drop-down list.

19 Save and then print **WMedS2-CRGHHeartDisease.docx**.

In Addition

Using Typefaces

A *typeface* is a set of characters with a common design and shape. A typeface can be decorative or plain and either monospaced or proportional. A monospaced typeface allots the same amount of horizontal space for each character, while a proportional typeface allots a varying amount of space for each character. Proportional typefaces are divided into two main categories: *serif* and *sans serif*. A serif is a small line at the end of a character stroke. Word refers to typeface as *font*. Consider using a serif font for text-intensive documents, since serifs help move the reader's eyes across the page. Use a sans serif font for headings and headlines.

Activity 2.2

Using the Font Dialog Box and Format Painter; Repeating a Command

In addition to buttons in the Font group, you can apply font formatting with options at the Font dialog box. With options at this dialog box, you can change the font, font size, font style, and font color; choose an underlining style; and apply formatting effects. Once you apply font formatting to text, you can copy that formatting to different locations in the document using the Format Painter. If you apply formatting to text in a document and then want to apply the same formatting to other text, apply the Repeat command by pressing the F4 function key.

Project The changes you made to the heart disease document have enhanced the readability and visual appeal of the text. Now you will turn your attention to the headings.

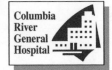

Columbia
River
General
Hospital

1. With **WMedS2-CRGHHeartDisease.docx** open, press Ctrl + Home to move the insertion point to the beginning of the page and then select the entire document by pressing Ctrl + A.

   Ctrl + A is the keyboard shortcut to select the entire document.

2. Click the Font group dialog box launcher [⬛].

   The dialog box launcher displays as a small button containing a diagonal arrow.

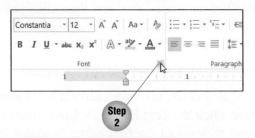

Step 2

3. At the Font dialog box, click *Cambria* in the *Font* list box (you will need to scroll up the list box to display this option) and then click *11* in the *Size* list box.

4. Click the down-pointing arrow at the right side of the *Font color* option and then click the *Black, Text 1* option (second column, first row in the *Theme Colors* section).

Step 3

Step 4

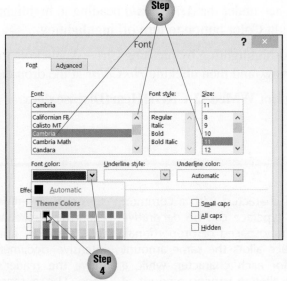

5 Click OK to close the Font dialog box.

6 Select the heading *HEART DISEASE* that displays towards the beginning of the document and then click the Font group dialog box launcher.

7 At the Font dialog box, click *Candara* in the *Font* list box (you will need to scroll down the list box to display this option), and then click *14* in the *Size* list box (you will need to scroll down the list box to display this option).

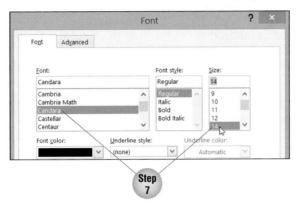

Step 7

8 Click OK to close the Font dialog box.

9 With the heading still selected, click the Format Painter button 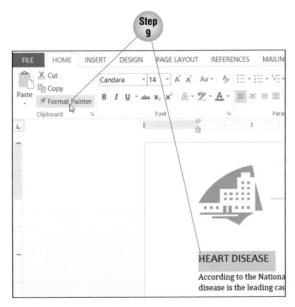 in the Clipboard group on the HOME tab.

> When Format Painter is active, the mouse pointer displays with a paintbrush attached.

Step 9

10 Scroll down the document and then select the heading *HEART DISEASE FACTS*.

> Selecting the heading applies the formatting from the first heading and also turns off Format Painter.

continues

11 Select the heading *Aortic disease* and then click the Font group dialog box launcher.

12 Click *Candara* in the *Font* list box (you will need to scroll down the list box to display this option), click *Bold* in the *Font style* list box, and then click *14* in the *Size* list box (you will need to scroll down the list box to display this option).

13 Click the down-pointing arrow at the right side of the *Underline style* option box and then click *(none)* at the drop-down list.

14 Click OK to close the dialog box and then deselect the heading.

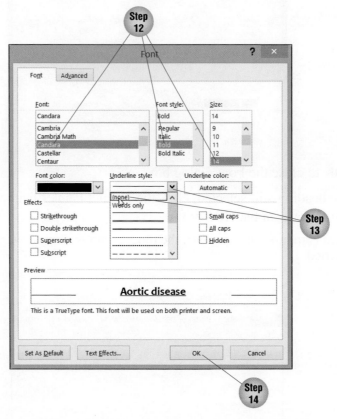

15 Click any character in the heading *Aortic disease* and then double-click the Format Painter button in the Clipboard group on the HOME tab.

16 Select the heading *Arrhythmia (abnormal heart rhythm)*.

Because you double-clicked the Format Painter button, the feature remains active even after you select the text and apply the formatting.

17 Select individually the remaining headings: *Cardiomyopathy (heart muscle disease), Congenital heart disease, Coronary artery disease, Heart failure, Heart valve disease, Pericardial disease*, and *Vascular disease*.

18 Click the Format Painter button in the Clipboard group to turn off Format Painter.

19 Select the text *National Center for Chronic Disease Prevention and Health Promotion*, located in the first paragraph.

20 Click the Text Effects and Typography button in the Font group, point to *Shadow*, and then click the *Offset Diagonal Bottom Right* option (first column, first row in the *Outer* section).

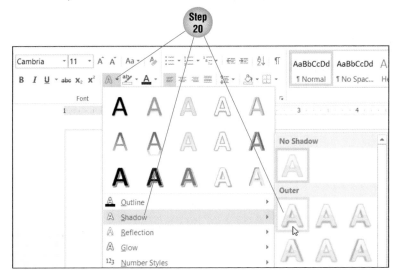

Step 20

In Brief

Change Font at Font Dialog Box
1. Click Font group dialog box launcher.
2. Click desired font in *Font* list box.
3. Click OK.

Apply Font Effects
1. Select text.
2. Click Font group dialog box launcher.
3. Click desired effect check box.
4. Click OK.

Apply Formatting with Format Painter
1. Apply formatting.
2. Position insertion point within formatted text.
3. Double-click Format Painter button.
4. Select text to be formatted.
5. Click Format Painter button.

21 Select the text *American Heart Association* that displays in the second paragraph and then press the F4 function key.

> Pressing F4 repeats the previous command and applies the shadow effect to the selected text.

22 Select the text *Marfan Syndrome* in the first paragraph in the *Aortic disease* section and then press F4.

23 Save **WMedS2-CRGHHeartDisease.docx**.

In Addition

Using Font Keyboard Shortcuts

Along with buttons in the Font group and the Font dialog box, you can apply font formatting by using the following keyboard shortcuts:

Font Group Button	Keyboard Shortcut
Font	Ctrl + Shift + F
Font Size	Ctrl + Shift + P
Increase Font Size	Ctrl + Shift + >
Decrease Font Size	Ctrl + Shift + <
Change Case	Shift + F3
Bold	Ctrl + B
Italic	Ctrl + I
Underline	Ctrl + U
Subscript	Ctrl + =
Superscript	Ctrl + Shift + +

Activity 2.3

Aligning Text in Paragraphs

Paragraphs of text in a document are aligned at the left margin by default. This default alignment can be changed to center (used for titles, headings, or other text you want centered), right (used for addresses, dates, times, or other text you want aligned at the right margin), and justified (used for text you want aligned at both the left and right margins, such as text in a report or an article). Change paragraph alignment with buttons in the Paragraph group on the HOME tab, the *Alignment* option at the Paragraph dialog box, or with keyboard shortcuts. You can use the keyboard shortcut Ctrl + Q to remove formatting from the paragraph in which the insertion point is positioned. If you want to remove character formatting and paragraph formatting from selected text, click the Clear All Formatting button in the Font group on the HOME tab.

Project

You decide to improve the appearance of the heart disease document by changing the text alignment.

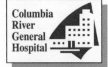

Columbia River General Hospital

1. With **WMedS2-CRGHHeartDisease.docx** open, center the heading *HEART DISEASE* by clicking anywhere within the title and then clicking the Center button in the Paragraph group on the HOME tab.

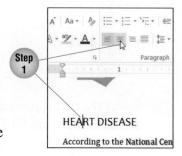

2. Click any character in the heading *HEART DISEASE FACTS* (located toward the middle of page 2, after the *HEART DISEASE* section) and then click the Center button.

3. Press Ctrl + Home to move the insertion point to the beginning of the document and then select from the middle of the paragraph *Heart disease is actually a number of* (third paragraph in the document) to the end of the document.

   The entire third paragraph does not have to be selected, only a portion.

4. Click the Justify button in the Paragraph group.

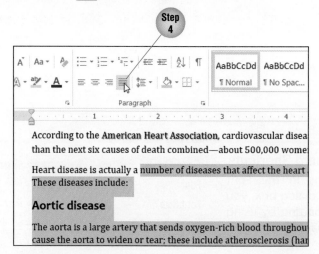

5. Move the insertion point to any character in the heading *HEART DISEASE FACTS* and then click the Center button.

   When you justified the text, the *HEART DISEASE FACTS* title was moved to the left.

6. Press Ctrl + End to move the insertion point to the end of the document and then press the Enter key.

7 Click the Center button in the Paragraph group.

8 Click the Bold button in the Font group to turn on bold formatting and then type your first and last names.

9 Press Shift + Enter.

10 Type Date:, press the spacebar, and then press Alt + Shift + D.

> Alt + Shift + D is the keyboard shortcut to insert the current date.

11 Press Shift + Enter, type Time:, press the spacebar, and then press Alt + Shift + T.

> Alt + Shift + T is the keyboard shortcut to insert the current time.

12 Press the Enter key.

13 Return paragraph alignment back to the default (left alignment) by pressing the shortcut key Ctrl + Q.

> Pressing Ctrl + Q returns all paragraph formatting to the default.

14 After looking at the centered text you just typed, you decide to remove the formatting and apply different formatting. To do this, first select the three lines of text you just typed.

15 Click the Clear All Formatting button in the Font group on the HOME tab.

> Clicking the Clear All Formatting button returns all paragraph and character formatting to the default.

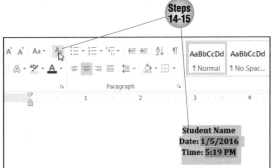

16 With the three lines still selected, click the Align Right button ≡ in the Paragraph group, click the Font button arrow, click *Cambria* at the drop-down gallery, click the Font Size button arrow, and then click *10* at the drop-down gallery.

17 Deselect the text and then save **WMedS2-CRGHHeartDisease.docx**.

In Addition

Understanding Methods for Changing Alignment

You can change paragraph alignment with the *Alignment* option box at the Paragraph dialog box. Display the Paragraph dialog box by clicking the Paragraph group dialog box launcher. At the Paragraph dialog box, click the down-pointing arrow at the right of the *Alignment* option box and then click the desired alignment at the drop-down list. You can also change alignment by using the following keyboard shortcuts:

Alignment	Keyboard Shortcut
Left	Ctrl + L
Center	Ctrl + E
Right	Ctrl + R
Justified	Ctrl + J

Activity 2.4

Indenting Text

To draw attention to specific text in a document, consider *indenting* the text, which means to increase the margin(s) of one or more lines. Indenting might include the first line of text in a paragraph, all lines of text in a paragraph, or the second and subsequent lines of a paragraph (called a *hanging indent*). Several methods are available for indenting text, including buttons in the Paragraph group on the HOME tab, markers on the horizontal ruler, options at the Paragraph dialog box with the Indents and Spacing tab selected, and keyboard shortcuts.

Project

You want to emphasize certain paragraphs of information in the heart disease document, and you have decided to accomplish this by indenting.

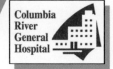

1. With **WMedS2-CRGHHeartDisease.docx** open, click anywhere in the paragraph below the *Aortic disease* heading.

2. Position the mouse pointer on the Left Indent marker on the horizontal ruler, shown in Figure W2.1, hold down the left mouse button, drag the marker to the 0.5-inch mark on the ruler, and then release the mouse button.

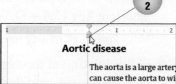

> The text *Left Indent* displays in a ScreenTip when you position the mouse pointer on the Left Indent marker. To position a marker at a precise measurement on the horizontal ruler, hold down the Alt key while dragging the marker.

3. Drag the Right Indent marker to the 6-inch mark on the horizontal ruler.

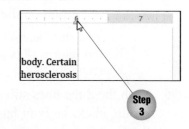

4. Click anywhere in the paragraph below the *Arrhythmia (abnormal heart rhythm)* heading and then click the Increase Indent button ⧢ in the Paragraph group on the HOME tab.

> This indents text 0.5 inches from the left margin.

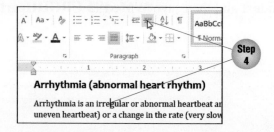

5. Drag the Right Indent marker to the 6-inch mark on the horizontal ruler.

6. Click anywhere in the paragraph below *Cardiomyopathy (heart muscle disease)* and then click the PAGE LAYOUT tab. In the *Indent* section of the Paragraph group, click in the *Left* measurement box and then type **0.5**. Click the up-pointing arrow at the right side of the *Right* measurement box until *0.5"* displays in the box.

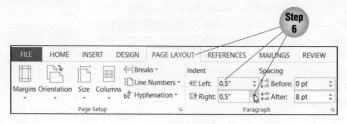

7 Click anywhere in the paragraph below the *Congenital heart disease* heading and then use the Paragraph dialog box to change the left and right indents. Begin by clicking the Paragraph group dialog box launcher.

8 At the Paragraph dialog box, click the up-pointing arrow at the right of the *Left* measurement box in the *Indentation* section until *0.5"* displays in the box.

9 Click the up-pointing arrow at the right of the *Right* measurement box in the *Indentation* section until *0.5"* displays in the box.

10 Click OK to close the Paragraph dialog box.

11 Click anywhere in the paragraph below the *Coronary artery disease* heading and then press F4.

12 Indent the paragraph of text below each of the headings *Heart failure, Heart valve disease, Pericardial disease,* and *Vascular disease* by clicking in each paragraph and then pressing F4.

13 Click anywhere in the first paragraph of text below the title *HEART DISEASE* (the paragraph that begins *According to the National Center for Chronic Disease*).

14 Drag the First Line Indent marker to the 0.5-inch mark on the horizontal ruler and then drag the Hanging Indent marker to the 1-inch mark on the ruler.

> This creates a hanging indent in the paragraph.

15 Click anywhere in the second paragraph of text below the heading *HEART DISEASE*, click the HOME tab, click the Increase Indent button in the Paragraph group, and then press Ctrl + T.

> Ctrl + T is the keyboard shortcut to create a hanging indent. For additional keyboard shortcuts, refer to the In Addition at the bottom of this page.

16 Save **WMedS2-CRGHHeartDisease.docx**.

FIGURE W2.1 Indent Markers on the Horizontal Ruler

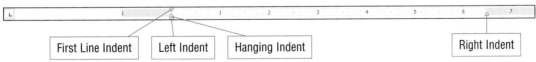

First Line Indent   Left Indent   Hanging Indent   Right Indent

In Addition

Indenting Text Using Keyboard Shortcuts

Indent text by using the following keyboard shortcuts:

Indentation	Keyboard Shortcut
Indent text from left margin	Ctrl + M
Decrease indent from left margin	Ctrl + Shift + M
Create a hanging indent	Ctrl + T
Remove hanging indent	Ctrl + Shift + T

Activity 2.5

Changing Line and Paragraph Spacing

By default, line spacing in Word is set at 1.08. Line spacing can be changed with the Line and Paragraph Spacing button in the Paragraph group on the HOME tab, with keyboard shortcuts, or with the *Line spacing* and *At* options at the Paragraph dialog box. Control spacing above and below paragraphs with options at the Line and Paragraph Spacing button drop-down gallery, the *Before* and *After* measurement boxes in the Paragraph group on the PAGE LAYOUT tab, or with the *Before* and *After* measurement boxes in the *Spacing* section of the Paragraph dialog box with the Indents and Spacing tab selected.

Project

Your supervisor needs the heart disease document in a few hours. You decide to make a few spacing changes in the document before printing the final version.

Columbia River General Hospital

1. With **WMedS2-CRGHHeartDisease.docx** open, select the entire document by pressing Ctrl + A.

2. Click the Line and Paragraph Spacing button in the Paragraph group on the HOME tab and then click *1.5* at the drop-down gallery.

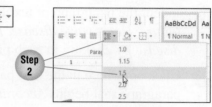

Step 2

3. Deselect the text and then scroll through the document. After viewing the document, you decide to decrease the line spacing to 1.3. To begin, press Ctrl + A to select the entire document, click the Line and Paragraph Spacing button, and then click *Line Spacing Options* at the drop-down gallery.

Step 4

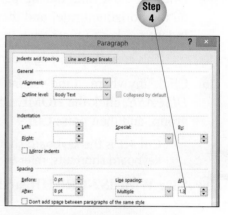

4. Type **1.3** in the *At* measurement box in the *Spacing* section of the Paragraph dialog box.

   The Paragraph dialog box also contains a *Line spacing* option box. Click the down-pointing arrow at the right side of this option box and a drop-down list displays with line spacing options.

5. Click OK to close the dialog box and then deselect the text.

6. You decide to single-space the text in the *HEART DISEASE FACTS* section. To do this, select from the beginning of the heading *HEART DISEASE FACTS* to the end of the document.

   and Paragraph Spacing button and then click *1.0* at the drop-down

   this option changes the line spacing to single for the selected paragraphs. change line spacing with keyboard shortcuts. Press Ctrl + 1 to change acing, Ctrl + 2 to change to double spacing, and Ctrl + 5 to change to cing.

   in the *Aortic disease* heading and then click the PAGE LAYOUT tab.

   inting arrow at the right of the *After* x in the Paragraph group. (The text lay.) Click in the *Before* measurement 0 pt), type **15**, and then press Enter. should display.)

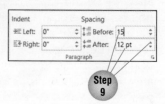

Step 9

10 After looking at the extra spacing before and after the heading, you decide to remove it. To do this, make sure the insertion point is positioned in the heading *Aortic disease* and then click the Paragraph group dialog box launcher.

11 At the Paragraph dialog box, click three times on the down-pointing arrow at the right of the *Before* measurement box in the *Spacing* section and then click twice on the down-pointing arrow at the right of the *After* measurement box.

> Both the *Before* and *After* measurement boxes should now display *0 pt*.

12 Click OK to close the Paragraph dialog box.

13 Click anywhere in the heading *Arrhythmia (abnormal heart rhythm)* and then press F4.

> Pressing F4 repeats the command, applying the same paragraph spacing you applied in Step 11.

14 Continue clicking in each of the remaining headings [*Cardiomyopathy (heart disease), Congenital heart disease, Coronary artery disease, Heart failure, Heart valve disease, Pericardial disease,* and *Vascular disease*] and pressing F4.

15 You decide to change the justified paragraph to left alignment. To do this, select all the text in the *HEART DISEASE* section except the title, click the HOME tab, and then click the Align Left button ≡ in the Paragraph group.

16 Select all of the text in the *HEART DISEASE FACTS* section, except the title and the right-aligned text, and then click the Align Left button in the Paragraph group.

17 You also decide to remove the hanging indents. To do this, select the two paragraphs of text below the *HEART DISEASE* title, press Ctrl + Shift + T, and then click the Decrease Indent button ≣ in the Paragraph group.

> Ctrl + Shift + T is the keyboard shortcut to remove a hanging indent.

18 Scroll down the page and notice that the heading *Coronary artery disease* displays at the bottom of the first page while the paragraph that follows it displays at the top of the second page. To keep the heading with the paragraph of text, begin by clicking in the heading *Coronary artery disease* and then clicking the Paragraph group dialog box launcher.

19 At the Paragraph dialog box, click the Line and Page Breaks tab, click the *Keep with next* check box to insert a check mark, and then click OK.

20 Save, print, and then close **WMedS2-CRGHHeartDisease.docx**.

In Brief
Change Line Spacing
1. Click Line and Paragraph Spacing button.
2. Click desired line spacing option at drop-down gallery.

OR

1. Click Line and Paragraph Spacing button.
2. Click *Line Spacing Options.*
3. Type desired line spacing in *At* measurement box.
4. Click OK.

Step 11

Step 19

In Addition

Adjusting Spacing Before and After Paragraphs

Spacing before or after paragraphs is added in points. (A vertical inch contains approximately 72 points.) To add 9 points of spacing after selected paragraphs, click the PAGE LAYOUT tab or display the Paragraph dialog box with the Indents and Spacing tab selected. Select the current measurement in the *After* measurement box and then type 9. You can also click the up- or down-pointing arrows at the right sides of the measurement boxes to increase or decrease the amount of spacing before or after paragraphs.

Activity 2.6

Inserting Bullets and Numbering

If you want to draw the reader's attention to a list of items, consider inserting a bullet before each item. Click the Bullets button in the Paragraph group on the HOME tab to insert bullets before items in a list. If a list of items is organized in a sequence, consider inserting numbers before each item with the Numbering button in the Paragraph group. Create multiple-level bulleted or numbered lists with options at the Multilevel List button drop-down list in the Paragraph group.

Project

Dr. St. Claire has asked you to edit and format a document on diabetes. The medical staff will provide this informational document to patients who have been diagnosed with diabetes or are interested in learning more about diabetes. To improve the readability of the document, you decide to add numbering and bullets to specific paragraphs.

1 Open **NSMCDiabetes.docx** and then save it with the name **WMedS2-NSMCDiabetes**.

2 Select the three paragraphs of text below the *Types of Diabetes* heading and then click the Numbering button in the Paragraph group on the HOME tab.

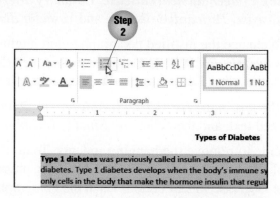

3 Position the insertion point at the end of the third numbered paragraph and then press the Enter key.

Pressing the Enter key automatically inserts the number *4.* and indents the position of the insertion point.

4 Type the first four words, Other types of diabetes, as shown in Figure W2.2, click the Bold button in the Font group to turn off bold formatting, and then type the remaining text shown in Figure W2.2.

Because the first words of the existing numbered paragraphs are bold, Word automatically turned on bold when you started a new numbered paragraph.

diabetes have a 20 to 50 percent chance of developing diabetes in the following 5- to 10-year period.
4. **Other types of diabetes** result from specific genetic conditions (such as maturity-onset diabetes of youth), surgery, drugs, malnutrition, infections, and other illnesses. Such types of diabetes may account for 1 to 5 percent of all diagnosed cases of diabetes.

FIGURE W2.2 Step 4

Other types of diabetes result from specific genetic conditions (such as maturity-onset diabetes of youth), surgery, drugs, malnutrition, infections, and other illnesses. Such types of diabetes may account for 1 to 5 percent of all diagnosed cases of diabetes.

5 Select the four lines of text below the *Heart Disease and Stroke* heading and then click the Bullets button ⊟ ▾ in the Paragraph group.

    Clicking the Bullets button in the Paragraph group inserts a round bullet before each paragraph.

Step 5

Heart Disease and Stroke
Heart disease is the leading cause of diabetes
death rates about 2 to 4 times higher than ad
The risk for stroke is 2 to 4 times higher amor
About 65% of deaths among people with diab

6 With the text still selected, replace the round bullets with custom bullets by clicking the Bullets button arrow and then clicking a bullet that you like in the *Bullet Library* section of the drop-down gallery.

    The choices at the Bullets button drop-down gallery vary depending on the most recent bullets selected.

7 Select the text below the *High Blood Pressure* heading and then press F4.

    Pressing F4 repeats the last command (inserting bullets).

8 Continue selecting text below each of the remaining headings (*Blindness*, *Kidney Disease*, *Nervous System Disease*, *Amputations*, *Dental Disease*, *Complications of Pregnancy*, and *Other Complications* [except for the text in parentheses]) and pressing F4 to insert bullets.

9 Save **WMedS2-NSMCDiabetes.docx**.

In Addition

Inserting Multilevel List Numbering

Use the Multilevel List button in the Paragraph group on the HOME tab to specify the type of numbering for lists that have more than one level. Apply predesigned multilevel numbering to text in a document by clicking the Multilevel List button and then clicking the desired numbering style at the drop-down list.

Creating Numbered and Bulleted Text As You Type

If you type *1.* and then press the spacebar, Word indents the number approximately 0.25 inch from the left margin and then hang indents the text in the paragraph approximately 0.5 inch from the left margin. When you press Enter after typing text, *2.* is inserted 0.25 inch from the left margin at the beginning of the next paragraph. You can insert bullets as you type by beginning a paragraph with the symbol *, >, or -. Type one of the symbols and then press the spacebar and the symbol is replaced

with a bullet. The type of bullet inserted depends on the type of character entered. For example, if you use the asterisk symbol (*), a round bullet is inserted, and if you type the greater than symbol (>), an arrow bullet is inserted.

Turning Off the Automatic Numbering and Bulleting Feature

If you do not want automatic numbering or bulleting in a document, turn off the features at the AutoCorrect dialog box with the AutoFormat As You Type tab selected. Display this dialog box by clicking the FILE tab and then clicking *Options*. At the Word Options dialog box, click the *Proofing* option and then click the AutoCorrect Options button. At the AutoCorrect dialog box, click the AutoFormat As You Type tab. Click the *Automatic numbered lists* check box and/or *Automatic bulleted lists* check box to remove the check mark.

Inserting Symbols and Special Characters

Insert special symbols such as é, ö, and Å with options at the Symbol button drop-down list or at the Symbol dialog box. Display the Symbol button drop-down list by clicking the INSERT tab and then clicking the Symbol button in the Symbols group. Click the desired symbol to insert it in the document. To display additional symbols, click the Symbol button and then click the *More Symbols* option to display the Symbol dialog box with the Symbols tab selected. Click the desired symbol at the dialog box, click the Insert button, and then click the Close button. The Symbols tab also provides options for changing the font to display different symbols. Click the Special Characters tab and a list displays containing common special characters and the keyboard shortcuts you can use to insert them.

Project

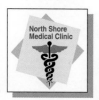

North Shore Medical Clinic

You need to include a registered trademark symbol after the organization name *American Diabetes Association* and insert Spanish text indicating that the diabetes document is also available in Spanish. You will use the Symbol dialog box to insert the registered trademark symbol and the necessary Spanish characters.

1. With **WMedS2-NSMCDiabetes.docx** open, move the insertion point to the end of the document.

2. Position the insertion point immediately after the word *Association*, located within the parentheses.

3. Click the INSERT tab, click the Symbol button Ω in the Symbols group, and then click *More Symbols* at the bottom of the drop-down list.

4. At the Symbol dialog box, click the Special Characters tab.

5. At the Symbol dialog box with the Special Characters tab selected, click the ® symbol in the *Character* list box.

6. Click the Insert button and then click the Close button.

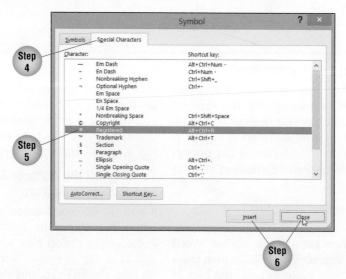

7. Press Ctrl + End to move the insertion point to the end of the document and then press the Enter key.

8. Type the text shown in Figure W2.3 up to the *é* in *También*. To insert the é symbol, begin by clicking the Symbol button and then clicking *More Symbols*.

The text in Figure W2.3 is in Spanish and translates as *(Also available in Spanish.)*

9 At the Symbol dialog box with the Symbols tab selected, click the down-pointing arrow at the right of the *Font* option box and then click *(normal text)* at the drop-down list, if it is not already selected. (You may need to scroll up to see this option.)

10 Scroll down the list box and then click the *é* symbol (the location of this symbol may vary).

11 Click the Insert button and then click the Close button.

12 Type the text shown in Figure W2.3 up to the *ñ* symbol, click the Symbol button, and then click *More Symbols* at the drop-down list.

13 At the Symbol dialog box, click the *ñ* symbol (the location of this symbol may vary).

14 Click the Insert button and then click the Close button.

15 Type the remaining text shown in Figure W2.3.

16 Save **WMedS2-NSMCDiabetes.docx**.

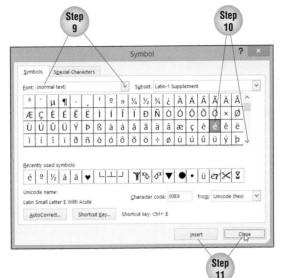

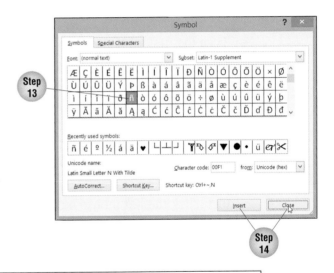

In Brief

Insert Symbol
1. Click INSERT tab.
2. Click Symbol button.
3. Click *More Symbols*.
4. Click desired symbol.
5. Click Insert button.
6. Click Close button.

Insert Special Character
1. Click INSERT tab.
2. Click Symbol button.
3. Click *More Symbols*.
4. Click Special Characters tab.
5. Click desired character.
6. Click Insert button.
7. Click Close button.

FIGURE W2.3 Steps 8–15

(También disponible en español.)

In Addition

Inserting Symbols with Keyboard Shortcuts

Another method for inserting symbols in a document is to use a keyboard shortcut. Click a symbol at the Symbol dialog box and the keyboard shortcut displays toward the bottom of the dialog box. For example, click the ø symbol and the keyboard shortcut Ctrl+/,O displays. To insert the ø symbol in a document using the keyboard shortcut, hold down the Ctrl key and then press the / key. Release the Ctrl key and then press the o key. Not all symbols can be inserted using a keyboard shortcut.

Inserting Symbols Using the Symbol Button Drop-down List

When you click the Symbol button in the Symbols group, a drop-down list displays with symbol choices. The list displays the most recently used symbols. If the list contains the desired symbol, click the symbol to insert it in the document.

Activity 2.8

Setting Tabs

Word offers a variety of default settings, including left tabs set every 0.5 inch in a document. You can set your own tabs using the horizontal ruler or the Tabs dialog box. The default tabs display as tiny vertical lines along the bottom of the horizontal ruler. With a left tab, text aligns at the left edge of the tab. The other types of tabs that can be set on the horizontal ruler are center, right, decimal, and bar. Switch between these tab types by clicking the Alignment button at the left side of the horizontal ruler. To set a tab, display the desired alignment symbol on the Alignment button and then click the horizontal ruler at the position where you want to set the tab.

You can also add leaders to every type of tab except bar tabs. Leaders are useful for directing the reader's eyes across the page and can be periods, hyphens, or underlines. Tabs with leaders are set with options at the Tabs dialog box. At the Tabs dialog box, you can choose the type of tab, the type of leader, and the tab position measurement.

Project

Dr. St. Claire has done some additional research on diabetes and has asked you to include the information in the document. You think that the information would be easiest to read if it were set in three columns and decide to set tabs to create this formatting.

1. With **WMedS2-NSMCDiabetes.docx** open, move the insertion point to the end of the paragraph of text below the *Statistics on Diabetes* heading and then press the Enter key twice.

2. Type the first sentence shown in Figure W2.4 and then press the Enter key twice.

3. Make sure the left tab symbol ⌊L⌋ displays in the Alignment button at the left side of the horizontal ruler.

   If the horizontal ruler is not visible, click the VIEW tab and then click the *Ruler* check box in the Show group.

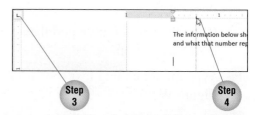

4. Position the arrow pointer below the 0.5-inch mark on the horizontal ruler and then click the left mouse button.

5. Click the Alignment button to display the center tab symbol ⊥, position the arrow pointer below the 3.25-inch mark on the ruler, and then click the left mouse button.

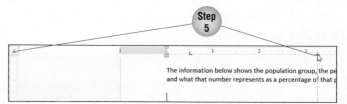

6. Click the Alignment button to display the right tab symbol ⌐, position the arrow pointer below the 6-inch mark on the ruler, and then click the left mouse button.

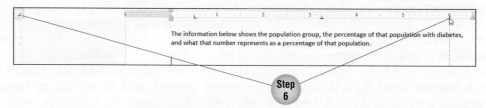

7. Type the rest of the text shown in Figure W2.4, pressing the Tab key before typing each entry, including those in the first column. Make sure to bold and underline the text as shown in the figure.

FIGURE W2.4 Steps 2–7

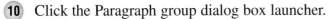

The information below shows the population group, the percentage of that population with diabetes, and what that number represents as a percentage of that population.

Population	Number with diabetes	Percentage
Under 20	210 thousand	0.26%
20 and older	18 million	8.70%
Men 20 and older	8.7 million	8.70%
Women 20 and older	9.3 million	8.70%

In Brief

Set Tab
1. Display desired alignment symbol on Alignment button.
2. Click horizontal ruler at desired position.

OR

1. Click Paragraph group dialog box launcher.
2. Click Tabs button.
3. Type tab measurement.
4. Click desired alignment.
5. Click desired leader (optional).
6. Click Set.
7. Click OK.

8 After typing the last entry in the third column, press the Enter key and then press Ctrl + Q, the keyboard shortcut to remove paragraph formatting.

  Pressing Ctrl + Q removes the tabs you set from the ruler.

9 You decide to add leaders to the center and right tabs. To begin, select all the text you typed at the left, center, and right tabs *except* the headings (***Population***, ***Number with diabetes***, and ***Percentage***).

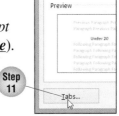

10 Click the Paragraph group dialog box launcher.

11 At the Paragraph dialog box, click the Tabs button that displays in the lower left corner.

12 At the Tabs dialog box, click *3.25"* in the *Tab stop position* section, click *2....* in the *Leader* section, and then click the Set button.

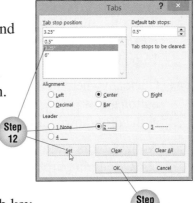

13 Click *6"* in the *Tab stop position* section, click *2....* in the *Leader* section, and then click the Set button.

14 Click OK to close the dialog box.

15 Position the insertion point immediately to the right of the last *8.70%* in the ***Percentage*** column and then press the Enter key.

16 Press the Tab key, type **60 and older**, press the Tab key, type **8.6 million**, press the Tab key, and then type **18.30%**.

17 Save **WMedS2-NSMCDiabetes.docx**.

In Addition

Moving a Tab
Move a tab on the horizontal ruler by positioning the mouse pointer on the tab symbol on the ruler, holding down the left mouse button, dragging the symbol to the new location on the ruler, and then releasing the mouse button.

Setting a Decimal Tab
Set a decimal tab for column entries you want aligned at the decimal point. To set a decimal tab, click the Alignment button located at the left side of the horizontal ruler until the decimal tab symbol displays and then click the desired position on the horizontal ruler.

Deleting a Tab
Delete a tab from the horizontal ruler by positioning the arrow pointer on the tab symbol. Hold down the left mouse button, drag the symbol down into the document screen, and then release the mouse button.

Clearing Tabs at the Tabs Dialog Box
At the Tabs dialog box, you can clear an individual tab or all tabs. To clear all tabs, click the Clear All button. To clear an individual tab, specify the tab position and then click the Clear button.

Activity 2.9

Adding Borders and Shading

Insert a border around text and/or apply shading to selected text with the Borders button and the Shading button in the Paragraph group on the HOME tab. You can also apply these effects at the Borders and Shading dialog box. At this dialog box with the Borders tab selected, specify the border type, style, color, and width. Click the Shading tab to display options for choosing a fill color and pattern style. Click the Page Border tab to display options for applying a page border.

Project

To add visual appeal and increase the readability of the diabetes document, you decide to add borders to specific text, apply shading behind the title, and apply shading and a border to the information in tabbed columns.

1. With **WMedS2-NSMCDiabetes.docx** open, select the numbered paragraphs of text below the heading *Types of Diabetes*.

2. Click the Borders button arrow in the Paragraph group on the HOME tab and then click *Outside Borders* at the drop-down gallery.

   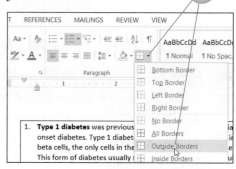

   The button image changes depending on the most recently selected option at the drop-down gallery.

3. Select the title, *UNDERSTANDING DIABETES*; change the font size to 16 points; and then apply bold formatting.

4. Click anywhere in the title, click the Shading button arrow , and then click *More Colors* at the drop-down gallery.

   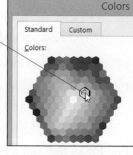

5. At the Colors dialog box with the Standard tab selected, click the light purple color as shown at the right.

6. Click OK to close the Colors dialog box.

7. Select text from the sentence that begins *The information below shows the population group* through the line of text containing the column entries *60 and older*, *8.6 million*, and *18.30%*.

8. Click the Borders button arrow and then click *Borders and Shading* at the bottom of the drop-down gallery.

9. At the Borders and Shading dialog box with the Borders tab selected, click the down-pointing arrow at the right of the *Style* list box until the first double-line option displays and then click the double-line option.

   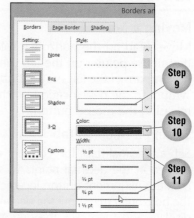

10. Click the down-pointing arrow at the right of the *Color* option box and then click the *Dark Blue* option (second option from the right in the *Standard Colors* section).

11. Click the down-pointing arrow at the right of the *Width* option box and then click *¾ pt* at the drop-down list.

12 Click the Shading tab.

13 Click the down-pointing arrow at the right of the *Fill* option box and then click *More Colors* at the drop-down list.

14 At the Colors dialog box, click the same light purple color you selected in Step 5.

15 Click OK to close the Colors dialog box.

16 With the Borders and Shading dialog box displayed, insert a page border around all pages in the document. Begin by clicking the Page Border tab.

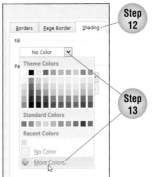

Step 12
Step 13
Step 16
Step 17
Step 18

You can also display the Borders and Shading dialog box with the Page Border tab selected by clicking the DESIGN tab and then clicking the Page Borders button in the Page Background group.

17 Click the *Shadow* option in the *Setting* section. Click the down-pointing arrow at the right of the *Color* option box and then click the *Dark Blue* option in the *Standard Colors* section (second option from the right).

18 Click the down-pointing arrow at the right of the *Width* option box and then click 2 ¼ pt at the drop-down list.

19 Click OK to close the Borders and Shading dialog box.

20 Select the entire document and then change the font to Georgia.

21 Click in the heading *Dental Disease*, display the Paragraph dialog box with the Line and Page Breaks tab selected, click the *Keep with next* check box to insert a check mark, and then click OK.

22 Save, print, and then close **WMedS2-NSMCDiabetes.docx**.

In Addition

Applying Borders

Both the Borders tab and the Page Borders tab of the Borders and Shading dialog box contain a *Preview* section you can use to control exactly where borders display. Click the sides, top, or bottom of the diagram in the *Preview* section to insert or remove a border line. Buttons display around the diagram that you can also use to insert or remove borders.

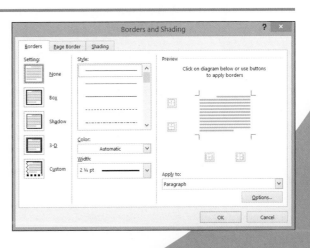

Activity 2.10

Applying Styles, Style Sets, and Themes

A Word document is based on a template with default formatting such as 11-point Calibri font, 1.08 line spacing, and 8 points of spacing after each paragraph. You can change these default formats with buttons and options on the ribbon, but you can also change them by applying styles. A style is a predesigned set of formatting instructions. To apply a style, click the desired style thumbnail in the Styles group on the HOME tab. Click the More button at the right side of the style thumbnails to display a drop-down gallery of additional styles. Word groups styles that apply similar formatting into style sets. Style sets are available in the Document Formatting group on the DESIGN tab. When you choose a different style set, the available styles in the Styles group on the HOME tab change to reflect the currently selected style set.

Another way to apply formatting to a document is by applying a theme. A theme is a set of formatting choices that includes a set of colors, a set of heading and body text fonts, and a set of lines and fill effects. Apply a theme with the Themes button in the Document Formatting group on the DESIGN tab. Customize a theme (or style set) with the Colors, Fonts, and Effects buttons, also located on the DESIGN tab.

Project

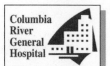

You have been asked by Douglas Brown, legal counsel, to format a document that explains records storage and maintenance at the hospital. You decide to apply styles and a theme to enhance the visual appeal of the document.

1. Open **CRGHRecords.docx** and then save it with the name **WMedS2-CRGHRecords**.

2. Apply a heading style to the title by clicking anywhere in the title *Maintaining Medical Records* and then clicking the *Heading 1* option in the Styles group on the HOME tab.

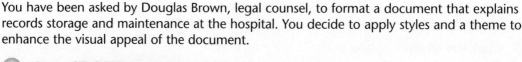

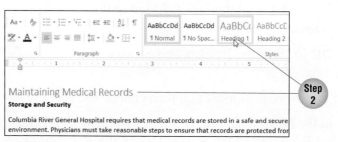

Step 2

3. Click anywhere in the heading *Storage and Security* and then click the *Heading 2* option.

> The Heading 1 and Heading 2 styles apply both paragraph and character formatting. Some styles apply only paragraph formatting and others apply only character formatting.

4. Apply the Heading 2 style to the headings *Creating a Patient Profile* and *Creating Progress Notes*.

5. Apply a different style set by clicking the DESIGN tab, clicking the More button at the right of the style set thumbnails in the Document Formatting group, and then clicking the *Lines (Stylish)* option.

Step 5

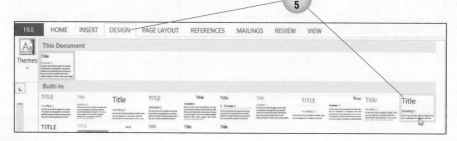

122　WORD Section 2

6 Change the paragraph spacing by clicking the Paragraph Spacing button in the Document Formatting group and then clicking *Relaxed* at the drop-down gallery.

7 Apply a theme by clicking the Themes button in the Document Formatting group and then clicking the *Organic* option.

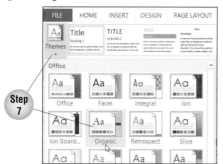

8 Change the theme colors by clicking the Colors button in the Document Formatting group and then clicking the *Green Yellow* option at the drop-down gallery.

9 Change the theme fonts by clicking the Fonts button in the Document Formatting group and then clicking the *Corbel* option at the drop-down gallery.

10 Save, print, and then close **WMedS2-CRGHRecords.docx**.

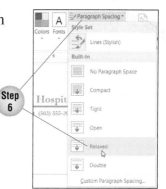

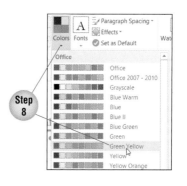

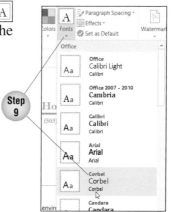

In Brief

Apply Style
1. Position insertion point at desired location.
2. Click style thumbnail in Styles group or click More button and then click desired style.

Change Style Set
1. Click DESIGN tab.
2. Click desired style set thumbnail in Document Formatting group.

Apply Paragraph Spacing
1. Click DESIGN tab.
2. Click Paragraph Spacing button in Document Formatting group.
3. Click desired option at drop-down gallery.

Apply Theme
1. Click DESIGN tab.
2. Click Themes button in Document Formatting group.
3. Click desired theme at drop-down gallery.

Change Theme Colors
1. Click DESIGN tab.
2. Click Colors button in Document Formatting group.
3. Click desired colors at drop-down gallery.

Change Theme Fonts
1. Click DESIGN tab.
2. Click Fonts button in Document Formatting group.
3. Click desired fonts at drop-down gallery.

In Addition

Applying the No Spacing Style

By default, a Word document contains line spacing of 1.08 and 8 points of spacing after paragraphs. The extra space between lines and paragraphs is designed to make text easier to read on a computer screen. You can change the line spacing to 1.0 and remove the spacing after paragraphs by clicking the *No Spacing* style in the Styles group on the HOME tab.

Collapsing and Expanding Headings

When you apply heading styles to text in a document, you can collapse text below the headings. By collapsing text, you can more easily use the headings to navigate to specific locations in the document. Collapse text by clicking the gray triangle that displays when you hover over a heading with a heading style applied. Expand collapsed text by clicking the white triangle before a heading with a heading style applied.

Applying Styles at the Styles Task Pane

The Styles task pane provides additional styles you can apply to text in a document. Display this task pane by clicking the Styles group task pane launcher. The styles in the currently selected style set display in the task pane followed by a paragraph symbol (¶), indicating that the style applies paragraph formatting, or a character symbol (a), indicating that the style applies character formatting. The Styles task pane also includes a Clear All style that clears all formatting from selected text.

Features Summary

Feature	Ribbon Tab, Group	Button	Keyboard Shortcut
1.5 line spacing	HOME, Paragraph		Ctrl + 5
align left	HOME, Paragraph		Ctrl + L
align right	HOME, Paragraph		Ctrl + R
bold	HOME, Font	**B**	Ctrl + B
borders	HOME, Paragraph		
bullets	HOME, Paragraph		
center	HOME, Paragraph		Ctrl + E
change case	HOME, Font	Aa	Shift + F3
clear all formatting	HOME, Font		
decrease indent	HOME, Paragraph		Ctrl + Shift + M
double line spacing	HOME, Paragraph		Ctrl + 2
font	HOME, Font		
font color	HOME, Font	A	
Font dialog box	HOME, Font		Ctrl + Shift + F
font size	HOME, Font		Ctrl + Shift + P
Format Painter	HOME, Clipboard		Ctrl + Shift + C
hanging indent			Ctrl + T
highlight	HOME, Font		
increase indent	HOME, Paragraph		Ctrl + M
italics	HOME, Font	*I*	Ctrl + I
justify	HOME, Paragraph		Ctrl + J
line and paragraph spacing	HOME, Paragraph		
numbering	HOME, Paragraph		
Paragraph dialog box	HOME, Paragraph		
remove hanging indent			Ctrl + Shift + T
shading	HOME, Paragraph		
single line spacing	HOME, Paragraph		Ctrl + 1

Feature	Ribbon Tab, Group	Button	Keyboard Shortcut
spacing after paragraphs	PAGE LAYOUT, Paragraph	‡⁼ After: 0 pt	
spacing before paragraphs	PAGE LAYOUT, Paragraph	↕⁼ Before: 0 pt	
styles	HOME, Styles		
style sets	DESIGN, Document Formatting		
symbols	INSERT, Symbols	Ω	
Tabs dialog box	HOME, Paragraph OR PAGE LAYOUT, Paragraph	⌐, Tabs	
theme colors	DESIGN, Document Formatting	◼	
theme fonts	DESIGN, Document Formatting	A	
themes	DESIGN, Document Formatting	Aa	
underline	HOME, Font	U ▾	Ctrl + U

Knowledge Check

Completion: In the space provided at the right, write in the correct term, command, or option.

1. The Bold button is located in this group on the HOME tab.
2. Use this keyboard shortcut to italicize selected text.
3. Repeat a command by pressing this function key.
4. Click this button in the Paragraph group on the HOME tab to align text at the right margin.
5. Click this button in the Font group on the HOME tab to remove paragraph formatting and character formatting from selected text.
6. Indent text from the left margin by dragging the Left Indent marker on this.
7. The Line and Paragraph Spacing button displays in this group on the HOME tab.
8. Display the Symbol button drop-down list by clicking this tab and then clicking the Symbol button in the Symbols group.
9. This is the name of the button that displays at the left side of the horizontal ruler.
10. Set tabs at the Tabs dialog box or using this.
11. When you set a tab, these can be added to help guide the reader's eyes across the page.
12. Insert a page border with options at this dialog box with the Page Border tab selected.
13. A document contains a number of predesigned formats combined into groups called this.
14. This is a set of formatting choices that includes colors, fonts, and effects.

Skills Review

Review 1   Applying Fonts; Using the Format Painter; Using the Repeat Command

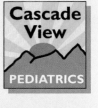

1. Open **CVPWell-Child.docx** and save it with the name **WMedS2-R-CVPWell-Child**.
2. Select the entire document and then change the font to Constantia.
3. Select the title, *WELL-CHILD APPOINTMENTS*, change the font to 16-point Candara, apply bold formatting, and then deselect the text.
4. Select the heading *Appointment Recommendations*, change the font to 14-point Candara, apply bold formatting, and then deselect the heading.
5. Using Format Painter, apply the same formatting you applied in Step 4 to the remaining headings (*Appointment Services, Appointment Suggestions, Immunizations,* and *Child Development Assessment*).
6. Select the last paragraph of text in the document (the text in parentheses), change the font size to 10 points, and then apply small caps formatting. ***Hint: The* Small caps *check box is located in the* Effects *section on the* Font *tab of the* Font *dialog box.**
7. Select *WELL-CHILD APPOINTMENTS* and then apply the Offset Diagonal Bottom Right text effect, located at the *Shadow* side menu of the Text Effects and Typography button drop-down list.
8. Select the heading *Appointment Recommendations* and then apply the Offset Diagonal Bottom Right text effect from the *Shadow* side menu of the Text Effects and Typography button drop-down list.
9. Use the Repeat command to apply the text effect from Step 8 to the remaining headings in the document (*Appointment Services, Appointment Suggestions, Immunizations,* and *Child Development Assessment*).
10. Save **WMedS2-R-CVPWell-Child.docx**.

Review 2   Aligning and Indenting Text; Changing Line and Paragraph Spacing; Inserting Bullets and Numbering

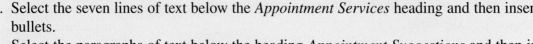

1. With **WMedS2-R-CVPWell-Child.docx** open, position the insertion point anywhere in the paragraph below the heading *Appointment Recommendations*, change the paragraph alignment to justify, and then indent the paragraph 0.25 inch from the left margin.
2. Position the insertion point anywhere in the last paragraph of text in the document (the text in parentheses) and then change the paragraph alignment to center.
3. Select the entire document and then change the line spacing to *1.15*.
4. Click anywhere in the heading *Appointment Recommendations* and then change the spacing after paragraphs to 6 points.
5. Use the Repeat command to change the paragraph spacing after the remaining headings (*Appointment Services, Appointment Suggestions, Immunizations,* and *Child Development Assessment*) to 6 points.
6. Select the seven lines of text below the *Appointment Services* heading and then insert bullets.
7. Select the paragraphs of text below the heading *Appointment Suggestions* and then insert numbering.

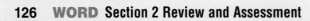

8. Move the insertion point to the end of the second numbered paragraph, press the Enter key, and then type **Bring snacks for young children in case you have to wait for your appointment.**

9. Save **WMedS2-R-CVPWell-Child.docx**.

Review 3 Setting Tabs; Adding Borders, Shading, and Symbols

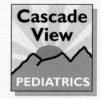

1. With **WMedS2-R-CVPWell-Child.docx** open, position the insertion point at the end of the paragraph that begins *Cascade View Pediatrics' schedule for immunizations*, press Enter two times, and then create the tabbed text shown in Figure W2.5 with the following specifications:
   a. Set a left tab at the 1.5-inch mark on the horizontal ruler.
   b. Set a right tab at the 5-inch mark on the horizontal ruler.
   c. Type the column headings (*Vaccine* and *Shots/Doses*) with bold and underline formatting at the appropriate tabs.
   d. Before typing the column entries, display the Tabs dialog box and add leaders to the right tab as shown in the figure.
   e. Type the remainder of the text as shown in the figure.

2. Select the tabbed text you just typed (including the blank line above the column headings, the sentences after the asterisks, and the blank line below the sentences) and then apply a border and shading of your choosing.

3. Click anywhere in the title *WELL-CHILD APPOINTMENTS* and then apply shading of your choosing. (The shading will span from the left to the right margin.)

4. Apply a page border of your choosing to the document. (If possible, match the color of the page border with the colors in the letterhead and/or title shading.)

5. Position the insertion point in the heading *Immunizations* and then keep the heading with the paragraph of text located on the next page. ***Hint: Use the* Keep with next *check box in the Paragraph dialog box.***

6. Move the insertion point to the end of the document.

7. Change the font to Candara and the line spacing to single. Type the following text at the left margin:
   ®2016 Cascade View Pediatrics
   Raphaël Severin, MD

8. Save, print, and then close **WMedS2-R-CVPWell-Child.docx**.

FIGURE W2.5 Review 3

Vaccine	Shots/Doses
Hepatitis B	3 shots
DTaP	5 shots
Hib	4 shots
Pneumococcal (PCV)	4 shots
Polio	4 shots
Measles-Mumps-Rubella	2 shots
Varicella (chickenpox)	1 shot
Influenza*	1 or 2 doses
Hepatitis A**	2 shots

*Two doses are recommended for children receiving the influenza vaccine for the first time.
**The hepatitis A vaccine is recommended only in certain areas where infection rates are highest.

Review 4 Applying Styles and a Theme

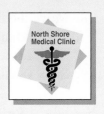

1. Open **CysticFibrosis.docx** and save it with the name **WMedS2-R-CysticFibrosis**.
2. Apply the Heading 1 style to the title *Cystic Fibrosis* and apply the Heading 2 style to the headings *Cause, Diagnosis,* and *Symptoms of Cystic Fibrosis.*
3. Apply the Lines (Simple) style set to the document.
4. Apply the Depth theme.
5. Apply the Blue theme colors.
6. Apply the Cambria theme fonts.
7. Apply to the document a page border of your choosing. Choose a color for the page border that matches or complements the theme colors.
8. Save, print, and then close **WMedS2-R-CysticFibrosis.docx**.

Skills Assessment

Assessment 1 Changing Fonts; Aligning and Indenting Text; Changing Paragraph Spacing

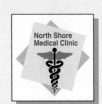

1. Open **NSMCRequest.docx** and save it with the name **WMedS2-A1-NSMCRequest**.
2. Select the entire document and then change the font to Cambria and the font size to 12 points.
3. Set the title, *MEDICAL RECORDS*, in 14-point Constantia and then apply bold formatting.
4. Set the heading *How to Request a Copy of Your Medical Records* in 12-point Constantia, apply bold formatting, add a shadow text effect, and then change the spacing after the paragraph to 6 points.
5. Use Format Painter to apply the same formatting you applied in Step 4 to the following headings in the document:
   Information from Your Medical Records
   Submitting a Request
   Additional Information about Medical Records
   Mailing Medical Records
   Reproduction Charges
   Sending Records to Another Medical Facility
   Processing Time
   Picking Up Medical Records
6. Select the title, *MEDICAL RECORDS*, center the text, and then apply paragraph shading of your choosing.
7. Select the four lines of text below the paragraph in the *How to Request a Copy of Your Medical Records* section (*AIDS/HIV* through *Fertility treatment*) and then apply bullets.
8. Select all the text in the *Submitting a Request* section *except* the first paragraph (the paragraph that begins *Once you have completed*) and then indent them 0.5 inch from the left margin.

9. Move the insertion point to the end of the document and then type the following text at the left margin (press Shift + Enter after typing the first line of text):

    ®2016 North Shore Medical Clinic
    Maria Cárdenas, MD

10. Save and then print **WMedS2-A1-NSMCRequest.docx**.

11. Apply the Heading 1 style to the title, *MEDICAL RECORDS*, and apply the Heading 2 style to the headings (*How to Request a Copy of Your Medical Records, Information from Your Medical Records, Submitting a Request, Additional Information about Medical Records, Mailing Medical Records, Reproduction Charges, Sending Records to Another Medical Facility, Processing Time,* and *Picking Up Medical Records*).

12. Apply the Basic (Elegant) style set, apply the Frame theme, and then change the theme colors to *Violet*.

13. Save, print, and then close **WMedS2-A1-NSMCRequest.docx**.

Assessment 2 Preparing and Formatting a Letter

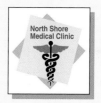

1. Open **NSMCLtrhd.docx** and save it with the name **WMedS2-A2-NSMCLtr**.

2. Click the *No Spacing* style. (This removes the 8 points of spacing after paragraphs and changes the line spacing to single.)

3. You have been asked by your supervisor to send a letter to the local community college indicating that a medical office assistant internship is available. Send the letter to Mrs. Janelle Meyers, Medical Assistant Program, Columbia River Community College, Third Avenue North, Portland, OR 97301, and include the following information:

    • In the first paragraph, tell Mrs. Meyers that your clinic has an opening for a medical office assistant intern for 15 hours a week. Note that the position pays minimum wage and has flexible hours.

    • In the second paragraph, tell Mrs. Meyers that the intern will be trained in specific areas and then include the following in a numbered list: registering patients, typing memos and correspondence, filing correspondence and some medical records, making photocopies, and scheduling appointments.

    • In the third paragraph, tell Mrs. Meyers that she can contact Lee Elliott at the clinic. Provide the clinic name, address, telephone number, and web address. ***Hint: This information can be found in the letterhead.***

    • End the letter with the complimentary close *Sincerely,* and then type your name four lines below it.

4. After typing the letter, select the text and then change the font to a font other than Calibri.

5. Change the numbered list to a bulleted list.

6. Save, print, and then close **WMedS2-A2-NSMCLtr.docx**.

Assessment 3 Setting Leader Tabs

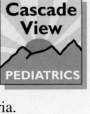

1. Open **CVPLtrhd.docx** and save it with the name **WMedS2-A3-CVPHours**.
2. Type the text shown in Figure W2.6. *Hint: Make sure to apply bold formatting to the title,* **CLINIC HOURS.**
3. After typing the text, select the document and then change the font to Cambria.
4. Save, print, and then close **WMedS2-A3-CVPHours.docx**.

FIGURE W2.6 Assessment 3

> ### CLINIC HOURS
>
> Monday .... 8:00 a.m. to 7:00 p.m.
>
> Tuesday .... 8:00 a.m. to 5:00 p.m.
>
> Wednesday .... 8:00 a.m. to 7:00 p.m.
>
> Thursday .... 8:00 a.m. to 5:00 p.m.
>
> Friday .... 8:00 a.m. to 3:00 p.m.
>
> Saturday .... 9:00 a.m. to 1:00 p.m.
>
> Sunday .... CLOSED

Assessment 4 Finding Information on Controlling Page Breaks

HELP

1. Your supervisor at North Shore Medical Clinic, Lee Elliott, has asked you to learn about how to prevent page breaks between paragraphs and how to make sure that at least two lines of a paragraph appear at the top or bottom of a page to prevent widows (when the last line of a paragraph appears by itself at the top of a page) and orphans (when the first line of a paragraph appears by itself at the bottom of a page). Use the Help feature in Word to locate the necessary information.
2. Your supervisor would like you to prepare a memo to all medical office staff about the information you have found. To do so, complete the following steps:
   a. Open **NSMCMemoForm.docx** and save it with the name **WMedS2-A4-NSMCMemoForm**.
   b. Create an appropriate subject for the memo.
   c. Write a paragraph discussing how to prevent page breaks between paragraphs in Word and list the steps required to complete the task.
   d. Write a paragraph discussing how to keep selected paragraphs together on a single page and list the steps required to complete the task.
   e. Write a paragraph discussing how to prevent widows and orphans and list the steps required to complete the task.
3. Save, print, and then close **WMedS2-A4-NSMCMemoForm.docx**.

Assessment 5 Locating Information and Writing a Memo

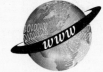

1. Visit the website of the American Association of Medical Assistants (AAMA) at www.aama-ntl.org. At the website, find the following information:
   - Mission of the AAMA
   - Administrative duties of a medical assistant
   - Salaries and benefits of a medical assistant
   - Any other information you find interesting
2. Using one of Word's memo templates, create a memo to your instructor explaining the information you found at the website.
3. Save the completed memo with the name **WMedS2-A5-AAMAMemo**.
4. Print and then close **WMedS2-A5-AAMAMemo.docx**.

Marquee Challenge

Challenge 1 Preparing a Job Announcement

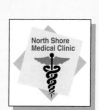

1. Open **NSMCLtrhd.docx** and save it with the name **WMedS2-C1-NSMCLtr**.
2. Click the *No Spacing* style, change the font to 12-point Cambria, and then type the job announcement shown in Figure W2.7 on page 132. Change the font size of the title to 14 points and apply paragraph shading as shown. ***Hint: Display the Colors dialog box to locate the purple shading color.***
3. Save, print, and then close **WMedS2-C1-NSMCLtr.docx**.

Challenge 2 Preparing a Flyer for a Diabetes Presentation

1. At a blank document, remove the spacing after paragraphs, change the font to Constantia, and then create the flyer shown in Figure W2.8 on page 133.
2. Save the completed flyer with the name **WMedS2-C2-Flyer**.
3. Print and then close **WMedS2-C2-Flyer.docx**.

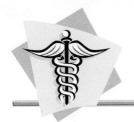

North Shore Medical Clinic
7450 Meridian Street, Suite 150
Portland, OR 97202
(503) 555-2330
www.emcp.net/nsmc

JOB ANNOUNCEMENT

JOB TITLE .... Medical Office Assistant
STATUS .... Full-time employment
SALARY .... Depending on experience
CLOSING DATE .... March 1, 2016

JOB SUMMARY
- Register new patients; assist with form completion
- Retrieve charts
- Enter patient data into computer database
- Maintain and file medical records
- Schedule patients
- Call patients with appointment reminders
- Answer telephones and route messages
- Call and/or fax pharmacy for prescription order refills
- Mail lab test results to patients
- Perform other clerical duties as required

REQUIRED SKILLS
- Keyboarding (35+ wpm)
- Knowledge of Microsoft Word, Excel, and PowerPoint
- Thorough understanding of medical terms
- Excellent grammar and spelling skills
- Excellent customer service skills

EDUCATION
- High school diploma
- Post-secondary training as a medical office assistant, CMA or RMA preferred
- CPR certification

For further information, contact Lee Elliott at (503) 555-2330.

Understanding

DIABETES

Please join Dr. Käri St. Claire from North Shore Medical Clinic as she presents *Understanding Diabetes.* At this informative presentation, she will discuss:

- Types of diabetes
- Statistics on diabetes
- Complications of diabetes
- Living with diabetes
- Developing self-management skills

When .... Wednesday, October 19
Time..7:00 p.m. to 8:30 p.m.
Where .... Columbia River General Hospital
Location... Room 224
Cost .... FREE!

Sponsored by the
Greater Portland Healthcare Workers Association

Word SECTION 3

Formatting and Enhancing a Document

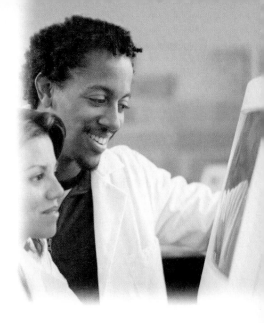

Skills

- Find and replace text and formatting
- Reveal formatting
- Cut, copy, and paste text
- Use the Clipboard task pane to copy and paste items
- Change page margins and orientation
- Customize the page and page background
- Insert page numbers, headers, and footers
- Insert a page break and a section break
- Create and modify columns
- Insert, size, and move images
- Insert, size, and move WordArt
- Insert the contents of one file into another file
- Insert and customize shapes and text boxes
- Prepare an envelope
- Prepare labels

Student Resources

Before beginning the activities in Word Section 3, copy to your storage medium the WordMedS3 folder from the Student Resources CD. This folder contains the data files you need to complete the projects in this Word section.

Projects Overview

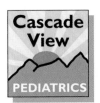

Edit, format, and reorganize a child development assessment form; format and add visual appeal to a monthly newsletter; enhance the visual appeal of a parenting class flyer; format and add visual appeal to a patient confidentiality document; prepare an envelope and mailing labels; prepare a notice and two announcements; and format a document on Fifth disease.

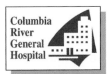

Format and add visual appeal to a document on writing and maintaining medical records.

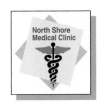

Prepare an envelope and mailing labels, format and add visual appeal to a document on fibromyalgia, and flip and copy shapes to create a clinic notice.

Activity 3.1

Finding and Replacing Text

Use the Find and Replace feature to find specific text and replace it with other text. For example, you can create a template for an agreement by using a generic name throughout the document. You can then find and replace the generic name with a real name later on. To avoid having to constantly re-type a long phrase that occurs often in a document, you can type an abbreviation instead and then replace the abbreviations with the full phrase when you are finished. You can also find and replace certain formatting. These options are available at the Find and Replace dialog box with the Replace tab selected.

Project

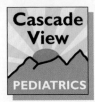

Sydney Larsen, the office manager at Cascade View Pediatrics, has asked you to proofread the Assessment of Child Development form that parents fill out before each well-child appointment. Your review identifies some spelling and grammar errors that you will correct using the Find and Replace feature.

1 Open **CDAssessment.docx** and then save it with the name **WMedS3-CDAssessment**.

2 After looking over the document, you realize that *development* is misspelled as *developement* throughout the document. You decide to use the Find and Replace feature to correct this spelling error. To begin, click the Replace button in the Editing group on the HOME tab.

3 At the Find and Replace dialog box with the Replace tab selected, type **developement** in the *Find what* text box and then press the Tab key.

> Pressing the Tab key moves the insertion point to the *Replace with* text box.

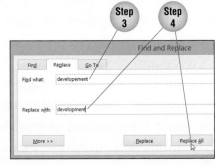

4 Type **development** in the *Replace with* text box and then click the Replace All button located toward the bottom of the dialog box.

> Clicking the Replace All button replaces all occurrences of the text in the document. If you want control over which instances in a document are replaced, use the Find Next and Replace buttons to move through the document and replace or skip over each instance individually.

5 At the message telling you that three replacements were made, click OK.

6 Click the Close button to close the Find and Replace dialog box.

7 Looking at the document, you realize that *well-baby* should be replaced with *well-child*. To begin, display the Find and Replace dialog box by clicking the Replace button in the Editing group.

8 At the Find and Replace dialog box with the Replace tab selected, type **well-baby** in the *Find what* text box.

9 Press the Tab key, type **well-child** in the *Replace with* text box, and then click the Replace All button.

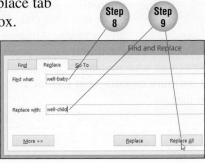

10 At the message telling you that two replacements were made, click OK.

11 Click the Close button to close the Find and Replace dialog box.

12 Select the title, *ASSESSMENT OF CHILD DEVELOPMENT*, change the font to 16-point Candara, apply bold formatting, change the alignment to center, and then add 12 points of spacing after the paragraph.

13 Select the subtitle *Ages Newborn to Three Years*, change the font to 14-point Candara, apply bold formatting, change the alignment to center, and then add 9 points of spacing after the paragraph.

14 Change the font of the headings *Child Development – Talking* and *Child Development – Hearing* to 12-point Candara and then apply bold formatting.

15 Save **WMedS3-CDAssessment.docx**.

In Brief

Find and Replace Text
1. Click Replace button in Editing group on HOME tab.
2. Type text in *Find what* text box.
3. Press Tab.
4. Type text in *Replace with* text box.
5. Click Replace All button.

In Addition

Using Options at the Expanded Find and Replace Dialog Box

The Find and Replace dialog box contains a variety of options from which you can choose when finding and replacing text. To display these options, click the More button at the bottom of the dialog box. This causes the dialog box to expand as shown at the right. The available options are described below.

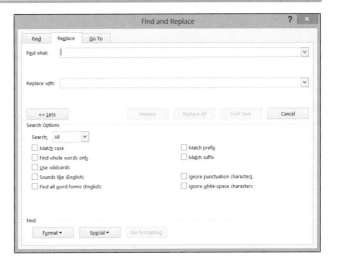

Option	Action
Match case	Exactly match the case of the search text. For example, if you search for *Book*, Word will stop at *Book* but not *book* or *BOOK*.
Find whole words only	Find a whole word, not a part of a word. For example, if you search for *her*, Word will stop at *her* but not t*her*e, *her*e, or *her*s.
Use wildcards	Search for wildcards, special characters, or special search operators. For example, search for le*s, and Word finds *less*, *leases*, and *letters*.
Sounds like	Find words that sound alike but are spelled differently, such as *know* and *no*.
Find all word forms	Find all forms of the word entered in the *Find what* text box. For example, if you search for *hold*, Word will stop at *held* and *holding*.
Match prefix	Find only those words that begin with the letters in the *Find what* text box. For example, if you search for *per*, Word will stop at words such as *perform* and *perfect* but skip over words such as *super* and *hyperlink*.
Match suffix	Find only those words that end with the letters in the *Find what* text box. For example, if you search for *ly*, Word will stop at words such as *accurately* and *quietly* but skip over words such as *catalyst* and *lyre*.
Ignore punctuation characters	Ignore punctuation within characters. For example, if you enter *US* in the *Find what* text box, Word will stop at *U.S.*
Ignore white-space characters	Ignore spaces between letters. For example, if you enter *F B I* in the *Find what* text box, Word will stop at *FBI*.

Activity 3.2

Revealing Formatting; Finding and Replacing Formatting

Display formatting applied to specific text in a document at the Reveal Formatting task pane. Display this task pane by pressing Shift + F1. The Reveal Formatting task pane displays font, paragraph, and section formatting that has been applied to the selected text or the text in which the insertion point is positioned. As mentioned in Activity 3.1, you can use options at the Find and Replace dialog box with the Replace tab selected to search for specific formatting or for text with specific formatting applied and replace it with different formatting.

Project

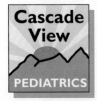

After reviewing the Assessment of Child Development form, you decide that the headings would look better in a different font and font color. To display the formatting applied to specific text, you will use the Reveal Formatting task pane. You will then use Find and Replace to change the font formatting.

1. With **WMedS3-CDAssessment.docx** open, press Ctrl + Home to move the insertion point to the beginning of the document and then press Shift + F1.

   Pressing Shift + F1 displays the Reveal Formatting task pane with information on the formatting applied to the title. Generally, a black triangle precedes *Font* and *Paragraph* and a white triangle precedes *Section* in the *Formatting of selected text* section. Clicking a black triangle hides items displayed below a heading and clicking a white triangle reveals them. Some items in the Reveal Formatting task pane are hyperlinks. For example, click the <u>FONT</u> hyperlink to display the Font dialog box. Use these hyperlinks to make changes to the document formatting.

2. Click anywhere in the paragraph of text below the subtitle and look at the Reveal Formatting task pane to determine the formatting.

3. Click anywhere in the heading *Child Development – Talking* and then notice the formatting applied to it.

4. Close the Reveal Formatting task pane by clicking the Close button in the upper right corner of the task pane.

5. You decide to change the font of all text in 12-point Candara bold to 13-point Cambria bold in a dark blue font color. Start by positioning the insertion point at the beginning of the document and then clicking the Replace button in the Editing group on the HOME tab.

6. At the Find and Replace dialog box, press the Delete key. (This deletes any text that displays in the *Find what* text box.)

7. Click the More button. (If a check mark displays in the *Find all word forms* check box, click to remove it.)

8. Click the Format button at the bottom of the dialog box and then click *Font* at the drop-down list.

9. At the Find Font dialog box, change the font to *Candara*, the font style to *Bold*, and the size to *12*. Click OK to close the dialog box.

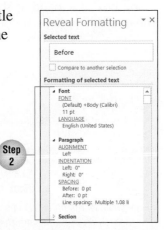

Step 2

Step 8

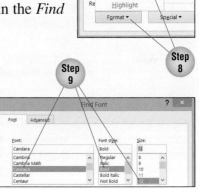

Step 9

10 At the Find and Replace dialog box, press the Tab key and then press the Delete key. (This removes any text in the *Replace with* text box.)

In Brief
Reveal Formatting
1. Click in desired text.
2. Press Shift + F1.

11 Click the Format button at the bottom of the dialog box and then click *Font* at the drop-down list.

12 At the Replace Font dialog box, change the font to *Cambria*, the font style to *Bold*, the size to *13*, and the font color to *Dark Blue*. Click OK to close the dialog box.

> To change the font size to *13*, select the existing text in the *Size* text box and then type **13**.

Step 12

13 At the Find and Replace dialog box, click the Replace All button. At the message telling you that the search of the document is complete and two replacements were made, click OK.

14 With the Find and Replace dialog box open and the insertion point positioned in the *Find what* text box, click the No Formatting button (located toward the bottom of the dialog box). Press the Tab key to move the insertion point to the *Replace with* text box and then click the No Formatting button. (This deletes any font formatting that displays in the *Find what* and *Replace with* text boxes.)

15 With the Find and Replace dialog box open, find all text set in 12-point Calibri bold and replace it with 11-point Cambria bold in Dark Blue.

> Twelve replacements should be made.

16 At the Find and Replace dialog box with the insertion point positioned in the *Find what* text box, click the No Formatting button. Press the Tab key and then click the No Formatting button. Click the Less button and then click the Close button.

17 Select the title, *ASSESSMENT OF CHILD DEVELOPMENT*, and the subtitle *Ages Newborn to Three Years* and then change the font to 16-point Cambria and apply the Dark Blue font color. (Make sure bold formatting is still applied to the title and subtitle.)

18 Save **WMedS3-CDAssessment.docx**.

In Addition

Comparing Formatting

Along with displaying formatting applied to text, you can use the Reveal Formatting task pane to compare formatting of two text selections to determine what is different. To compare formatting, display the Reveal Formatting task pane and then select the first instance of formatting to be compared. Click the *Compare to another selection* check box to insert a check mark and then select the second instance of formatting to compare. Any differences between the two selections will display in the *Formatting differences* list box.

Activity 3.3

Cutting, Copying, and Pasting Text; Using Paste Special

With the Cut, Copy, and Paste buttons in the Clipboard group on the HOME tab, you can move and/or copy words, sentences, or entire sections of text to other locations in a document. You can cut and paste text or copy and paste text within the same document or between documents. Specify the formatting of pasted text with options at the Paste Special dialog box.

Project

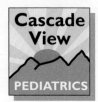

After consulting with Deanna Reynolds, the child development specialist at Cascade View Pediatrics, Sydney Larsen has asked you to reorganize the Assessment of Child Development form and include additional information from other sources.

1. With **WMedS3-CDAssessment.docx** open, move the *Child Development – Hearing* section above the *Child Development – Talking* section. Begin by selecting from the beginning of the *Child Development – Hearing* heading to the end of the document.

2. Click the Cut button ✂ in the Clipboard group on the HOME tab.

   This places the text in a location called the Clipboard.

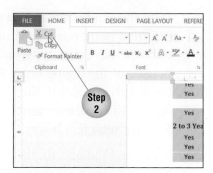

3. Position the insertion point at the beginning of the heading *Child Development – Talking* and then click the Paste button 📋 in the Clipboard group on the HOME tab.

   A Paste Options button 📋 (Ctrl) ▾ displays below the pasted text. Click this button and a drop-down list of buttons displays. Use these buttons to specify the formatting of the pasted text. By default, the Keep Source Formatting button (first button from the left) is selected. With this button selected, text is pasted with the formatting from the source location or document. You can also click the Merge Formatting button (middle button) to merge the pasted text with the destination formatting or click the Keep Text Only button (third button) to paste only the text and not the formatting.

4. Copy text from another document and paste it in the Assessment of Child Development document. To begin, open **CDSpecialistQuestions.docx**.

5. Select the line containing the text *Child's Name: _____* and the two lines of text below it and then click the Copy button 📋 in the Clipboard group.

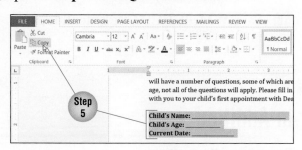

6. Click the Word button on the Taskbar and then click the **WMedS3-CDAssessment.docx** thumbnail.

7. Position the insertion point at the end of the first paragraph of text (the paragraph that begins *Before you bring your child to the next*) and then press Enter twice.

8. Click the Paste button in the Clipboard group.

9 Click the Paste Options button that displays in the lower right corner of the pasted text and then click the Merge Formatting button.

> The copied text and the heading below it should be separated by one blank line (a double space).

Step 9

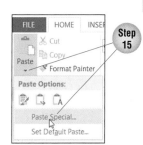

10 Click the Word button on the Taskbar and then click the **CDSpecialistQuestions.docx** thumbnail.

11 Move the insertion point to the end of the document and then select the heading *Additional Information* and the paragraph of text below it.

12 Click the Copy button in the Clipboard group.

13 Click the Word button on the Taskbar and then click the **WMedS3-CDAssessment.docx** thumbnail.

14 Move the insertion point to the end of the document and then press Enter twice. (The insertion point should be positioned a double space below the last line of text.)

15 Paste the copied text into the document without the formatting by clicking the Paste button arrow and then clicking *Paste Special* at the drop-down list.

16 At the Paste Special dialog box, click *Unformatted Text* in the *As* list box and then click OK.

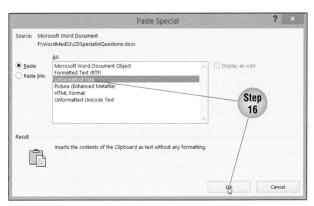

17 Set the heading *Additional Information* in 11-point Cambria and then apply bold formatting and the Dark Blue font color.

18 Save **WMedS3-CDAssessment.docx**.

In Brief

Cut and Paste Text
1. Select text.
2. Click Cut button in Clipboard group.
3. Move insertion point to desired position.
4. Click Paste button in Clipboard group.

Copy and Paste Text
1. Select text.
2. Click Copy button in Clipboard group.
3. Move insertion point to desired position.
4. Click Paste button in Clipboard group.

Use Paste Special Dialog Box
1. Cut or copy text.
2. Click Paste button arrow.
3. Click *Paste Special*.
4. Click desired format in *As* list box.
5. Click OK.

In Addition

Moving and Copying Text with the Mouse

You can move selected text using only the mouse. To do this, select the text and then move the I-beam pointer inside the selected text until the I-beam pointer turns into an arrow pointer. Hold down the left mouse button, drag the arrow pointer (displays with a gray box attached) to the location where you want to insert the selected text, and then release the mouse button. Copy and paste selected text by following similar steps, but hold down the Ctrl key as you drag the selected text with the mouse. When you hold down the Ctrl key, a box containing a plus symbol displays near the gray box attached to the arrow pointer.

Activity 3.4

Using the Clipboard Task Pane

Using the Clipboard task pane, you can collect up to 24 different items at one time and then paste them in various locations in a document. Display the Clipboard task pane by clicking the Clipboard group task pane launcher on the HOME tab.

Cut or copy an item and the item displays in the Clipboard task pane. Paste an item by positioning the insertion point at the desired location and then clicking the item in the Clipboard task pane. When all desired items have been inserted, click the Clear All button in the upper right corner of the task pane.

Project

Sydney Larsen wants you to include additional information from the Child Development Specialist Questionnaire in the Assessment of Child Development form. You will use the Clipboard task pane to copy sections of text from the questionnaire and paste them into the form.

1. Make sure **WMedS3-CDAssessment.docx** and **CDSpecialistQuestions.docx** are open.

2. Make **CDSpecialistQuestions.docx** active and then display the Clipboard task pane by clicking the Clipboard group task pane launcher on the HOME tab. If items display in the Clipboard task pane, click the Clear All button in the upper right corner of the task pane.

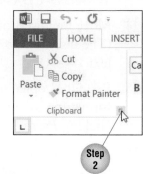

Step 2

3. Select from the beginning of the *Family Health History* heading to just above (on the blank line) the next heading (*Feeding/Oral Behavior*) and then click the Copy button in the Clipboard group.

   Notice how the copied item appears in the Clipboard task pane.

4. Select from the beginning of the *Feeding/Oral Behavior* heading to just above the *Sleep* heading and then click the Copy button.

5. Select from the beginning of the *Sleep* heading to just above the *Your Child's Health* heading and then click the Copy button.

6. Select from the beginning of the *Feelings and Moods* heading to just above the *Additional Information* heading and then click the Copy button.

7. Click the Word button on the Taskbar and then click the **WMedS3-CDAssessment.docx** thumbnail.

8. Click the Clipboard group task pane launcher to display the Clipboard task pane.

9. Move the insertion point to the blank line immediately above the heading *Additional Information* (located toward the end of the document) and then press Enter.

10. In the Clipboard task pane, click the item representing *Feelings and Moods*.

11. Click the Paste Options button that displays below the pasted text and then click the Merge Formatting button.

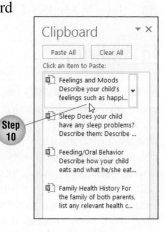

Step 10

12. With the insertion point positioned on the blank line immediately above the heading *Additional Information*, click the item in the Clipboard task pane representing *Feeding/Oral Behavior*.

13 Click the Paste Options button and then click the Merge Formatting button.

14 With the insertion point positioned on the blank line immediately above the heading *Additional Information*, paste the item representing *Sleep*.

15 Click the Paste Options button and then click the Merge Formatting button.

16 Click the Clear All button in the upper right corner of the Clipboard task pane.

17 Close the Clipboard task pane by clicking the Close button in the upper right corner of the task pane.

18 Click the Word button on the Taskbar, click the **CDSpecialistQuestions.docx** thumbnail, and then close the document.

> This displays **WMedS3-CDAssessment.docx**.

19 Set the headings *Feelings and Moods*, *Feeding/Oral Behavior*, and *Sleep* in 11-point Cambria bold and then apply the Dark Blue font color.

20 Select the title, *ASSESSMENT OF CHILD DEVELOPMENT*, and the subtitle *Ages Newborn to Three Years*, click the Shading button arrow, and then click the *Blue, Accent 5, Lighter 60%* option (ninth column, third row in the *Theme Colors* section).

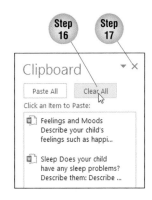

21 Apply Blue, Accent 5, Lighter 80% shading to the headings *Child Development – Hearing* and *Child Development – Talking*.

22 Save **WMedS3-CDAssessment.docx**.

In Brief

Use Clipboard Task Pane
1. Click Clipboard group task pane launcher.
2. Select text.
3. Click Copy button.
4. Select and copy any additional items.
5. Move insertion point to desired position.
6. Click desired item in Clipboard task pane.
7. Paste any other desired items from Clipboard task pane.
8. Click Clear All button.
9. Close task pane.

In Addition

Exploring Options at the Clipboard Task Pane

Click the Options button located toward the bottom of the Clipboard task pane and a pop-up menu displays with five options, as shown at the right. Click each option to toggle it on or off. Using these options, you can choose to display the Clipboard task pane automatically when you cut or copy text, display the Clipboard task pane by pressing Ctrl + C twice, cut and copy text without displaying the Clipboard task pane, display the Office Clipboard icon on the Taskbar when the Clipboard is active, and display a status message near the Taskbar when copying items to the Clipboard.

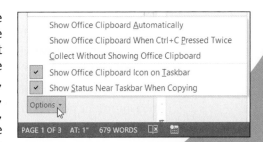

Activity 3.5

Customizing the Page Setup

In Word, a page contains a number of defaults such as a width of 8.5 inches and a depth of 11 inches; top, bottom, left, and right margins of one inch; portrait orientation; and a page break after approximately 9 inches of vertical text. Change these default settings with the buttons in the Page Setup group on the PAGE LAYOUT tab. Change the default margins with the Margins button. Use the Orientation button to change the orientation from portrait to landscape. Use the Size button to specify a paper size.

Project

To further improve the Assessment of Child Development form, you will change the document margins, orientation, and page size and then customize and add visual appeal to the document by applying a theme and changing the theme colors.

1. With **WMedS3-CDAssessment.docx** open, click the PAGE LAYOUT tab and then click the Margins button [ ] in the Page Setup group. Scroll down the drop-down list and then click the *Office 2003 Default* option.

    The *Office 2003 Default* option changes the left and right margins to 1.25 inches, which is the default setting for Word 2003.

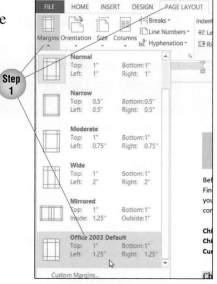

2. Change the page orientation by clicking the Orientation button [ ] in the Page Setup group on the PAGE LAYOUT tab and then clicking *Landscape* at the drop-down list.

    By default, a page is set in portrait orientation. At this orientation, the page is 8.5 inches wide and 11 inches tall. When you change to landscape orientation, the page is 11 inches wide and 8.5 inches tall. You can also change page orientation at the Page Setup dialog box with the Margins tab selected.

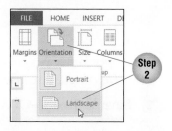

3. With the document in landscape orientation, you decide to make changes to the margins. To begin, click the Margins button in the Page Setup group on the PAGE LAYOUT tab and then click the text *Custom Margins* at the bottom of the drop-down list.

4. At the Page Setup dialog box with the Margins tab selected, click the down-pointing arrow at the right side of the *Bottom* measurement box until *1"* displays. Click the up-pointing arrow at the right side of the *Left* measurement box until *1.5"* displays.

    You can also change a margin by selecting the measurement and then typing the new measurement.

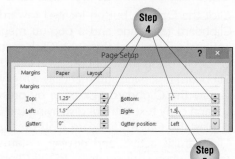

5. Select the current number in the *Right* measurement box and then type **1.5**.

6 Click OK to close the Page Setup dialog box.

7 You decide to experiment with paper size. Click the Size button in the Page Setup group and then click the *Legal* option at the drop-down list.

> Your drop-down list may display differently than what you see in the image at the right.

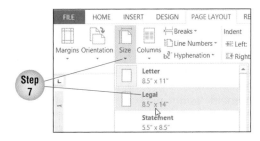

Step 7

8 Scroll through the document and notice how it is affected by changing the page size to *Legal*. Return the document to the default page size by clicking the Size button in the Page Setup group and then clicking *Letter* at the drop-down list.

9 Return the margins to the default setting by clicking the Margins button and then clicking *Normal* at the drop-down list.

10 Return to portrait orientation by clicking the Orientation button and then clicking *Portrait* at the drop-down list.

11 Apply a theme to the document by clicking the DESIGN tab, clicking the Themes button in the Document Formatting group, scrolling down the drop-down gallery, and then clicking the *Parallax* option.

12 Click the Colors button in the Document Formatting group and then click *Blue II* at the drop-down gallery.

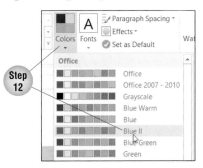

Step 12

13 Save **WMedS3-CDAssessment.docx**.

In Brief

Change Margins
1. Click PAGE LAYOUT tab.
2. Click Margins button.
3. Click desired option.

Change Orientation
1. Click PAGE LAYOUT tab.
2. Click Orientation button.
3. Click desired option.

Change Page Size
1. Click PAGE LAYOUT tab.
2. Click Size button.
3. Click desired option.

In Addition

Applying Landscape Orientation

Certain types of document content are better suited to landscape orientation than portrait orientation. Suppose you are preparing an annual report and you need to include a couple of tables that have several columns of text. If you use the default portrait orientation, the columns would need to be quite narrow, possibly so narrow that reading would become difficult. Changing the orientation to landscape provides three more inches of usable space. You are not committed to using landscape orientation for the entire document. To use both portrait and landscape orientation in the same document, select the text whose orientation you want to change, display the Page Setup dialog box, click the desired orientation, and then change the *Apply to* option to *Selected text*.

Activity 3.6

Customizing the Page and Page Background

The Page Background group on the DESIGN tab contains buttons you can use to insert a watermark, change the page color, and insert a page border. In an activity in Section 1, you applied a watermark to a document using options at the Building Blocks Organizer dialog box, but you can also apply a watermark with the Watermark button in the Page Background group on the DESIGN tab. In a project in Section 2, you applied a page border to a document by clicking the Borders button, but you can also apply a page border by using the Page Borders button in the Page Background group. The Pages group on the INSERT tab contains buttons for adding a cover page, a blank page, and a page break.

Project

To add visual interest to the Assessment of Child Development document, you will apply page color and a page border. You will add a cover page at the beginning of the document and identify the document as a draft by inserting a watermark.

Cascade View
PEDIATRICS

① With **WMedS3-CDAssessment.docx** open, press Ctrl + Home.

② Insert a watermark by clicking the DESIGN tab, clicking the Watermark button in the Page Background group, scrolling down the drop-down list, and then clicking the *DRAFT 1* option.

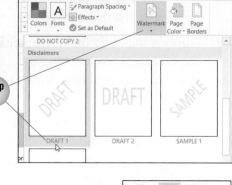

③ Apply a page color to the document by clicking the Page Color button in the Page Background group and then clicking the *Turquoise, Accent 3, Lighter 80%* option (seventh column, second row in the *Theme Colors* section).

> Page color is designed for viewing a document on the screen. The color does not print.

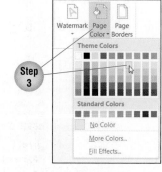

④ Click the Page Borders button in the Page Background group.

⑤ At the Borders and Shading dialog box with the Page Border tab selected, click the down-pointing arrow at the right side of the *Art* option box. Scroll down the list of page borders and then click the art border option shown at the right. Click OK to close the dialog box.

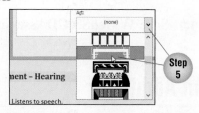

⑥ Move the insertion point to the beginning of the heading *Feelings and Moods* and then insert a hard page break by clicking the INSERT tab and then clicking the Page Break button in the Pages group.

> You can also insert a hard page break with the keyboard shortcut Ctrl + Enter or by clicking the PAGE LAYOUT tab, clicking the Breaks button in the Page Setup group, and then clicking *Page* at the drop-down list.

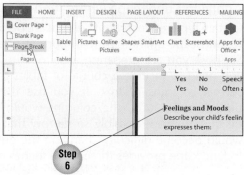

7. Save and then print **WMedS3-CDAssessment.docx**. (The page background color does not print.)

8. After looking at the printed document, you decide to make some changes. Remove the page color by clicking the DESIGN tab, clicking the Page Color button in the Page Background group, and then clicking *No Color*.

9. Remove the page border by clicking the Page Borders button, clicking *None* in the *Setting* section of the Borders and Shading dialog box, and then clicking OK.

10. Delete the page break you inserted by positioning the insertion point on the blank line a double-space below the line of text in the *2 to 3 Years* section at the bottom of page 2 and then pressing the Delete key twice.

11. Press Ctrl + Home to move the insertion point to the beginning of the document.

12. Insert a cover page by clicking the INSERT tab, clicking the Cover Page button in the Pages group, scrolling down the drop-down list, and then clicking the *Whisp* option.

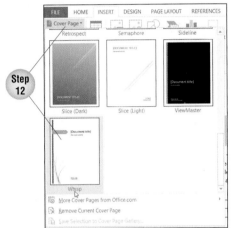

Step 12

13. Click in the placeholder text *[Date]*, click the down-pointing arrow at the right of the placeholder, and then click the Today button to insert the current date.

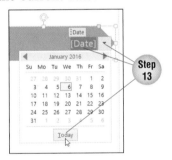

Step 13

14. Click in the placeholder text *[Document title]* and then type **Assessment of Child Development**.

15. Click in the placeholder text *[Document subtitle]* and then type **Ages Newborn to Three Years**.

16. Click in the placeholder text *[COMPANY NAME]* and then type **Cascade View Pediatrics**.

17. Select the name that displays above *CASCADE VIEW PEDIATRICS* and then type your first and last names.

18. Save **WMedS3-CDAssessment.docx**.

In Brief

Apply Watermark
1. Click DESIGN tab.
2. Click Watermark button.
3. Click desired watermark option.

Apply Page Color
1. Click DESIGN tab.
2. Click Page Color button.
3. Click desired color.

Insert Page Border
1. Click DESIGN tab.
2. Click Page Borders button.
3. Click desired options at Borders and Shading dialog box.
4. Click OK.

Insert Page Break
1. Click INSERT tab.
2. Click Page Break button.

Insert Cover Page
1. Click INSERT tab.
2. Click Cover Page button.
3. Click desired option.
4. Type text in appropriate placeholders.

In Addition

Inserting a Blank Page

The Pages group on the INSERT tab contains a Blank Page button. Click this button to insert a blank page at the position of the insertion point. Inserting a blank page can be useful as a placeholder in a document when you want to insert an illustration, graphic, or figure.

Activity 3.7

Inserting Page Numbering, Headers, and Footers

Insert page numbering in a document with options at the Page Number button drop-down list. Click the Page Number button in the Header & Footer group on the INSERT tab and a drop-down list displays with options for inserting page numbers at the top or bottom of the page or in the page margins, as well as options for removing and formatting page numbers. Text that appears in the top margin of a page is called a *header* and text that appears in the bottom margin of a page is referred to as a *footer*. Headers and footers are common in manuscripts, textbooks, reports, and other publications. Insert a predesigned header in a document with the Header button in the Header & Footer group on the INSERT tab. Insert a predesigned footer by clicking the Footer button. Predesigned headers and footers contain formatting that you can customize to suit your needs.

Project

Put the finishing touches on the Assessment of Child Development document by adding a header, footer, and page numbers.

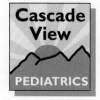

1. With **WMedS3-CDAssessment.docx** open, move the insertion point to the beginning of the title *ASSESSMENT OF CHILD DEVELOPMENT* at the top of the second page (*not* on the cover page).

   When a document contains a cover page, you generally insert elements such as page numbers, headers, and footers on the first page *after* the cover page.

2. Insert numbers at the bottom of each page by clicking the INSERT tab, clicking the Page Number button in the Header & Footer group, and then pointing to *Bottom of Page*.

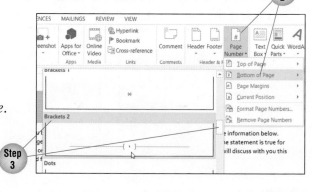

3. At the gallery of predesigned page numbers, scroll down and then click the *Brackets 2* option.

4. Double-click in the body of the document and then scroll through the document, observing how the page numbers display toward the bottom of each page except the cover page.

5. Remove page numbering by clicking the INSERT tab, clicking the Page Number button in the Header & Footer group, and then clicking *Remove Page Numbers* at the drop-down list.

6. Insert a header in the document by clicking the Header button in the Header & Footer group, scrolling down the drop-down list, and then clicking the *Motion (Even Page)* option.

   Notice how the document title you entered in the cover page is inserted in the header.

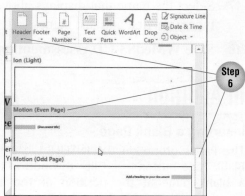

7 Double-click in the body of the document.

This makes the document active and dims the header.

8 Insert a footer in the document by clicking the INSERT tab, clicking the Footer button 🗋 in the Header & Footer group, scrolling down the drop-down list, and then clicking the *Motion (Odd Page)* option.

Notice how the date you entered in the cover page is inserted in the footer.

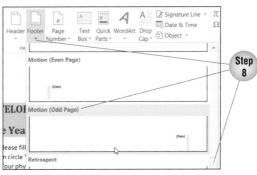

In Brief

Insert Page Numbers
1. Click INSERT tab.
2. Click Page Number button.
3. Point to desired location.
4. Click desired option at drop-down list.

Insert Header
1. Click INSERT tab.
2. Click Header button.
3. Click desired option at drop-down list.

Insert Footer
1. Click INSERT tab.
2. Click Footer button.
3. Click desired option at drop-down list.

9 Double-click in the body of the document and then scroll through the document, observing how the header and footer appear on each page except the cover page.

10 Save and then print **WMedS3-CDAssessment.docx**.

11 Remove the header by clicking the INSERT tab, clicking the Header button in the Header & Footer group, and then clicking *Remove Header* at the drop-down list.

12 Edit the footer by clicking the Footer button in the Header & Footer group and then clicking *Edit Footer* at the drop-down list.

13 Select the date in the footer, change the font to 10-point Calibri, and then apply bold formatting.

14 Double-click in the document.

15 Remove the Draft watermark by clicking the DESIGN tab, clicking the Watermark button, and then clicking *Remove Watermark* at the drop-down list.

16 Insert a page break at the beginning of the heading *Feelings and Moods*.

17 Save, print, and then close **WMedS3-CDAssessment.docx**.

In Addition

Creating Your Own Header or Footer

Create your own header or footer using the *Edit Header* or *Edit Footer* options at the Header and Footer button drop-down lists. For example, to create a header, click the INSERT tab, click the Header button, and then click *Edit Header* at the drop-down list. This displays the Header pane and the HEADER & FOOTER TOOLS DESIGN tab with buttons and options for editing the header. Make the desired edits to the header with options on the tab and then close the Header pane by clicking the Close Header and Footer button in the Close group on the HEADER & FOOTER TOOLS DESIGN tab.

Activity 3.8

Inserting a Section Break; Creating and Modifying Columns

To increase the ease with which a person can read and understand groups of words in a document (referred as *readability*), consider setting the text in columns. Columns reduce line length, thus making a large amount of content easier to read. Create columns with the Columns button in the Page Setup group on the PAGE LAYOUT tab or with options at the Columns dialog box. If you want to apply column formatting to only a portion of a document, insert a section break in the document by using the options at the Breaks button drop-down list in the Page Setup group on the PAGE LAYOUT tab.

Project

Sydney Larsen has asked you to format the monthly newsletter for Cascade View Pediatrics into columns and to apply formatting to improve the visual appeal of the newsletter.

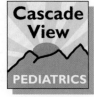

1. Open **CVPNewsltr.docx** and then save the document with the name **WMedS3-CVPNewsltr**.

2. Position the insertion point at the beginning of the first heading, *Pediatrician Joins CVP*.

3. Insert a continuous section break by clicking the PAGE LAYOUT tab, clicking the Breaks button in the Page Setup group, and then clicking *Continuous* in the *Section Breaks* section.

   A continuous section break separates the document into sections but does not insert a page break. Continuous section breaks are not visible in Print Layout view. Click one of the other three options in the *Section Breaks* section of the Breaks button drop-down list to insert a section break that begins a new page.

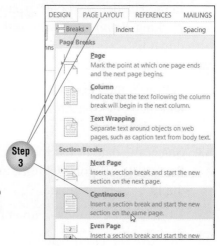

4. Click the VIEW tab and then click the Draft button in the Views group.

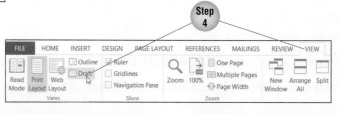

5. With the insertion point positioned below the section break, format the text below the section break into three columns by clicking the PAGE LAYOUT tab, clicking the Columns button in the Page Setup group, and then clicking *Three* at the drop-down list.

   Formatting text into columns automatically changes the view to Print Layout view.

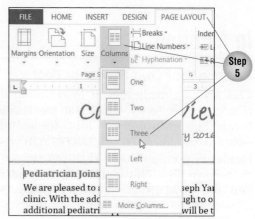

6 As you view the document, you notice that the three columns are pretty narrow, so you decide to set the text in two columns with a line between them. To do this, click in the heading *Pediatrician Joins CVP* and then display the Columns dialog box by clicking the Columns button in the Page Setup group and then clicking *More Columns* at the drop-down list.

7 At the Columns dialog box, click *Two* in the *Presets* section.

8 Slightly decrease the spacing between the two columns by clicking once on the down-pointing arrow at the right of the *Spacing* measurement box in the *Width and spacing* section.

> Make sure *0.4"* displays in the *Spacing* measurement box.

9 Make sure a check mark displays in the *Equal column width* check box. If not, click the check box to insert a check mark.

> This option, when activated, makes the two columns the same width.

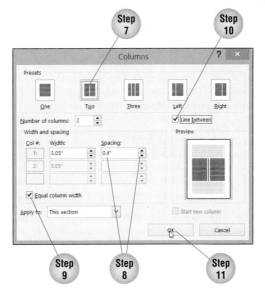

Step 7 · Step 10 · Step 9 · Step 8 · Step 11

10 Click the *Line between* check box to insert a check mark.

> Turning on the *Line between* option inserts a line between the two columns. The *Preview* section of the dialog box provides a visual representation of this.

11 Click OK to close the Columns dialog box.

12 Press Ctrl + End to move the insertion point to the end of the document. Balance the two columns by clicking the Breaks button in the Page Setup group and then clicking *Continuous* in the *Section Breaks* section.

13 Save, print, and then close **WMedS3-CVPNewsltr.docx**.

In Brief

Insert Continuous Section Break
1. Click PAGE LAYOUT tab.
2. Click Breaks button in Page Setup group.
3. Click *Continuous* in *Section Breaks* section.

Format Text into Columns
1. Click PAGE LAYOUT tab.
2. Click Columns button in Page Setup group.
3. Click desired number of columns.

Display Columns Dialog Box
1. Click PAGE LAYOUT tab.
2. Click Columns button in Page Setup group.
3. Click *More Columns*.

In Addition

Changing Column Width

One method for changing column width in a document is to drag the column marker on the horizontal ruler. To change the width of columns of text, position the arrow pointer on the left or right edge of a column marker on the horizontal ruler until it turns into a left-and-right-pointing arrow. Hold down the left mouse button, drag the column marker to the left or right to make the column of text wider or narrower, and then release the mouse button. To make more precise adjustments to column width, hold down the Alt key as you drag the column marker. Exact measurements will display on the horizontal ruler.

Activity 3.9

Inserting, Sizing, and Moving Images in a Document

Microsoft Office includes a gallery of media images (including clip art, photographs, and illustrations) that you can insert in a document. Use the Online Pictures button on the INSERT tab to search for and insert images from Office.com. Use the Pictures button if you want to insert a picture from your computer or network. You can move, size, and customize a picture with buttons on the PICTURE TOOLS FORMAT tab, which displays after you insert the image.

Project

Cascade View PEDIATRICS

Deanna Reynolds has asked you to enhance a document she created for her parenting classes. You decide to add clip art images to the document and apply some additional formatting to enhance the visual appeal.

1. Open **CVPClasses.docx** and then save the document with the name **WMedS3-CVPClasses**.

2. You know that adding images to a document can make it more engaging for readers, so you decide to insert an image of a parent and child. To begin, display the Insert Pictures window by clicking the INSERT tab and then clicking the Online Pictures button in the Illustrations group.

3. Click in the search box that displays to the right of the *Office.com Clip Art* option, type **toddler walking**, and then press Enter.

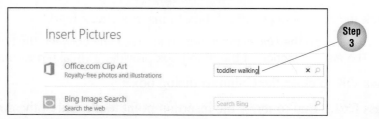

4. Double-click the image shown below. If this image is not available, choose another similar image.

   The image is inserted in the document, it is selected (sizing handles display around it), and the PICTURE TOOLS FORMAT tab displays as shown in Figure W3.1.

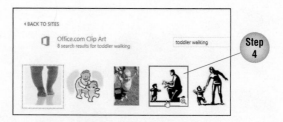

FIGURE W3.1 PICTURE TOOLS FORMAT Tab

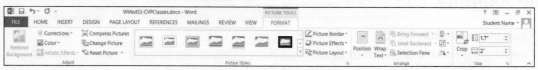

5 With the image selected, click the Wrap Text button 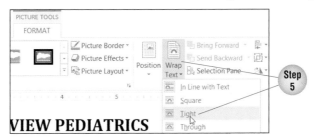 in the Arrange group on the PICTURE TOOLS FORMAT tab and then click *Tight* at the drop-down list.

6 Click in the *Shape Height* measurement box in the Size group, type **1.8**, and then press Enter.

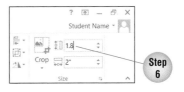

When you change the height measurement, the width measurement is automatically changed to maintain the proportions of the image.

7 Add a shadow effect to the image by clicking the More button that displays at the right side of the picture style thumbnails in the Picture Styles group and then clicking the *Center Shadow Rectangle* option (sixth column, second row).

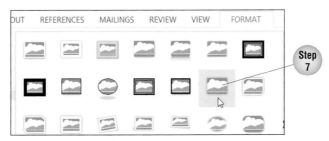

8 Move the image by positioning the mouse pointer on the image until the pointer displays with a four-headed arrow attached, holding down the mouse button, dragging the image so it is positioned as shown in Figure W3.2 on page 155, and then releasing the mouse button.

9 Click outside the image to deselect it.

10 Position the insertion point at the beginning of the bulleted list.

11 Click the INSERT tab and then click the Online Pictures button in the Illustrations group.

12 At the Insert Pictures window, type **toddler walking** in the *Office.com Clip Art* text box and then press Enter.

13 Double-click the image shown below. If this image is not available, choose another similar image.

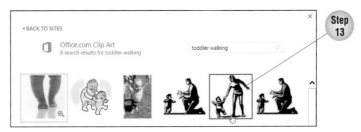

continues

14 With the image selected, click the Wrap Text button in the Arrange group and then click *Square* at the drop-down list.

15 Click the down-pointing arrow at the right side of the *Shape Height* measurement box in the Size group until *1.1"* displays in the box.

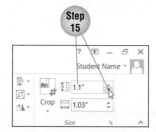

16 Add a shadow effect to the image by clicking the More button that displays at the right side of the picture style thumbnails in the Picture Styles group and then clicking the *Center Shadow Rectangle* option (sixth column, second row).

17 Move the image by positioning the arrow pointer on the image until the pointer displays with a four-headed arrow attached, holding down the left mouse button, dragging the image so it is positioned as shown in Figure W3.2, and then releasing the mouse button.

18 Click outside the image to deselect it.

19 Move the insertion point to the end of the document and then insert the Cascade View Pediatrics logo. To begin, click the INSERT tab and then click the Pictures button [icon] in the Illustrations group.

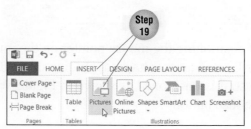

20 At the Insert Picture dialog box, navigate to the WordMedS3 folder on your storage medium and then double-click *CVPLogo.jpg*.

21 With the image selected in the document, click the Wrap Text button in the Arrange group and then click *Tight* at the drop-down list.

22 With the image still selected, hold down the Shift key and then drag one of the corner sizing handles to reduce the size of the logo so it displays as shown in Figure W3.2. Move the logo to the position shown in the figure.

> Holding down the Shift key while increasing or decreasing the size of an image maintains the proportions of the image. When you insert the image, it will display on the second page. Make sure you decrease the size so the logo fits on the first page.

23 Save, print, and then close **WMedS3-CVPClasses.docx**.

FIGURE W3.2 Completed WMedS3-CVPClasses Document

CASCADE VIEW PEDIATRICS
Basic Parenting Course

Presented by Deanna Reynolds
Child Development Specialist

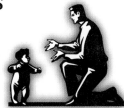

Parenting is a full-time job and wondering about your child's behaviors and your responsibilities as a parent are normal. You may have asked yourself:

- What can I do when my child misbehaves?
- Is my child's development and behavior "normal"?
- What is the different between punishment and discipline?
- How can I improve the way I communicate with my child?
- How can I help my child learn to make good choices?

Deanna Reynolds, Child Development Specialist at Cascade View Pediatrics, will cover these questions as well as others in a four-week course designed to help you better handle the challenges of parenting.

When .... Monday and Wednesday
Beginning .... Monday, March 7
Ending .... Wednesday, March 30
Time .... 7:00 p.m. to 8:30 p.m.
Where .... Cascade View Pediatrics
Location .... Suite 150, Room 3
Cost $85

For more information on this important parenting course and to sign up for the class, call (503) 555-7753. You can also read more about the course and register online by visiting the Cascade View Pediatrics website at www.emcp.net/cvp.

Cascade View
PEDIATRICS

In Brief

Insert Image from Office.com
1. Click INSERT tab.
2. Click Online Pictures button.
3. Type search text in search box and then press Enter.
4. Double-click desired image.

Insert Picture
1. Click INSERT tab.
2. Click Pictures button.
3. Navigate to desired folder.
4. Double-click desired picture file.

In Addition

Formatting an Image with Buttons on the PICTURE TOOLS FORMAT Tab

Images inserted in a document can be formatted in a variety of ways, including adding fill color and border lines, increasing or decreasing the brightness or contrast, choosing a wrapping style, and cropping the image. Format an image with buttons on the PICTURE TOOLS FORMAT tab (shown in Figure W3.1 on page 152). With buttons in the Adjust group you can correct the brightness and contrast of the image; change the image color; change to a different image; reset the image to its original size, position, and color; and compress the image. Compressing an image reduces file size to save room on the hard drive and reduce download time. Use buttons in the Picture Styles group to apply a predesigned style, insert a picture border, or apply a picture effect. The Arrange group contains buttons for positioning the image, wrapping text around the image, and aligning and rotating the image. Use options in the Size group to crop the image and specify the height and width of the image.

Activity
3.10

Inserting, Sizing, and Moving
WordArt in a Document; Inserting a File

Use the WordArt feature to distort or modify text to conform to a variety of shapes. Consider using WordArt to create a company logo, letterhead, flyer title, or heading. With WordArt, you can change the font, style, and alignment of text; use different fill patterns and colors; customize border lines; and add shadow and three-dimensional effects. You can size and move selected WordArt text as desired.

In some situations, you may want to insert the contents of one file into another. Do this at the Insert File dialog box, which you display by clicking *Text from File* at the Object button drop-down list in the Text group on the INSERT tab.

Project

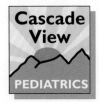

The Health Insurance Portability and Accountability Act of 1996 (HIPAA) requires that healthcare providers adopt and adhere to policies and procedures that protect the patient's privacy regarding disclosure of sensitive health information. Cascade View Pediatrics has established clear guidelines for patient confidentiality. Sydney Larsen has asked you to compile a document with information on patient confidentiality and enhance the document with WordArt for more impact.

1. Open **CVPHIPAA.docx** and then save the document with the name **WMedS3-CVPHIPAA**.

2. Press Ctrl + End to move the insertion point to the end of the document.

3. Insert a file into the current document by clicking the INSERT tab, clicking the Object button arrow 🔲 in the Text group, and then clicking *Text from File* at the drop-down list.

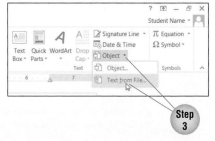

Step 3

4. At the Insert File dialog box, navigate to the WordMedS3 folder on your storage medium and then double-click *CVPRules.docx*.

5. Select the paragraphs of text in the document (excluding the title) and then insert bullets by clicking the Bullets button in the Paragraph group on the HOME tab.

6. Move the insertion point to the beginning of the document and then insert WordArt by clicking the INSERT tab and then clicking the WordArt button 🅰 in the Text group.

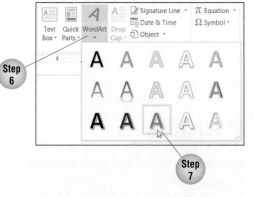

Step 6

Step 7

7. At the WordArt button drop-down list, click the *Fill - Blue, Accent 1, Outline - Background 1, Hard Shadow - Accent 1* option (third column, third row).

8. Type **Important**.

   This inserts the WordArt text *Important* in the document, selects the WordArt text box, and displays the DRAWING TOOLS FORMAT tab. (See the In Addition on the next page for more information.)

9. Increase the width of the WordArt text by clicking in the *Shape Width* measurement box in the Size group on the DRAWING TOOLS FORMAT tab, typing **5**, and then pressing Enter.

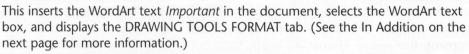

Step 9

10 Change the shape of the WordArt by clicking the Text Effects button [A▾] in the WordArt Styles group on the DRAWING TOOLS FORMAT tab, pointing to *Transform* at the drop-down list, and then clicking the *Square* option (first column, first row in the *Warp* section).

11 Click the Text Fill button arrow [A▾] in the WordArt Styles group on the DRAWING TOOLS FORMAT tab and then click the *Gold, Accent 4* option at the drop-down gallery (eighth column, first row in the *Theme Colors* section).

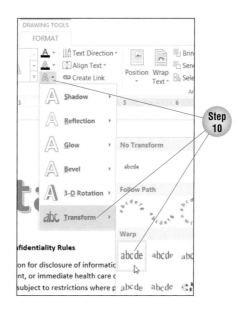

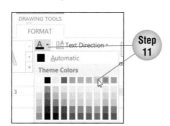

In Brief

Insert File
1. Click INSERT tab.
2. Click Object button arrow in Text group.
3. Click *Text from File*.
4. At Insert File dialog box, double-click desired document.

Insert WordArt
1. Click INSERT tab.
2. Click WordArt button.
3. Click desired option at drop-down list.
4. Type desired text.

12 Click the Text Outline button arrow [A▾] in the WordArt Styles group and then click the *Dark Red* option in the *Standard Colors* section of the drop-down gallery.

13 Position the WordArt text so it is centered between the left and right margins. To do this, position the mouse pointer on the WordArt text until the pointer displays with a four-headed arrow attached. Hold down the left mouse button, drag the WordArt text to the desired position, and then release the mouse button.

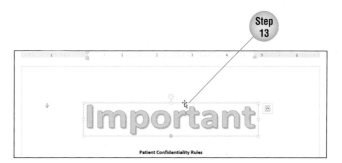

14 Click outside the WordArt text box to deselect it.

15 Save **WMedS3-CVPHIPAA.docx**.

In Addition

Using the DRAWING TOOLS FORMAT Tab

When WordArt is selected, the DRAWING TOOLS FORMAT tab displays, as shown below. Use options in the Insert Shapes group to draw a shape or text box. With options in the Shape Styles group, you can apply a predesigned style, change the shape fill color and the shape outline color, and apply shape effects. Change the style of the WordArt text with options in the WordArt Styles group, specify the layering of the WordArt text with options in the Arrange group, and specify the height and width of the WordArt text with options in the Size group.

Activity 3.11

Inserting and Customizing Shapes and Text Boxes

With the Shapes button on the INSERT tab, you can draw a variety of shapes and lines and then customize them with options on the DRAWING TOOLS FORMAT tab. Use the Text Box button on the INSERT tab to draw a box into which you can then type text. Customize a text box with buttons on the DRAWING TOOLS FORMAT tab. You can size and move a drawn object or text box in the same manner as you would size and move an image or WordArt text.

Project

To further enhance the patient confidentiality rules document and to emphasize the priority of maintaining confidentiality, you decide to add a shape containing text at the bottom of the document.

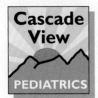

1. With **WMedS3-CVPHIPAA.docx** open, press Ctrl + End to move the insertion point to the end of the document.

2. Draw the banner shape shown in Figure W3.3. To do this, click the INSERT tab, click the Shapes button in the Illustrations group, and then click the *Up Ribbon* option (first column, second row in the *Stars and Banners* section).

3. Position the mouse pointer (displays as crosshairs) below the text at approximately the 1-inch mark on the horizontal ruler and the 6.5-inch mark on the vertical ruler. Hold down the left mouse button, drag down and to the right until the banner is approximately 5 inches wide and 1.5 inches high, and then release the mouse button.

   This inserts the shape in the document and makes active the DRAWING TOOLS FORMAT tab.

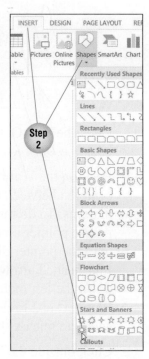

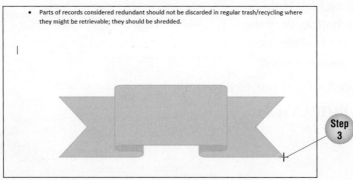

4. Apply a shape style by clicking the More button at the right of the thumbnails in the Shape Styles group and then clicking the *Subtle Effect - Gold, Accent 4* option (fifth column, fourth row).

5. Draw a text box inside the shape by clicking the INSERT tab, clicking the Text Box button in the Text group, and then clicking *Draw Text Box* at the drop-down list.

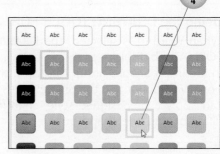

6 Position the mouse pointer (displays as crosshairs) inside the banner, hold down the left mouse button, drag to create a text box similar to the one shown at the right, and then release the mouse button.

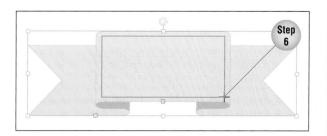

In Brief

Draw Shape
1. Click INSERT tab.
2. Click Shapes button.
3. Click desired shape.
4. Drag with mouse to draw shape.

Draw Text Box
1. Click INSERT tab.
2. Click Text Box button.
3. Click *Draw Text Box* option at drop-down list.
4. Drag with mouse to draw text box.

7 Change the font size to 14 points, turn on bold formatting, change to center alignment, and then type **Patient confidentiality is a top priority at Cascade View Pediatrics!**

8 Vertically align text within the text box by clicking the DRAWING TOOLS FORMAT tab, clicking the Align Text button ⬍, and then clicking *Middle* at the drop-down list.

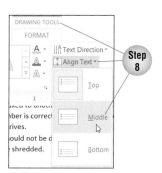

9 Remove fill from the text box by clicking the DRAWING TOOLS FORMAT tab, clicking the Shape Fill button arrow 🖌, and then clicking *No Fill* at the drop-down gallery.

10 Remove the outline from the text box by clicking the Shape Outline button arrow 🖉 and then clicking *No Outline* at the drop-down gallery.

> When you remove the fill and outline from the text box, the text box looks as if it is part of the shape.

11 Deselect the text box by clicking outside the banner and text box.

12 Save, print, and then close **WMedS3-CVPHIPAA.docx**.

FIGURE W3.3 Up Ribbon Banner Shape with Text Box

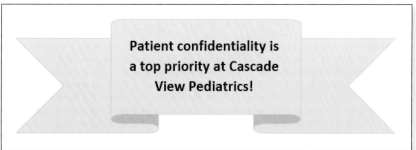

In Addition

Drawing Lines and Enclosed Shapes

With options at the Shapes button drop-down list, you can draw lines as well as enclosed shapes. To draw a line, click an option in the *Lines* section. The mouse pointer changes to crosshairs. Position the crosshairs in the document and then drag with the mouse to draw the line. To draw a perfectly straight horizontal or vertical line, hold down the Shift key while dragging the mouse.

If you choose an option in the other sections of the drop-down list, the shape you draw is considered an enclosed shape. When drawing an enclosed shape, you can maintain the proportions of the shape by holding down the Shift key while dragging with the mouse to create the shape.

Activity 3.12

Preparing an Envelope

Word simplifies the creation of envelopes with options at the Envelopes and Labels dialog box with the Envelopes tab selected. At this dialog box, all you have to do is type a delivery address and a return address. If you open the Envelopes and Labels dialog box in a document that already contains a name and address, that name and address are inserted automatically as the delivery address. If you enter a return address, Word will ask you before printing if you want to save the new return address as the default return address. Click Yes if you want to use the return address for future envelopes or click No if you will use a different return address for future envelopes.

Project

Deanna Reynolds has asked you to mail a Basic Parenting Course flyer to Lowell Quasim, Education Coordinator at Columbia River General Hospital.

Cascade View PEDIATRICS

1. Press Ctrl + N to display a blank document.

   You can also display a blank document by clicking the FILE tab, clicking the *New* option, and then clicking the *Blank document* template. Another method is to insert the New button on the Quick Access toolbar and then click the button to display a blank document. To insert New the button on the Quick Access toolbar, click the Customize Quick Access Toolbar button that displays at the right side of the toolbar and then click *New* at the drop-down list.

2. Click the MAILINGS tab and then click the Envelopes button in the Create group.

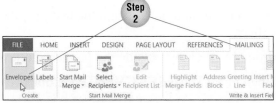

Step 2

3. At the Envelopes and Labels dialog box with the Envelopes tab selected, type the following name and address in the *Delivery address* text box. (Press Enter at the end of each line except the last line [contains the city name, state, and ZIP code.])

   Mr. Lowell Quasim
   Education Coordinator
   Columbia River General Hospital
   4550 Fremont Street
   Portland, OR 97045

4. Click in the *Return address* text box and then type the following name and address, pressing Enter at the end of each line except the last one. (If any text displays in the *Return address* text box, select and then delete it before you begin typing.)

   Deanna Reynolds
   Cascade View Pediatrics
   350 North Skagit
   Portland, OR 97505

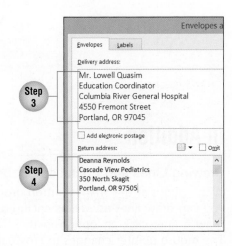

Step 3

Step 4

5 Click the Add to Document button.

Clicking the Add to Document button inserts the envelope in the document. You can also send the envelope directly to the printer by clicking the Print button.

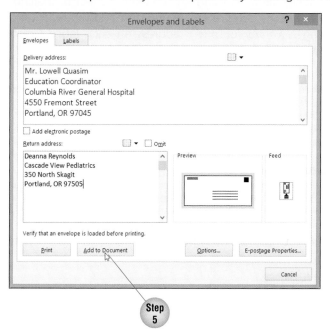

Step 5

In Brief

Prepare Envelope
1. Click MAILINGS tab.
2. Click Envelopes button.
3. Type delivery address.
4. Type return address.
5. Click either Add to Document button or Print button.

6 At the message asking if you want to save the new return address as the default address, click No.

7 Save the document with the name **WMedS3-CVPEnv**.

8 Print and then close **WMedS3-CVPEnv.docx**. *Note: Manual feed of the envelope into the printer may be required. Please check with your instructor before printing.*

In Addition

Customizing Envelopes

With options at the Envelope Options dialog box, shown at the right, you can customize an envelope to suit your needs. Display this dialog box by clicking the Options button at the Envelopes and Labels dialog box with the Envelopes tab selected. At the Envelope Options dialog box, you can change the envelope size, change the font for the delivery and return addresses, and specify the positioning of the addresses in relation to the left and top edges of the envelope.

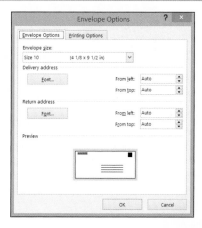

Activity
3.13

Preparing Mailing Labels

Use Word's labels feature to print text on mailing labels, file labels, and disc labels, among others. You can create labels for printing using a variety of pre-defined label templates, which correspond to the different types of labels you can purchase at an office supply store. With the labels feature, you can create a sheet of mailing labels with the same name and address or enter a different name and address on each label. Create labels with options at the Envelopes and Labels dialog box with the Labels tab selected.

Project

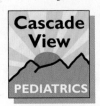

You will create a sheet of return-address mailing labels containing the Cascade View Pediatrics name and address and then create mailing labels for sending the Basic Parenting Course flyer to various professionals and clinics in the area.

1. Press Ctrl + N to display a blank document.

2. Click the MAILINGS tab and then click the Labels button in the Create group.

3. Type the following information in the *Address* text box. (Press Enter at the end of each line except the last line.)

> **Cascade View Pediatrics**
> **350 North Skagit**
> **Portland, OR 97505**

4. Click the Options button.

5. At the Label Options dialog box, click the down-pointing arrow at the right side of the *Label vendors* option box and then click *Avery US Letter* at the drop-down list.

6. Scroll down the *Product number* list box, click *5630 Easy Peel Address Labels* in the list box, and then click OK to close the dialog box.

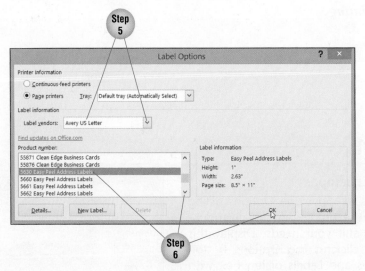

7. Click the New Document button at the Envelopes and Labels dialog box.

8. Save the document with the name **WMedS3-CVPLabels**.

9 Print and then close **WMedS3-CVPLabels.docx**.

The number of labels printed on the page varies depending on the label selected at the Label Options dialog box.

10 Click the MAILINGS tab and then click the Labels button in the Create group.

11 At the Envelopes and Labels dialog box, click the New Document button.

12 In the first label, type the first name and address shown in Figure W3.4. Press the Tab key twice to move the insertion point to the next label and then type the second name and address shown in Figure W3.4. Continue in this manner until you have typed all of the names and addresses shown in Figure W3.4.

13 Save the document with the name **WMedS3-CVPContactLabels**.

14 Print and then close **WMedS3-CVPContactLabels.docx**.

15 Close the blank document.

In Brief

Prepare Return-address Mailing Labels
1. Click MAILINGS tab.
2. Click Labels button.
3. Type name and address in *Address* text box.
4. Click New Document button or Print button.

Prepare Mailing Labels with Different Names and Addresses
1. Click MAILINGS tab.
2. Click Labels button.
3. Click New Document button.
4. At document screen, type names and addresses.

FIGURE W3.4 Mailing Labels for Step 12

Paul Watanabe Division Street Clinic 5330 Division Street Portland, OR 97255	Nora Reeves Community Counseling 1235 North 122nd Avenue Portland, OR 97230
Dr. Thomas Wickstrom Columbia Mental Health Center 550 Columbia Boulevard Portland, OR 97305	Christina Fuentes Parenting Services 210 Martin Luther King Way Portland, OR 97403

In Addition

Customizing Labels

Click the Options button at the Envelopes and Labels dialog box with the Labels tab selected and the Label Options dialog box displays as shown at the right. At this dialog box, choose the type of printer, the desired label vendor, and the product number. This dialog box also displays information about the selected label such as type, height, width, and paper size. When you select a label, Word automatically determines the label margins. To customize these default settings, click the Details button at the Label Options dialog box.

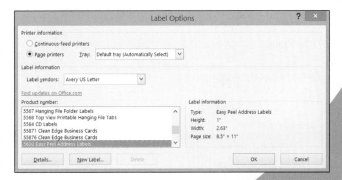

Features Summary

Feature	Ribbon Tab, Group	Button	Keyboard Shortcut
Clipboard task pane	HOME, Clipboard		
continuous section break	PAGE LAYOUT, Page Setup		
copy selected text	HOME, Clipboard		Ctrl + C
cut selected text	HOME, Clipboard		Ctrl + X
Envelopes and Labels dialog box with Envelopes tab selected	MAILINGS, Create		
Envelopes and Labels dialog box with Labels tab selected	MAILINGS, Create		
Find and Replace dialog box with Replace tab selected	HOME, Editing		Ctrl + H
footer	INSERT, Header & Footer		
header	INSERT, Header & Footer		
Insert Picture dialog box	INSERT, Illustrations		
Insert Pictures window	INSERT, Illustrations		
page border	DESIGN, Page Background		
page break	INSERT, Pages		Ctrl + Enter
page color	DESIGN, Page Background		
page margins	PAGE LAYOUT, Page Setup		
page number	INSERT, Header & Footer		
page orientation	PAGE LAYOUT, Page Setup		
Page Setup dialog box	PAGE LAYOUT, Page Setup		
page size	PAGE LAYOUT, Page Setup		
paste selected text	HOME, Clipboard		Ctrl + V
Paste Special dialog box	HOME, Clipboard	, *Paste Special*	
Reveal Formatting task pane			Shift + F1
shape	INSERT, Illustrations		
text box	INSERT, Text		
watermark	DESIGN, Page Background		
WordArt	INSERT, Text		

Knowledge Check

Completion: In the space provided at the right, write in the correct term, command, or option.

1. Click this button at the Find and Replace dialog box to replace all occurrences of text. _____
2. Click this button at the Find and Replace dialog box to display additional options. _____
3. Use this keyboard shortcut to display the Reveal Formatting task pane. _____
4. The Cut button is located in this group on the HOME tab. _____
5. Click this button to insert selected text into the document. _____
6. Click this to display the Clipboard task pane. _____
7. Click this tab to display the Margins button. _____
8. This is the default measurement for the top, bottom, left, and right margins. _____
9. This is the default page orientation. _____
10. This is the default page size. _____
11. Use this keyboard shortcut to insert a page break. _____
12. The Breaks button is located in this group on the PAGE LAYOUT tab. _____
13. Insert a footer by clicking the Footer button in this group on the INSERT tab. _____
14. The Online Pictures button displays in this group on the INSERT tab. _____
15. Click this button on the PICTURE TOOLS FORMAT tab to choose a text wrapping style. _____
16. Click this button on the INSERT tab to display the Insert Picture dialog box. _____
17. When changing the size of an image, maintain the image proportions by holding down this key while dragging a corner sizing handle. _____
18. To display the Envelopes and Labels dialog box, click this tab and then click the Envelopes button or the Labels button. _____

Skills Review

Review 1 Finding and Replacing Text; Cutting and Pasting Text

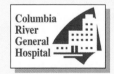

1. Open **CRGHMedRecs.docx** and then save the document with the name **WMedS3-R-CRGHMedRecs**.
2. Find every occurrence of *crgh* and replace it with *Columbia River General Hospital*.
3. Select the heading *Modifying Medical Records*, the paragraph of text below it, and the blank line below the paragraph and then move the selected text to the end of the document.
4. Save **WMedS3-R-CRGHMedRecs.docx**.

Review 2 Copying and Pasting Text

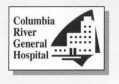

1. With **WMedS3-R-CRGHMedRecs.docx** open, open **CRGHRecMaint.docx**.
2. Display the Clipboard task pane and make sure it is empty.
3. At **CRGHRecMaint.docx**, select and then copy text from the beginning of the heading *Storage and Security* to the blank line just above the heading *Creating a Patient Profile*.
4. Select and then copy text from the beginning of the heading *Creating a Patient Profile* to the blank line just above the heading *Creating Progress Notes*.
5. Select and then copy text from the heading *Creating Progress Notes* to the end of the document.
6. Make **WMedS3-R-CRGHMedRecs.docx** the active document.
7. Display the Clipboard task pane.
8. Move the insertion point to the end of the document and then paste the text (merge formatting) that begins with the heading *Creating Progress Notes*.
9. With the insertion point positioned at the end of the document, paste the text (merge formatting) that begins with the heading *Creating a Patient Profile*.
10. With the insertion point positioned at the end of the document, paste the text (merge formatting) that begins with the heading *Storage and Security*.
11. Clear the contents of the Clipboard task pane and then close the task pane.
12. Save **WMedS3-R-CRGHMedRecs.docx**.
13. Make **CRGHRecMaint.docx** the active document and then close it.

Review 3 Inserting Page Numbers; Changing Margins; Changing Page Orientation

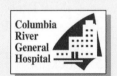

1. With **WMedS3-R-CRGHMedRecs.docx** open, insert page numbers that print at the bottom of each page using the *Plain Number 2* option.
2. Change the page orientation to landscape.
3. Change the top and bottom margins to 1.5 inches.
4. Save and then print **WMedS3-R-CRGHMedRecs.docx**.

Review 4 Inserting a Footer; Applying a Theme

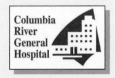

1. With **WMedS3-R-CRGHMedRecs.docx** open, change the page orientation to portrait and then change the left and right margins to 1 inch.
2. Remove the page numbering. ***Hint: Do this with the* Remove Page Numbers *option at the Page Number button drop-down list.***
3. Insert the Ion (Dark) footer. When the footer is inserted in the document, click the placeholder text *[DOCUMENT TITLE]* and then type **Creating and Maintaining Medical Records**. Type your first and last names in the *[AUTHOR NAME]* placeholder. ***Hint: Double-click in the document to make it active.***
4. Apply the Heading 1 style to the title *COLUMBIA RIVER GENERAL HOSPITAL* and apply the Heading 2 style to the following headings: *Legal Department, Creating and Maintaining Medical Records, Creating Medical Records, Modifying Medical Records, Creating Progress Notes, Creating a Patient Profile,* and *Storage and Security*.
5. Apply the Lines (Simple) style set to the document.
6. Apply the Organic theme to the document.

7. Change the theme colors to *Blue*.
8. Save **WMedS3-R-CRGHMedRecs.docx**.

Review 5 Inserting WordArt; Drawing a Shape and a Text Box

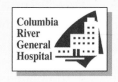

1. With **WMedS3-R-CRGHMedRecs.docx** open, move the insertion point to the beginning of the document, press Enter twice, move the insertion point back to the beginning of the document, and then click the Clear All Formatting button in the Font group.
2. Insert the WordArt shown in Figure W3.5. *Hint: Click the* **Fill - White, Outline - Accent 1, Glow - Accent 1** *option.*
3. With the WordArt selected, type **0.6** in the *Shape Height* measurement box, type **6** in the *Shape Width* measurement box, and then press Enter. Apply the Square text effect. (Find this effect by clicking the Text Effects button on the DRAWING TOOLS FORMAT tab and then pointing to *Transform*.) Move the WordArt so it is positioned as shown in Figure W3.5.
4. Change the paragraph alignment to center for the headings *COLUMBIA RIVER GENERAL HOSPITAL* and *Legal Department*.
5. Move the insertion point to the end of the document and then draw a Bevel shape as shown in Figure W3.6. Change the height of the shape to 1.5 inches, the width to 4 inches, and apply the Subtle Effect - Blue, Accent 1 shape style (second column, fourth row).
6. Draw a text box inside the shape, remove the shape fill and outline from the text box, and then type the text shown in Figure W3.6. Change the font size to 12 points and then center the text within the shape. If necessary, move the shape and the text box so they are centered between the left and right margins.
7. Save **WMedS3-R-CRGHMedRecs.docx**.

FIGURE W3.5 WordArt for Review 5

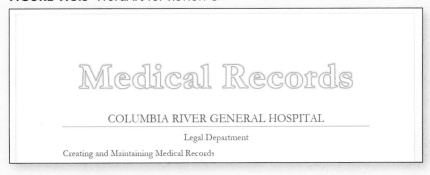

FIGURE W3.6 Shape for Review 5

Review 6 Formatting Text in Columns

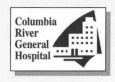

1. With **WMedS3-R-CRGHMedRecs.docx** open, move the insertion point to the blank line below the last paragraph of text (above the shape) and then insert a continuous section break.
2. Move the insertion point to the beginning of the first paragraph of text (the text that begins *At Columbia River General Hospital, physicians are*) and then insert a continuous section break.
3. Format text into two columns with a line and 0.4-inch line spacing between them.
4. Save, print, and then close **WMedS3-R-CRGHMedRecs.docx**.

Review 7 Inserting an Image

1. Open **NSMCPreCare.docx** and then save the document with the name **WMedS3-R-NSMCPreCare**.
2. Insert a clip art image of a pregnant woman as shown in Figure W3.7. (If this image is not available, choose another similar image.) Change the text wrapping for the image to *Tight*, change the height of the image to *2.5"*, and apply the Drop Shadow Rectangle picture style to the image. (This style is the fourth thumbnail from the left in the Picture Styles group on the PICTURE TOOLS FORMAT tab.) Position the clip art as shown in Figure W3.7.
3. Save, print, and then close **WMedS3-R-NSMCPreCare.docx**.

Review 8 Preparing an Envelope

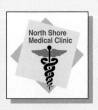

1. At a blank document, prepare an envelope with the return and delivery addresses shown in Figure W3.8 and add the envelope to the document.
2. Save the document with the name **WMedS3-R-NSMCEnv**.
3. Print and then close **WMedS3-R-NSMCEnv.docx**. (You may need to manually feed the envelope into the printer.)

Review 9 Preparing Mailing Labels

1. At a blank document, prepare a sheet of return-address mailing labels for the following name and address using the Avery US Letter 5630 Easy Peel Address Labels:

   North Shore Medical Clinic
   7450 Meridian Street
   Suite 150
   Portland, OR 97202
2. Save the mailing label document with the name **WMedS3-R-NSMCLabel**.
3. Print and then close **WMedS3-R-NSMCLabel.docx**.

FIGURE W3.7 Review 7

North Shore Medical Clinic
7450 Meridian Street, Suite 150
Portland, OR 97202
(503) 555-2330
www.emcp.net/nsmc

TAKING CARE OF YOURSELF

Prenatal Care Guidelines

- Stop smoking and avoid consistent or prolonged exposure to second-hand smoke.
- Stop all alcohol and recreational drug use.
- Limit your caffeine intake to the equivalent of one cup of coffee a day.
- Eat a healthy, well-balanced diet.
- Drink approximately eight glasses of water daily.
- Participate in moderate exercise regularly.
- Sleep seven to eight hours a night.
- Take your prenatal vitamins daily.
- Avoid taking any over-the-counter or prescribed medication unless your physician knows you are taking them.
- Avoid contact with noxious chemicals such as household cleaners, paint, varnish, and hair dye.
- Avoid changing kitty litter and wear gloves when gardening to decrease exposure to infections that may be present in cat litter and soil.
- All meat, poultry, fish, and seafood should be well cooked.
- Limit your intake of fish purchased in stores and restaurants to six to twelve ounces per week.

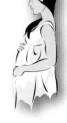

FIGURE W3.8 Review 8

North Shore Medical Clinic
7450 Meridian Street
Suite 150
Portland, OR 97202

Jennifer Cruz
Women's Health Center
142 Southeast Powell Boulevard
Portland, OR 97334

Skills Assessment

Assessment 1 Formatting a Document on Fibromyalgia

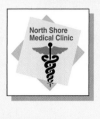

1. Open **Fibromyalgia.docx** and then save the document with the name **WMedS3-A1-FM**.
2. Open **FM.docx** and then copy individually the three sections (*Triggers and Metabolism*, *Symptoms*, and *Diagnosing Fm*), including the blank line below each section, to the Clipboard task pane.
3. Make **WMedS3-A1-FM.docx** the active document and then paste the sections from **FM.docx** into **WMedS3-A1-FM.docx**, merging the formatting so the sections are in the following order: *What Is Fibromyalgia?*, *Symptoms*, *Diagnosing Fm*, *Causes of Fm*, *Triggers and Metabolism*, and *Treatment*.
4. Make **FM.docx** the active document and then close it.
5. With **WMedS3-A1-FM.docx** the active document, search for all occurrences of *fm* and replace them with *fibromyalgia*. (Make sure the *Match case* check box at the expanded Find and Replace dialog box does not contain a check mark.)
6. Select the heading *What Is Fibromyalgia?*, click the Bold button, and then change the spacing after paragraphs to 6 points.
7. Use Format Painter to apply bold formatting and 6 points of space after paragraphs to the remaining headings: *Symptoms*, *Diagnosing Fibromyalgia*, *Causes of Fibromyalgia*, *Triggers and Metabolism*, and *Treatment*.
8. Search for all occurrences of 11-point Candara bold formatting and replace them with 12-point Corbel bold formatting.
9. Change the left and right margins to 1.5 inches.
10. Delete the title *FACTS ABOUT FIBROMYALGIA* and then create the title *Facts about Fibromyalgia* as WordArt with the following specifications: use the *Fill - White, Outline - Accent 2, Hard Shadow - Accent 2* option, change the text wrapping to *Top and Bottom*, change the width to 5.7 inches, apply the Wave 1 transform effect, and center the WordArt between the left and right margins.
11. Insert the Integral footer and then type your first and last names in the *Author* placeholder.
12. Move the insertion point to the end of the document and then insert a continuous section break.
13. Move the insertion point to the beginning of the heading *What Is Fibromyalgia?* and then insert a continuous section break.
14. Format the text into two columns with a line and 0.3-inch spacing between them.
15. Save, print, and then close **WMedS3-A1-FM.docx**.

Assessment 2 Creating an Announcement

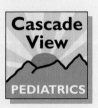

1. Open **CVPLtrhd.docx** and then save the document with the name **WMedS3-A2-CVPEOTM**.
2. Draw a shape of your choosing in the middle of the document and then insert the following information inside a text box in the shape (you determine the font and font size of the text):

Congratulations!
Lindsay Levy
Employee of the Month

3. Remove the shape fill and outline from the text box and then add a fill to the shape. The shape fill color should be complementary to the letterhead image.

4. Save, print, and then close **WMedS3-A2-CVPEOTM.docx**.

Assessment 3 Preparing a Notice

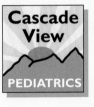

1. Open **CVPLtrhd.docx** and then save the document with the name **WMedS3-A3-CVPSupport**.
2. Use the information in Figure W3.9 to create a notice of a support group with the following specifications:
   a. Set the text in a font and font color that is complementary to the font style and color in the letterhead.
   b. To make it stand out, format the heading *Support Group for New Moms* differently than the paragraph that follows it.
   c. Set the text regarding dates, times, and location in tabbed columns. Consider using leaders to make the information more readable.
   d. Insert a clip art image related to mothers and babies.
3. Save, print, and then close **WMedS3-A3-CVPSupport.docx**.

FIGURE W3.9 Assessment 3

Support Group for New Moms

You and your baby are invited to meet other new moms and learn about parenting your newborn. Discussion topics include infant feeding, sleep patterns, newborn personalities, and child development. Support activities and educational sessions are coordinated by Deanna Reynolds, Child Development Specialist at Cascade View Pediatrics. The support group for new moms will provide you with opportunities to meet other new moms while sharing the joys, frustrations, successes, and challenges of motherhood. Join us weekly until your baby is six months old.

       When: Monday evenings
       Time: 7:00 p.m. to 8:30 p.m.
       Location: Cascade View Pediatrics
       Room: Conference Room 3B
       Cost: $25 per month

Assessment 4 Preparing Mailing Labels

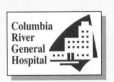

1. Prepare return-address mailing labels with the following information:
   Columbia River General Hospital
   Education Department
   4550 Fremont Street
   Portland, OR 97045
2. Save the labels document with the name **WMedS3-A4-CRGHLabel**.
3. Print and then close **WMedS3-A4-CRGHLabel.docx**.

Assessment 5 Finding Information on Flipping and Copying Objects

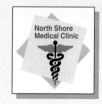

1. Use Word's Help feature to learn how to flip and copy objects.
2. At a blank document, re-create the content of Figure W3.10. Create the arrow at the left by clicking the Shapes button and then clicking the *Striped Right Arrow* option in the *Block Arrows* section. Format the arrow with dark red fill as shown. Copy and flip the arrow to create the arrow at the right side. Create the text in a text box.
3. Save the completed document with the name **WMedS3-A5-NSMCClose**.
4. Print and then close **WMedS3-A5-NSMCClose.docx**.

FIGURE W3.10 Assessment 5

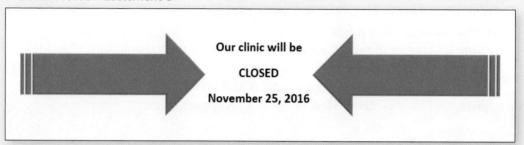

Assessment 6 Locating Information and Creating a Banner

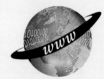

1. Using the Internet, search for a hospital near you. When you find the website for the hospital, locate the hospital address and telephone number.
2. Create a banner using a shape and insert the hospital name, address, and telephone number inside the banner.
3. Save the banner document with the name **WMedS3-A6-Banner**.
4. Print and then close **WMedS3-A6-Banner.docx**.

Assessment 7 Locating Information on Chickenpox

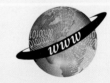

1. Using the Internet, search for information on chickenpox. Find information on the symptoms, treatment, incubation period, and infectious period of chickenpox.
2. Using the information you find, create a document that contains information on the four areas listed above: symptoms, treatment, incubation period, and infectious period.
3. Add any enhancements you feel will improve the visual appeal of the document. You might include a clip art image, WordArt, or a shape.
4. Save the document with the name **WMedS3-A7-Chickenpox**.
5. Print and then close **WMedS3-A7-Chickenpox.docx**.

Marquee Challenge

Challenge 1 Preparing a Class Announcement Document

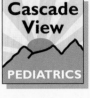

1. Open **CVPLtrhd.docx** and then save the document with the name **WMedS3-C1-CVPBabyCare**.
2. Create the class announcement shown in Figure W3.11 on page 174. Set the text in 12-point Constantia and the title in 18-point Constantia. *Hint: Search for images matching the words* **baby** *and* **parents** *to find the clip art image shown in Figure W3.11. If this image is not available, choose another image related to babies and parents.*
3. Save, print, and then close **WMedS3-C1-CVPBabyCare.docx**.

Challenge 2 Preparing a Fact Sheet on Fifth Disease

1. Open **FifthDisease.docx** and then save the document with the name **WMedS3-C2-CVPFifth**.
2. Format the document so it appears as shown in Figure W3.12 on page 175. Insert the page border, the WordArt (Fill - White, Outline - Accent 1, Glow - Accent 1 with the Gold, Accent 4, Lighter 80% text fill applied), and clip art image as shown. (To insert the clip art, search for images related to *wash hands*. If this image is not available, choose a similar clip art image.)
3. Save, print, and then close **WMedS3-C2-CVPFifth.docx**.

Challenge 3 Preparing a Cascade View Pediatrics Newsletter

1. Open **CVPNewsltr.docx** and then save the document with the name **WMedS3-C3-CVPNewsltr**.
2. Format the document so it appears as shown in Figure W3.13 on page 176. Choose similar images if the pediatrician clip art images are not available. The page border can be found in the *Art* drop-down list (about two-thirds of the way down the list) at the Borders and Shading dialog box with the Page Border tab selected. Change the page border color to an aqua color. *Hint: You will need to display the Colors dialog box with the Standard tab selected to locate an aqua color.*
3. Save, print, and then close **WMedS3-C3-CVPNewsltr.docx**.

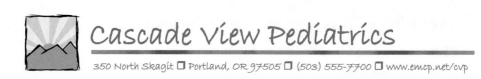

Cascade View Pediatrics

350 North Skagit ☐ Portland, OR 97505 ☐ (503) 555-7700 ☐ www.emcp.net/cvp

BABY CARE CLASS

Deanna Reynolds, Child Development Specialist for Cascade View Pediatrics, is offering a one-day class on basic baby care. This five-hour class offers basic survival techniques to care for your newborn. During this informative class, you will learn about newborn characteristics, infant milestones, bathing and hygiene, diapering, crying and comforting, sleeping, and recognizing signs of illness in your newborn. This class is ideal for first-time parents.

Date ....Saturday, April 9

Time ....9:00 a.m. to 2:00 p.m.

Location ....Cascade View Pediatrics

Room....................................... Conference Room 2

Cost $70

**For more information, contact
Deanna Reynolds at (503) 555-7705**

Fifth Disease

Fifth disease (also called *erythema infectiosum*) is an infection common in children between the ages of 5 and 15. It produces a red rash on the face that spreads to the trunk, arms, and legs. Fifth disease is actually a viral illness caused by a virus called parvovirus B19. Most children recover from Fifth disease in a short time with no complications.

Symptoms

Fifth disease begins with a low-grade fever, headache, body aches, and mild cold-like symptoms such as a stuffy or runny nose. These symptoms pass and the illness seems to be gone but in 7 to 10 days a red rash on the cheeks appears, making the face look like it has been slapped. (This is why the disease is also called *slapped cheek syndrome.*) The rash spreads to other parts of the body and red blotches expand down the trunk, arms, and legs. The rash may last from one to three weeks and may recur over weeks to months.

Contagiousness

A person with Fifth disease is most contagious before the rash appears and probably no longer contagious after the rash begins. Fifth disease spreads easily from person to person in fluids from the nose, mouth, and throat of someone with the infection and especially through large droplets from coughs and sneezes. It can also spread through sharing a drinking glass and from mother to fetus. Once someone is infected with the virus, they develop immunity to it and more than likely will not become infected again.

Treatment

Since a virus causes Fifth disease, it cannot be treated with antibiotics. Antiviral medicines do exist but none that will treat Fifth disease. No specific medication or vaccine is available and treatment is limited to relieving the symptoms.

Complications

Most children with Fifth disease recover without any complications and usually feel well by the time the rash appears. The infection, however, is more serious for children with HIV or blood disorders such as sickle cell anemia or hemolytic anemia. The virus can temporarily slow down or stop the body's production of the oxygen-carrying red blood cells, causing anemia.

Prevention

To help prevent your child from being infected with the virus, encourage your child to use good hygiene including frequent hand washing, disposing of tissues, and not sharing eating utensils with a sick person.

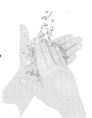

Cascade View Pediatrics

January 2016 Newsletter

Pediatrician Joins CVP

We are pleased to announce that Dr. Joseph Yarborough, Pediatric Specialist, has joined our clinic. With the addition of Dr. Yarborough to our staff, we are able to accommodate additional pediatric appointments. He will be taking appointments Monday through Friday from 8:00 a.m. to 4:00 p.m. Tuesdays and Thursdays have been reserved for well-child checkup appointments. Evening hours for well-child checkup appointments with Dr. Yarborough will be available next month.

Bring Your Insurance Card

At CVP, we deal with over 25 different insurance plans! No insurance plan is the same as the other and each has different co-pays, allowables, and deductibles. We do our best to assist you with insurance questions but you are responsible for knowing what your insurance covers. To help us with insurance issues, please bring your insurance card with you every time you visit the clinic. This may seem inconvenient but when we do not check insurance coverage with every visit, our billing accuracy declines by 10 percent.

Benefits of Lycopene

Lycopene is an antioxidant that is abundant in red tomatoes and processed tomato products. Antioxidants like lycopene neutralize free radicals, which can damage cells in the body. Research has shown that lycopene may help prevent macular degeneration (a common cause of blindness in the elderly), prostate cancer and some other forms of cancer, and heart disease.* To consume the recommended amount of at least 5 to 10 mg of lycopene per day, consider eating the following foods:

- Spaghetti sauce, ½ cup, approximately 28.1 mg of lycopene
- Tomato juice, 1 cup, approximately 25.0 mg of lycopene
- Tomato paste, 2 tablespoons, approximately 13.8 mg of lycopene
- Tomato soup, 1 cup, approximately 9.7 mg of lycopene

Other foods to consider that contain lycopene include watermelon, pink grapefruit, chili sauce, seafood sauce, and ketchup.

*Discuss medical conditions or problems with your doctor. Good nutrition is not a substitute for medical treatment and a doctor's care.

Well-Child Appointments

When you bring your child for a well-child checkup appointment, the doctor will be checking your child's progress and growth. During the visit, your doctor will weigh your child, measure his or her length and head circumference, and plot the information on your child's own growth chart. The doctor will perform a physical examination, paying special attention to any previous problems. You will be able to ask your doctor questions about how you are doing with your child and to seek advice on what to expect during the coming months. Your child will receive immunizations during some visits.

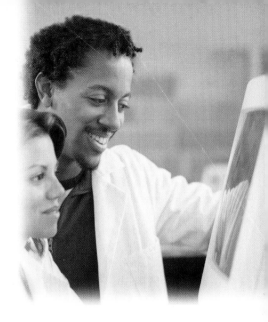

Word SECTION 4
Formatting with Special Features

Skills

- Create, edit, and modify merged documents
- Sort and filter records in a data source
- Merge envelopes
- Create, format, and modify a table
- Create a form for handwritten entries
- Create a form and save it as a template
- Fill in and print a form document
- Edit a form template
- Create and fill in a form with a drop-down list field

Student Resources

Before beginning the activities in Word Section 4, copy to your storage medium the WordMedS4 folder from the Student Resources CD. This folder contains the data files you need to complete the projects in this Word section.

Projects Overview

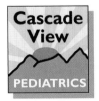

Prepare a main document reminding parents to schedule a well-child checkup appointment and create a data source using the Mail Merge feature; edit the main document and input text during a merge; and create and format a calendar.

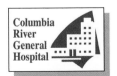

Prepare a main document advising clients of upcoming parent education classes and create a data source using the Mail Merge feature; merge envelopes; and prepare a template document for gathering information on secondary payer information.

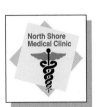

Sort and filter data source records by ZIP code and by last name; filter records in a data source and then print a letter for patients living in Lake Oswego; prepare and print merged envelopes; insert a table in a fact sheet on caffeine and then format the table; create a patient post-operative call sheet using tables; prepare a template document for updating patient information; prepare a main document advising patients of childbirth education classes and create a data source using the Mail Merge feature; create and format a medical questionnaire; create and format a table containing information on airfare from Portland to Chicago; create a treadmill test form; and prepare a pre-op questions document.

Activity 4.1

Merging Documents

If you need to mail the same basic yet personalized letter to a number of clients or customers, consider using the Mail Merge feature to make the job easier. Click the MAILINGS tab to display buttons for preparing a mail merge document. Generally, performing a mail merge requires two documents—the **data source document** and the **main document**. The data source document contains the variable information about each client or customer that will be inserted into the main document to personalize it. Before creating a data source document, determine what type of correspondence you will be creating and the type of information you will need to include. Variable information in a data source document is saved as a *record*. A record contains all of the information for one unit (for example, a person, family, customer, client, or business). A series of fields compose a record, and a series of records compose a data source document. Use buttons on the MAILINGS tab to create main documents and data source documents for merging.

Project

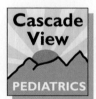

Your supervisor, Sydney Larsen, has asked you to create both a main document reminding parents to schedule a well-child checkup appointment and a data source document containing parent and patient information.

1 At a blank document, click the MAILINGS tab, click the Select Recipients button in the Start Mail Merge group, and then click *Type a New List* at the drop-down list.

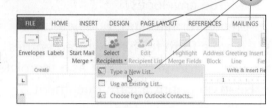

Step 1

> This displays the New Address List dialog box with predesigned fields. You can use these predesigned fields and/or create your own custom fields.

2 Delete the fields you do not need. Begin by clicking the Customize Columns button located toward the bottom of the dialog box.

> The predesigned fields cover most of the information you need for your data source document, but you decide to delete seven fields you do not need and add one of your own custom fields.

3 At the Customize Address List dialog box, click *First Name* in the *Field Names* list box and then click the Delete button.

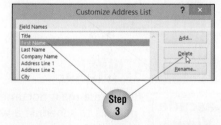

Step 3

4 At the message asking if you are sure you want to delete the field, click Yes.

5 Complete steps similar to those in Steps 3 and 4 to delete the following fields from the *Field Names* list box: *Company Name, Address Line 2, Country or Region, Home Phone, Work Phone,* and *E-mail Address.*

6 Click the Add button.

> If the New Address List dialog box does not contain fields for all the variable information you need to include, create your own custom field.

Step 7

7 At the Add Field dialog box, type **Child** and then click OK.

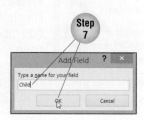

8 Click OK to close the Customize Address List dialog box.

9 At the New Address List dialog box with the insertion point positioned in the *Title* field, type **Mr. and Mrs.** and then press the Tab key.

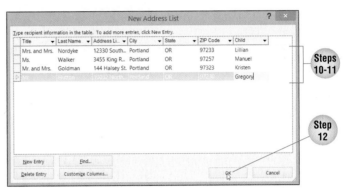

Step 9

> Pressing the Tab key moves the insertion point to the *Last Name* field. Press the Tab key to move the insertion point to the next field and press Shift + Tab to move the insertion point to the previous field.

10 Type **Nordyke** and then press the Tab key. Type **12330 South 32nd** and then press the Tab key. Type **Portland** and then press the Tab key. Type **OR** and then press the Tab key. Type **97233** and then press the Tab key. Type **Lillian** and then press the Tab key.

11 With the insertion point positioned in the *Title* column, complete steps similar to those in Steps 9 and 10 to enter the information for the three other patients shown in Figure W4.1.

Steps 10-11

Step 12

12 After entering all of the patient information in Figure W4.1, click OK to close the New Address List dialog box.

> After typing **Gregory** for the Mr. Hutton record, do not press the Tab key. If you do, a new blank client record will be created. If you accidentally create a new blank record, click the Delete Entry button at the New Address List dialog box and then click the Yes button.

13 At the Save Address List dialog box, navigate to your WordMedS4 folder. Click in the *File name* text box, type **CVPPatients**, and then press Enter.

FIGURE W4.1 Patient Information

Title	Mr. and Mrs.	*Title*	Ms.
Last Name	Nordyke	*Last Name*	Walker
Address Line 1	12330 South 32nd	*Address Line 1*	3455 King Road
City	Portland	*City*	Portland
State	OR	*State*	OR
ZIP Code	97233	*ZIP Code*	97257
Child	Lillian	*Child*	Manuel
Title	Mr. and Mrs.	*Title*	Mr.
Last Name	Goldman	*Last Name*	Hutton
Address Line 1	144 Halsey St.	*Address Line 1*	10032 North 23rd
City	Portland	*City*	Portland
State	OR	*State*	OR
ZIP Code	97323	*ZIP Code*	97230
Child	Kristen	*Child*	Gregory

continues

Activity 4

14 At the blank document, click the HOME tab and then click the *No Spacing* style in the Styles group. Press the Enter key six times, type **February 8, 2016** as shown in Figure W4.2, and then press the Enter key four times.

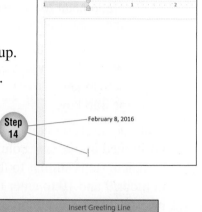

Step 15

15 Insert the address block field by clicking the MAILINGS tab and then clicking the Address Block button in the Write & Insert Fields group.

16 At the Insert Address Block dialog box, click OK.

> This inserts the field code that will eventually be replaced by the client name and address.

Step 14

February 8, 2016

17 Press the Enter key twice and then click the Greeting Line button in the Write & Insert Fields group.

18 At the Insert Greeting Line dialog box, click the down-pointing arrow at the right of the option box containing the comma (appears to the right of the option box containing *Mr. Randall*) and then click the colon at the drop-down list.

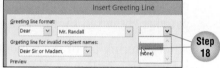

Step 18

19 Click OK to close the dialog box.

20 Press the Enter key twice and then begin to type the letter shown in Figure W4.2. Stop when you get to the location of the *Child* field. Insert the field by clicking the Insert Merge Field button arrow and then clicking *Child* at the drop-down list.

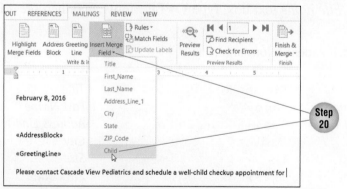

Step 20

21 Type the remainder of the letter as shown in Figure W4.2. *Note: Type your initials in place of the* **xx** *located toward the end of the letter.*

Step 22

22 When you are finished typing the letter, merge the letter with the records in the data source. Begin by clicking the Finish & Merge button in the Finish group on the MAILINGS tab and then clicking *Edit Individual Documents* at the drop-down list.

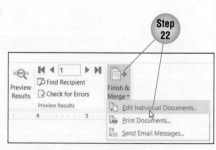

FIGURE W4.2 Main Document

February 8, 2016

«AddressBlock»

«GreetingLine»

Please contact Cascade View Pediatrics and schedule a well-child checkup appointment for «Child». At Cascade View Pediatrics, we recommend that children are seen by a pediatrician at the ages of 2 weeks and 2, 4, 6, 12, 18, and 24 months. Your child may require immunizations so plan at least 60 minutes for the appointment.

Your child's well-child appointment consists of a routine physical examination; vision, hearing, and speech screening; testing for anemia and lead poisoning; and immunizations. Additional services may include development testing, nutrition and social assessment, and guidance and parenting education.

To schedule a well-child appointment, please call our clinic at (503) 555-7700 or stop by our clinic at 350 North Skagit.

Sincerely,

Sydney Larsen
Office Manager

xx
WMedS4-Well-ChildMainDoc.docx

23. At the Merge to New Document dialog box, make sure *All* is selected and then click OK.

    The letters are merged with the records and displayed in a new document.

24. Save the merged letters in the normal manner with the name **WMedS4-Well-ChildApptLtrs**.

25. Print and then close **WMedS4-Well-ChildApptLtrs.docx**.

    Four letters will print.

26. Save the main document in the normal manner with the name **WMedS4-Well-ChildMainDoc**.

27. Close **WMedS4-Well-ChildMainDoc.docx**.

In Addition

Using the Mail Merge Wizard

The Mail Merge feature includes a Mail Merge wizard to guide you through the merge process. To access the wizard, click the MAILINGS tab, click the Start Mail Merge button in the Start Mail Merge group, and then click the *Step-by-Step Mail Merge Wizard* option at the drop-down list. The first of six Mail Merge task panes displays at the right of the screen. Once you complete the tasks at one task pane, the next task pane displays. The options in each task pane may vary depending on the type of merge you are performing.

Activity 4.2

Editing Merged Documents; Inputting Text during a Merge

When you complete a mail merge, you create a data source document and a main document. The data source document is associated with the main document. If you need to edit the main document, open it in the normal manner and make the required changes. To make changes to the data source document, click the Edit Recipient List button in the Start Mail Merge group on the MAILINGS tab. Changes you make to the data source document are saved automatically. To save edits made to the main document, you must do so manually. In some situations, you may not want to store all variable information in the data source file. If you want to input certain variable information directly into the main document during a merge, insert a fill-in field at the appropriate location in the main document.

Project

Sydney Larsen has asked you to customize the well-child checkup appointments letters to include an area to identify the specific type of appointment.

1. Open **WMedS4-Well-ChildMainDoc.docx**. If a message displays telling you that opening the document will run an SQL command, click Yes.

2. Click the MAILINGS tab.

3. Edit the first paragraph so it displays as shown in Figure W4.3. To insert the *Child* field, click the Insert Merge Field button arrow in the Write & Insert Fields group and then click *Child* at the drop-down list. Do not type the text *(Checkup)*. You will insert this as a fill-in field in the next step.

4. To insert a fill-in field for *(Checkup)*, click the Rules button [?] in the Write & Insert Fields group and then click *Fill-in* at the drop-down list.

   > Insert a fill-in field in those locations in a main document where you want to enter specific information during a merge.

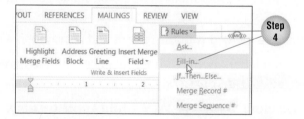

5. At the Insert Word Field: Fill-in dialog box, type **Insert specific well-child checkup appointment** in the *Prompt* text box and then click OK.

   > The text you type in the *Prompt* text box will display during a merge to indicate what information the user should type.

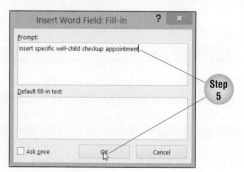

FIGURE W4.3 Edited Paragraph

According to our records, «Child» is due for (Checkup). Please contact Cascade View Pediatrics and schedule the well-child checkup appointment. Your child may require immunizations so plan at least 60 minutes for the appointment.

6 At the Microsoft Word dialog box with *Insert specific well-child checkup appointment* displayed in the upper left corner, type **(Checkup)** and then click OK. Type or edit the remainder of the paragraph so it displays as shown in Figure W4.3.

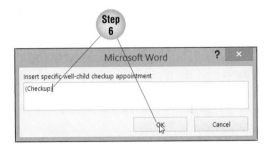

7 You need to edit some of the records in the data source. To begin, click the Edit Recipient List button in the Start Mail Merge group.

8 At the Mail Merge Recipients dialog box, click the file name ***CVPPatients.mdb*** in the *Data Source* list box and then click the Edit button below the list box.

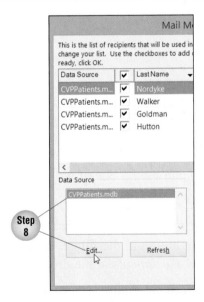

9 At the Edit Data Source dialog box, click any character in the address *3455 King Road* (in the record for Ms. Walker) and then type **6795 32nd Street**.

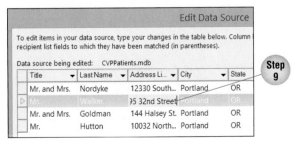

continues

10 Click any character in the ZIP code *97257* in the same record and then type **97239**.

11 Click the New Entry button and then type the following in the specified fields:

Title	**Mrs.**
Last Name	**Milovich**
Address Line 1	**19443 144th Place**
City	**Portland**
State	**OR**
ZIP Code	**97340**
Child	**Paulina**

12 Delete the record for Mr. Hutton by clicking in the gray square at the left of the record for Mr. Hutton and then clicking the Delete Entry button.

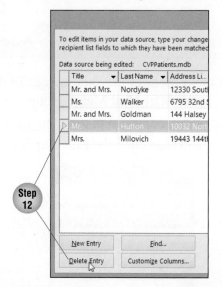

Step 12

13 At the message asking if you want to delete the entry, click Yes.

14 At the Edit Data Source dialog box, click OK. At the message asking if you want to update your recipient list, click Yes.

15 Click OK to close the Mail Merge Recipients dialog box.

16 Click the Finish & Merge button in the Finish group on the MAILINGS tab and then click *Edit Individual Documents* at the drop-down list.

17 At the Merge to New Document dialog box, make sure *All* is selected and then click OK.

18 When Word merges the main document with the first record, the text *(Checkup)* is selected in the document and a dialog box displays with the message *Insert specific well-child checkup appointment.* At this dialog box, type **her two-week checkup** and then click OK.

In Brief
Edit Data Source
1. Open main document.
2. Click MAILINGS tab.
3. Click Edit Recipient List button.
4. Click data source file name in *Data Source* list box.
5. Click Edit button.
6. At Edit Data Source dialog box, make necessary changes.
7. Click OK.
8. Click Yes at message.
9. Click OK.

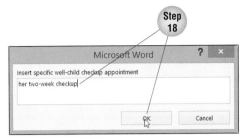

Step 18

19 At the next dialog box, type **his 18-month checkup** (over *her two-week checkup*) and then click OK.

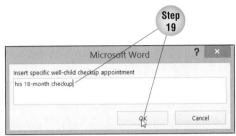

Step 19

20 At the next dialog box, type **her 12-month checkup** and then click OK.

21 At the next dialog box, type **her four-month checkup** and then click OK.

22 Save the merged letters in the normal manner in the WordMedS4 folder on your storage medium and name the document **WMedS4-Well-ChildEditedLtrs**.

23 Print and then close **WMedS4-Well-ChildEditedLtrs.docx**.

> This document will print four letters.

24 Save and then close **WMedS4-Well-ChildMainDoc.docx**.

In Addition

Editing a Data Source Using the Mail Merge Wizard

In addition to editing a data source by opening the main document and then clicking the Edit Recipient List button, you can edit a data source by using the Mail Merge wizard. To do so, open a main document, click the MAILINGS tab, click the Start Mail Merge button, and then click the *Step-by-Step Mail Merge Wizard* option. This series of actions causes the Mail Merge wizard to open at the third step. At this step, click the <u>Edit recipient list</u> hyperlink. At the Mail Merge Recipients dialog box, click the data source file name in the *Data Source* list box, click the Edit button, and then make the necessary edits to the fields in the records at the Edit Data Source dialog box.

Activity 4.3

Sorting Records in a Data Source

To organize records in a data source, you can sort them in ascending or descending order. To do this, click the MAILINGS tab, click the Select Recipients button, and then click *Use an Existing List*. At the Select Data Source dialog box, navigate to the folder that contains the data source file you want to use and then double-click the file. Click the Edit Recipient List button in the Start Mail Merge group on the MAILINGS tab and the Mail Merge Recipients dialog box displays. Click a column heading to sort data in ascending order by that field. To perform additional sorts, click the down-pointing arrow at the right of a field column heading and then click the desired sort order. You can refine a sort with options at the Filter and Sort dialog box.

Project

Lee Elliott has asked you to sort data source records by last name, city, and ZIP code.

North Shore Medical Clinic

1. Open **NSMCMainDoc.docx**. If a message displays telling you that opening the document will run an SQL command, click Yes.

   If a message displays telling you that Word cannot find the data source, proceed to Step 2.

2. Click the MAILINGS tab, click the Select Recipients button in the Start Mail Merge group, and then click *Use an Existing List* at the drop-down list. At the Select Data Source dialog box, navigate to the WordMedS4 folder on your storage medium and then double-click **NSMCPatientsDS.mdb**.

3. Sort records alphabetically in the data source attached to this main document. To begin, click the Edit Recipient List button in the Start Mail Merge group on the MAILINGS tab.

4. At the Mail Merge Recipients dialog box, click the *Last Name* column heading.

   This sorts the last names in ascending alphabetical order.

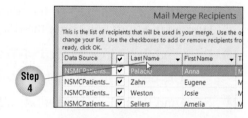

Step 4

5. Scroll to the right to display the *City* field, click the down-pointing arrow at the right of the *City* column heading, and then click *Sort Descending* at the drop-down list.

   This sorts the city names in descending alphabetical order.

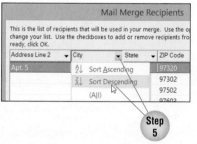

Step 5

6. Sort by ZIP code and then by last name. To begin, click the Sort hyperlink located in the *Refine recipient list* section.

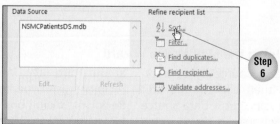

Step 6

(7) At the Filter and Sort dialog box with the Sort Records tab selected, click the down-pointing arrow at the right of the *Sort by* option box and then click *ZIP Code* at the drop-down list.

> You will need to scroll down the list to display *ZIP Code*.

(8) Make sure *Last Name* displays in the *Then by* option box.

(9) Click OK to close the Filter and Sort dialog box.

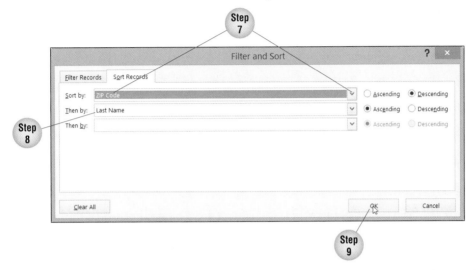

(10) Click OK to close the Mail Merge Recipients dialog box.

(11) Preview each letter by clicking the Preview Results button in the Preview Results group on the MAILINGS tab and then clicking the Next Record button in the Preview Results group. Keep clicking the Next Record button until the last letter (the tenth letter) displays.

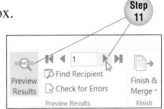

(12) Click the Finish & Merge button in the Finish group on the MAILINGS tab and then click *Edit Individual Documents* at the drop-down list.

(13) At the Merge to New Document dialog box, click OK.

(14) Save the merged letters document with the name **WMedS4-NSMCApptLtrs**.

(15) Print only the first page of **WMedS4-NSMCApptLtrs.docx**.

(16) Close **WMedS4-NSMCApptLtrs.docx**.

(17) Close **NSMCMainDoc.docx** without saving the changes.

In Addition

Clearing Sort Data

If you sort data in a data source file by clicking a column heading, the sort information will display when you open the Filter and Sort dialog box. Also, if you identify fields for sorting at the Filter and Sort dialog box, that information will display the next time you open the dialog box. To complete a new sort at the Filter and Sort dialog box, first click the Clear All button that displays in the lower left corner of the dialog box to remove any existing sort information.

In Brief
Complete Sort
1. Open main document.
2. Click MAILINGS tab.
3. Click Edit Recipient List button.
4. Click desired column heading.

OR

1. Open main document.
2. Click MAILINGS tab.
3. Click Edit Recipient List button.
4. Click *Sort* hyperlink.
5. Specify fields for sorting.
6. Click OK.

Filtering Records

Once you have created a main document and a data source document to produce personalized form letters, situations may arise in which you want to merge the main document with only certain records in the data source. For example, you may want to send a letter to patients living in a particular city or patients seeing a specific doctor. Filtering allows you to identify records that meet specific criteria and include only those records in the merge. One method for filtering records is to display the Mail Merge Recipients dialog box and then insert or remove check marks next to specific records. If you only need to select a few records, start by clicking the check box at the right of the *Data Source* column heading. This removes the check marks from all of the check boxes, making it easier for you to select only those few records that you need.

Project

You need to send a letter to only those patients living in Lake Oswego. Select the appropriate records and then merge and print the patient letters.

1. Open **NSMCMainDoc.docx**. If a message displays telling you that opening the document will run an SQL command, click Yes.

   If a message displays telling you that Word cannot find the data source, proceed to Step 2.

2. Click the MAILINGS tab, click the Select Recipients button in the Start Mail Merge group, and then click *Use an Existing List* at the drop-down list. At the Select Data Source dialog box, navigate to the WordMedS4 folder on your storage medium and then double-click **NSMCPatientsDS.mdb**.

3. Click the MAILINGS tab and then click the Edit Recipient List button in the Start Mail Merge group.

4. At the Mail Merge Recipients dialog box, click the check box at the right of the *Data Source* column heading.

   This removes the check mark from the check box preceding each record.

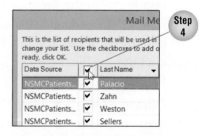

5. Select the records of those individuals coming to the clinic for dermatology reasons by clicking the check boxes preceding the names *Zahn*, *Sellers*, *Higgins*, *Koehler*, and *Coburn*.

6. Click OK to close the Mail Merge Recipients dialog box.

7. Click the Preview Results button and then click the Next Record and/or Previous Record buttons to view the merged letters.

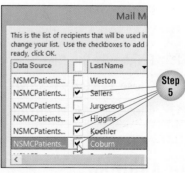

8. Select the records of those patients living in the city of Lake Oswego. Begin by clicking the Edit Recipient List button in the Start Mail Merge group.

9. At the Mail Merge Recipients dialog box, click the check box at the right of the *Data Source* column heading.

10 Click the check boxes preceding the patient names *Koehler* and *Lockard* to insert check marks.

11 Click OK to close the Mail Merge Recipients dialog box.

12 View the merged letter and then click the Previous Record button to view the other merged letter.

13 Send the merged letters directly to the printer by clicking the Finish & Merge button in the Finish group on the MAILINGS tab and then clicking *Print Documents* at the drop-down list.

14 Click OK at the Merge to Printer dialog box and then click OK at the Print dialog box.

Two letters will print.

15 Close **NSMCMainDoc.docx** without saving the changes.

In Brief
Filter Records
1. Open main document.
2. Click MAILINGS tab.
3. Click Edit Recipient List button.
4. At Mail Merge Recipients dialog box, select specific records by inserting/ removing check marks.
5. Click OK.

In Addition

Filtering Records Using the Filter and Sort Dialog Box

Using check boxes to select specific records is useful in a data source that contains a limited number of records, but it may not be practical when you are working with a larger data source. When a data source contains many different records, filter records with options at the Filter and Sort dialog box with the Filter Records tab selected, as shown below. Display this dialog box by clicking the Filter hyperlink in the *Refine recipient list* section of the Mail Merge Recipients dialog box. When you select a field from the *Field* drop-down list, Word automatically inserts *Equal to* in the *Comparison* option box, but you can make other comparisons.

Clicking the down-pointing arrow at the right of the *Comparison* option box causes a drop-down list to display with these additional options: *Not equal to, Less than, Greater than, Less than or equal, Greater than or equal, Is blank, Is not blank, Contains,* and *Does not contain.* Use one of these options to create a filter equation. For example, select all customers with a ZIP code higher than 97439 by clicking *ZIP Code* at the *Field* drop-down list, clicking *Greater than* at the *Comparison* option box, and then typing *97439* in the *Compare to* text box.

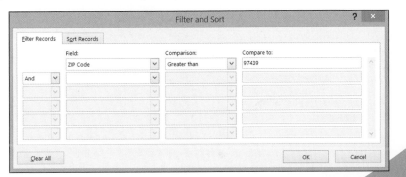

Activity 4.5

Preparing and Merging Envelopes

When you create a letter as a main document and then merge it with a data source document, you will most likely need properly addressed envelopes in which to send the letters. Create and print envelopes with options on the MAILINGS tab.

Project

Before mailing letters to clinic patients, you need to prepare and print the envelopes.

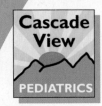

1. At a blank document, click the MAILINGS tab, click the Start Mail Merge button, and then click *Envelopes* at the drop-down list.

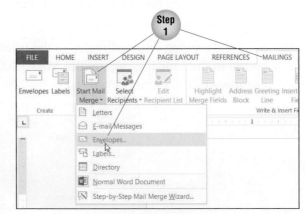

2. At the Envelope Options dialog box, make sure the envelope size is set to *10* and then click OK.

3. Click the Select Recipients button in the Start Mail Merge group and then click *Use an Existing List* at the drop-down list.

4. At the Select Data Source dialog box, navigate to the WordMedS4 folder on your storage medium.

5. Double-click **CVPPatients.mdb** in the *Select Data Source* list box.

   Notice that an Access icon displays before **CVPPatients.mdb**, indicating that it is an Access database file.

6. In the document window, click in the approximate location in the envelope where the recipient's name and address will appear.

   This causes a box with a dashed gray border to display. If you do not see this box, try clicking in a different location in the envelope.

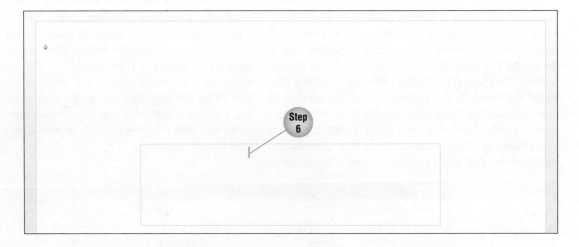

(7) Click the Address Block button in the Write & Insert Fields group.

(8) At the Insert Address Block dialog box, click OK.

This inserts the field «AddressBlock» inside the box in the envelope.

(9) Click the Finish & Merge button in the Finish group and then click *Edit Individual Documents* at the drop-down list.

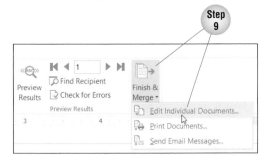

(10) At the Merge to New Document dialog box, make sure *All* is selected and then click OK.

(11) Save the merged envelopes in the normal manner in the WordMedS4 folder on your storage medium and name the document **WMedS4-CVPPatientEnvs**.

(12) Print **WMedS4-CVPPatientEnvs.docx**.

This document will print four envelopes. Check with your instructor about specific steps for printing envelopes. You may need to hand-feed envelopes into your printer.

(13) Close **WMedS4-CVPPatientEnvs.docx**.

(14) Save the envelope main document in the normal manner in the WordMedS4 folder and name it **WMedS4-CVPEnvMainDoc**.

(15) Close **WMedS4-CVPEnvMainDoc.docx**.

In Brief

Merge Envelopes
1. Click MAILINGS tab, click Start Mail Merge button, and then click *Envelopes*.
2. At Envelope Options dialog box, click OK.
3. Click Select Recipients button and then click *Use an Existing List*.
4. Navigate to folder containing data source and then double-click data source document name.
5. Click in document window at approximate location of recipient's name and address.
6. Click Address Block button.
7. At Insert Address Block dialog box, click OK.
8. Click Finish & Merge button.
9. Click *Edit Individual Documents*.
10. At Merge to New Document dialog box, click OK.

In Addition

Preparing a Directory Using the Mail Merge Feature

When merging letters, envelopes, or mailing labels, a new form is created for each record. For example, if a data source document containing eight records is merged with a letter main document, eight letters are created. If a data source document containing 20 records is merged with a mailing label main document, 20 labels are created. However, in some situations, you may want merged information to remain on the same page. This is useful, for example, when creating a directory or address list. To create a merged directory, click the Start Mail Merge button and then click *Directory* at the drop-down list. Create or identify an existing data source file and then insert the desired fields in the directory document. Set tabs if you want to insert the text in columns.

Activity 4.6

Creating and Modifying a Table

Insert a table when you want to display data in columns and rows. This data may be text, numbers, and/or formulas. You can create a table using the Table button on the INSERT tab or with options at the Insert Table dialog box. Once you specify the desired numbers of rows and columns, the table displays and you are ready to enter information in the cells. A *cell* is the "box" created by the intersection of a row and a column. Cells are designated with a letter-number label representing the column and row intersection. Columns are lettered from left to right, beginning with A, and rows are numbered from top to bottom, beginning with 1, so the first cell in every table is known as cell A1. You can modify the structure of the table by inserting or deleting columns and/or rows and by merging cells.

Project

Lee Elliott has asked you to edit a fact sheet on caffeine. You will open the fact sheet and then insert additional information about caffeine in a table for easy viewing.

1. Open **NSMCCaffeine.docx** and then save it with the name **WMedS4-NSMCCaffeine**. (If necessary, change the zoom to *100%*.)

2. Press Ctrl + End to move the insertion point to the end of the document.

3. Display the Insert Table dialog box by clicking the INSERT tab, clicking the Table button ▦ in the Tables group, and then clicking *Insert Table* at the drop-down list.

4. At the Insert Table dialog box, type **2** in the *Number of columns* measurement box, press the Tab key, type **11** in the *Number of rows* measurement box, and then click OK to close the dialog box.

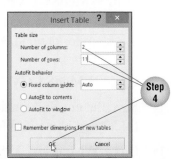

5. Type the text in the cells as shown in Figure W4.4. Press the Tab key to move the insertion point to the next cell or press Shift + Tab to move the insertion point to the previous cell. To move the insertion point to different cells within the table using the mouse, click in the desired cell. After typing the last entry in the table, *20 mg*, do not press the Tab key. This action will insert another row. If this happens, immediately click the Undo button.

6. After typing the table, you realize that you need to include a column that identifies the specific amount of the drink or food. To do this, click in the cell containing the text *Amount of Caffeine*, click the TABLE TOOLS LAYOUT tab, and then click the Insert Left button ▦ in the Rows & Columns group.

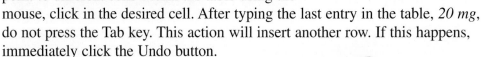
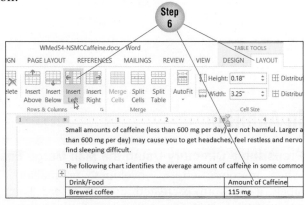

7. Click in the top cell of the new column, type **Amount of Drink/Food**, and then press the Down Arrow key. Type the amounts in the remaining cells as shown in Figure W4.5. (Press the Down Arrow key to move to the next cell down.)

FIGURE W4.4 Step 5

Drink/Food	Amount of Caffeine
Brewed coffee	115 mg
Pepsi	38 mg
Coca-Cola	34 mg
Diet Coke	45 mg
Mountain Dew	55 mg
Tea (leaf or bag)	50 mg
Iced tea	70 mg
Cocoa beverage	4 mg
Milk chocolate	6 mg
Dark chocolate	20 mg

In Brief

Insert Table
1. Click INSERT tab.
2. Click Table button.
3. Click *Insert Table*.
4. At Insert Table dialog box, type desired number of columns.
5. Press Tab key.
6. Type desired number of rows.
7. Click OK.

OR

1. Click INSERT tab.
2. Click Table button.
3. Drag in grid to select desired number of columns and rows.

8. Delete the *Cocoa beverage* row. To do this, click anywhere in the text *Cocoa beverage*, click the TABLE TOOLS LAYOUT tab, click the Delete button in the Rows & Columns group, and then click *Delete Rows* at the drop-down list.

9. Insert a row above *Drink/Food* by clicking anywhere in the text *Drink/Food* and then clicking the Insert Above button in the Rows & Columns group.

10. With the new top row selected, merge the cells by clicking the Merge Cells button in the Merge group.

FIGURE W4.5 Step 7

Amount of Drink/Food	Amount
5 ounces	115 mg
12 ounces	38 mg
12 ounces	34 mg
12 ounces	45 mg
12 ounces	55 mg
8 ounces	50 mg
12 ounces	70 mg
5 ounces	4 mg
1 ounce	6 mg
1 ounce	20 mg

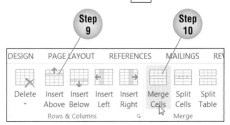

11. Type **CAFFEINE CHART** in the top row.

12. Select all cells in the table by clicking the table move handle that displays in the upper left corner of the table (square with a four-headed arrow inside).

You can also select all cells in a table by clicking the TABLE TOOLS LAYOUT tab, clicking the Select button in the Table group, and then clicking *Select Table* at the drop-down list.

Step 12

The following chart iden[...]

CAFFEINE CHART
Drink/Food
Brewed coffee
Pepsi
Coca-Cola
Diet Coke
Mountain Dew
Tea (leaf or bag)
Iced tea
Milk chocolate
Dark chocolate

13. Click the HOME tab, change the font to Cambria, change the font size to 12 points, and then click outside the table to deselect it.

14. Save **WMedS4-NSMCCaffeine.docx**.

In Addition

Other Methods for Creating a Table

You can also create a table using the Table button drop-down grid. To do so, click the INSERT tab, click the Table button, and then drag the mouse pointer down and to the right until the desired number of columns and rows are selected and the numbers above the grid display the desired numbers of columns and rows. Another method for creating a table is to draw a table by clicking the Table button and then clicking *Draw Table* at the drop-down list. The mouse pointer changes to a pencil. Drag in the document screen to create the desired number of columns and rows.

Activity 4.7

Changing the Table Layout

In the previous activity, you added a column and a row and deleted a row using buttons on the TABLE TOOLS LAYOUT tab. This tab contains additional buttons for customizing the table layout, such as changing cell size, alignment, direction, and margins; sorting data; and converting a table to text. You can also vertically and horizontally center a table on the page with options at the Table Properties dialog box. When you create a table, columns are all the same width and rows are all the same height. The width of the columns depends on how many there are, as well as the document margins. You can change column widths and row heights using a variety of methods, including dragging the table gridlines. You can apply formatting to text in cells by selecting the text or by selecting multiple cells and then applying formatting.

Project

The Caffeine Chart table needs adjustments to improve its appearance. You will increase and decrease the column widths, increase the height of a row, and apply formatting to both the entire table and specific cells within the table.

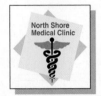

1. With **WMedS4-NSMCCaffeine.docx** open, position the mouse pointer on the gridline between the first and second columns until the pointer turns into a left-and-right-pointing arrow with a short double line in the middle. Hold down the left mouse button, drag to the left until the table column marker displays at the 1.5-inch mark on the horizontal ruler, and then release the mouse button.

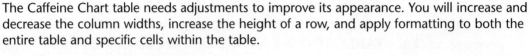

Step 1

2. Following the same procedure, drag the gridline between the second and third columns to the left until the table column marker displays at the 3.5-inch mark on the horizontal ruler.

3. Drag the gridline at the far right side of the table to the left until the table column marker displays at the 5.25-inch mark on the horizontal ruler.

4. Position the mouse pointer on the gridline between the first and second rows until the pointer turns into an up-and-down-pointing arrow with a short double line in the middle. Hold down the left mouse button, drag down approximately 0.25 inch on the vertical ruler, and then release the mouse button.

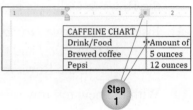

Step 4

5. Click in the top cell (contains the text *CAFFEINE CHART*), click the Select button in the Table group on the TABLE TOOLS LAYOUT tab, and then click *Select Cell* at the drop-down list.

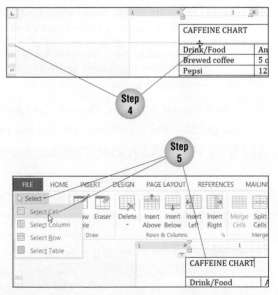

Step 5

6. Apply character formatting by clicking the HOME tab, clicking the Bold button in the Font group, clicking the Font Size button arrow, and then clicking *16* at the drop-down list.

7 With the cell still selected, horizontally and vertically center the text in the cell by clicking the TABLE TOOLS LAYOUT tab and then clicking the Align Center button in the Alignment group.

8 Increase the height of the top row by clicking the up-pointing arrow at the right side of the *Table Row Height* measurement box in the Cell Size group on the TABLE TOOLS LAYOUT tab until *0.5″* displays.

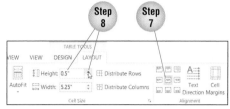

In Brief
Increase/Decrease Column/Row
1. Position mouse pointer on gridline until it turns into double-headed arrow.
2. Hold down left mouse button, drag to desired position, and then release mouse button.

9 Click in the cell containing the text *Drink/Food*.

10 Click the Select button in the Table group and then click *Select Row* at the drop-down list.

11 Apply bold formatting to the text in the row by pressing Ctrl + B and then click the Align Bottom Center button in the Alignment group on the TABLE TOOLS LAYOUT tab.

12 Position the mouse pointer in the cell containing the first occurrence of the text *5 ounces*, hold down the left mouse button, drag down and to the right to the cell containing the text *20 mg*, and then release the mouse button.

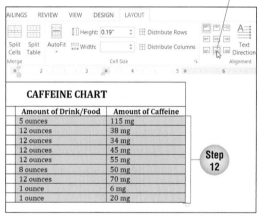

13 With the cells selected, click the Align Bottom Center button in the Alignment group.

14 Click anywhere in the table to deselect the cells.

15 Center the table between the left and right margins. To begin, click the Properties button in the Table group on the TABLE TOOLS LAYOUT tab.

16 At the Table Properties dialog box with the Table tab selected, click the *Center* option in the *Alignment* section.

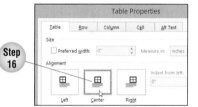

17 Click OK to close the dialog box.

18 Save **WMedS4-NSMCCaffeine.docx**.

In Addition

Selecting Cells with the Keyboard

Besides using the mouse, you can also select cells using the following keyboard shortcuts:

To select	Press
the next cell's contents	Tab
the preceding cell's contents	Shift + Tab
the entire table	Alt + 5 (on the numeric keypad with Num Lock off)
adjacent cells	Hold down the Shift key and then press an arrow key repeatedly.
a column	Position the insertion point in the top cell of a column, hold down the Shift key, and then press the Down Arrow key until the column is selected.

Activity 4.8

The TABLE TOOLS DESIGN tab contains a number of options for enhancing the appearance of the table. With options in the Table Styles group, apply predesigned color and border lines to a table. You can also apply shading to cells in a table with the Shading button in the Table Styles group. Maintain further control over the predesigned style formatting applied to columns and rows with options in the Table Style Options group. For example, if your table contains a row for totals, insert a check mark in the *Total Row* check box. With options in the Borders group, you can display a list of predesigned border lines; change the line style, width, and color; add or remove borders; and use the Border Painter button to apply the same border style formatting to other cells within the table.

Project

You will add final touches to the Caffeine Chart table by applying border, shading, and style formatting.

North Shore Medical Clinic

1. With **WMedS4-NSMCCaffeine.docx** open, click anywhere in the table and then select the entire table by clicking the table move handle that displays in the upper left corner of the table.

2. With the table selected, click the TABLE TOOLS DESIGN tab, click the Borders button arrow in the Borders group, and then click *Borders and Shading* at the drop-down list.

   This displays the Borders and Shading dialog box with the Borders tab selected.

3. At the Borders and Shading dialog box, click the *Grid* option in the *Setting* section, scroll down the *Style* list box, and then click the first thick/thin option as shown at the right.

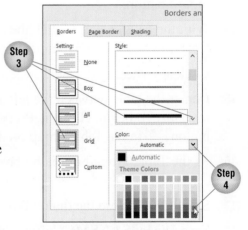

4. Click the down-pointing arrow at the right of the *Color* option box and then click the *Green, Accent 6, Darker 25%* option at the drop-down list (tenth column, fifth row in the *Theme Colors* section).

5. Click OK to close the Borders and Shading dialog box.

6. Select the second row in the table, click the Shading button arrow in the Table Styles group, and then click the *Gold, Accent 4, Lighter 80%* option at the drop-down list (eighth column, second row in the *Theme Colors* section).

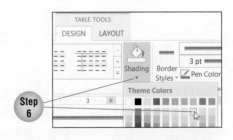

7. Save and then print **WMedS4-NSMCCaffeine.docx**.

8. Make sure the insertion point is positioned in the table and then apply a table style. Begin by clicking the More button that displays at the right of the table style thumbnails in the Table Styles group on the TABLE TOOLS DESIGN tab.

   This displays a drop-down gallery of style choices.

9 Click the *Grid Table 4 - Accent 1* option (second column, fourth row in the *Grid Tables* section).

> Notice the color and border style formatting and how applying the style changed the border and shading formatting you applied earlier.

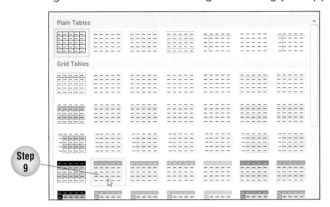

Step 9

10 Experiment with an additional style by clicking the More button at the right of the table style thumbnails in the Table Styles group and then clicking the *Grid Table 6 Colorful - Accent 5* option (sixth column, sixth row in the *Grid Tables* section).

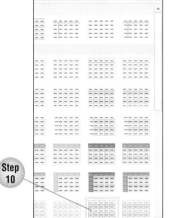

Step 10

11 Change the formatting by clicking the *Header Row* check box in the Table Style Options group to remove the check mark and then clicking the *First Column* check box to remove the check mark.

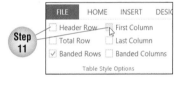

Step 11

12 Applying the table styles removed the horizontal alignment of the table. Reapply this formatting by clicking the TABLE TOOLS LAYOUT tab, clicking the Properties button, clicking the *Center* option in the *Alignment* section, and then clicking OK to close the dialog box.

13 Save, print, and then close **WMedS4-NSMCCaffeine.docx**.

In Brief

Display Borders and Shading Dialog Box
1. Click in cell, select cells, or select table.
2. Click TABLE TOOLS DESIGN tab.
3. Click Borders button arrow.
4. Click *Borders and Shading*.

Apply Table Style
1. Click in cell in table.
2. Click desired table style thumbnail in Table Styles group.

OR

1. Click in cell in table.
2. Click More button at right side of table style thumbnails.
3. Click desired table style at drop-down gallery.

In Addition

Sorting in a Table

Sort text in a table alphabetically, numerically, or by date with options at the Sort dialog box. Display this dialog box by positioning the insertion point in a cell in the table and then clicking the Sort button in the Data group on the TABLE TOOLS LAYOUT tab. Make sure the column you want to sort is selected in the *Sort by* option box and then click OK. If the first row in the table contains data, such as headings, that you do not want to include in the sort, click the *Header row* option in the *My list has* section of the Sort dialog box. If you want to sort specific cells in a table, select the cells first and then click the Sort button.

Inserting a Row Using the Mouse

You can use the mouse to insert a row by moving the mouse pointer immediately left of the row where you want the new row inserted. As you move the mouse pointer to the left side of a row, a plus symbol inside a circle displays along with thin, blue, double lines across the top or bottom of the row. Move the symbol and lines to the bottom of the row and then click the plus symbol to insert a new row below the current row. Move the symbol and lines to the top of the row and then click the plus symbol to insert a new row above the current row.

Activity 4.9

Creating a Form for Handwritten Entries

Forms are a major part of a patient's medical records. They come in a variety of types in a medical office or hospital and include those that require patients to enter handwritten information and those that require a medical office assistant or hospital worker to enter information at the computer. When creating forms for entering handwritten information, consider using tables to improve readability.

Project

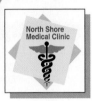

One of your job duties is to make follow-up calls to patients after they have received day surgery. You realize that creating a form will improve the clarity and completeness of the information you gather from the patients. You decide to create a table in which you can handwrite the patients' responses to your questions as you conduct your follow-up calls.

1. Open **NSMCLtrhd.docx** and then save it with the name **WMedS4-NSMCCallRecord**.

2. Click the *No Spacing* style in the Styles group on the HOME tab, change the font to 12-point Cambria, and then press the Enter key twice.

3. Create the form shown in Figure W4.6. To begin, type the title, **POST-OPERATIVE CALL RECORD**, select the text, change the paragraph alignment to center, and then apply bold formatting.

4. Press the Enter key twice and then change the paragraph alignment back to left.

5. Create a table with four rows and four columns by clicking the INSERT tab, clicking the Table button, dragging the mouse pointer down and to the right until four rows and four columns are selected in the grid and *4x4 Table* displays above it, and then releasing the left mouse button.

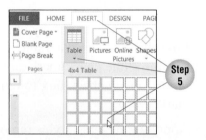

6. Type the text in the cells as shown in Figure W4.6. Bold and center the column heading text and apply Blue, Accent 1, Lighter 60% shading as shown.

7. After creating the first table, press Ctrl + End to move the insertion point below the table.

8. Press the Enter key and then type the text below the first table as shown in Figure W4.6.

9. Create the second table with four columns and six rows columns as shown in the figure.

10. Decrease or increase the size of the columns so they match what you see in the figure.

11. Type the text in the cells, bold and center the column heading text as shown in the figure, and then apply Blue, Accent 1, Lighter 60% shading as shown.

12. Press Ctrl + End to move the insertion point below the table and then press the Enter key.

13. Create the remaining two tables as shown in Figure W4.6.

14. Save, print, and then close **WMedS4-NSMCCallRecord.docx**.

FIGURE W4.6 Form for Handwritten Entries

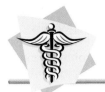

North Shore Medical Clinic
7450 Meridian Street, Suite 150
Portland, OR 97202
(503) 555-2330
www.emcp.net/nsmc

POST-OPERATIVE CALL RECORD

CALLER	DATE	TIME	ANSWERED

Person contacted: _____

General condition as relayed by person contacted: _____

EXPERIENCE	YES	NO	COMMENTS
Nausea			
Vomiting			
Dizziness			
Pain			
Elevated temperature			

COMPLIANCE	YES	NO	COMMENTS
Written instructions			
Elevated temperature			

REMINDER	YES	NO	COMMENTS
Sleep instructions			
Incision care			
Medication monitoring			
Physical restrictions			
Return appointment			

In Addition

Customizing Cell Size

When you first create a table, the column widths are equal, as are the row heights. You can customize the width of columns and the height of rows with buttons in the Cell Size group on the TABLE TOOLS LAYOUT tab. Use the *Table Row Height* measurement box to increase or decrease the height of rows and use the *Table Column Width* measurement box to increase or decrease the width of columns. The Distribute Rows button distributes equally the height of selected rows and the Distribute Columns button distributes equally the width of selected columns. You can also change column width using the move table column markers on the horizontal ruler. To do this, position the mouse pointer on a column marker until the pointer turns into a left-and-right-pointing arrow and then drag the marker to the desired position. Hold down the Shift key while dragging a column marker and the horizontal ruler remains stationary while the column marker moves. Hold down the Alt key while dragging a column marker and precise measurements display on the horizontal ruler.

Activity 4.10

Creating a Form and Saving It as a Template

Many hospitals and clinics purchase and use preprinted forms that are generally filled in by hand or using a computer. You can use Word create your own forms, eliminating the need for preprinted ones. You can insert text boxes, check boxes, and drop-down lists. Forms created in Word are saved as templates so that when someone fills in the form, they are working on a copy of the form, not the original. The original is the template that is saved as a protected document. When a form is created from the protected template, information can be typed only in certain designated fields. Use options in the Controls group on the DEVELOPER tab to insert text content controls, check box content controls, or other form content controls into a form template document. Turn on the display of the DEVELOPER tab at the Word Options dialog box. Generally, a form is created based on the default template document (called the Normal template).

Project

You are responsible for checking in patients as they arrive at the clinic and for updating their records, if necessary. You decide to create a form with fields that can be used to enter revised patient data at the computer.

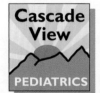

Cascade View
PEDIATRICS

1. To begin creating a form, you first need to display the DEVELOPER tab. Begin by clicking the FILE tab and then clicking *Options*.

2. At the Word Options dialog box, click *Customize Ribbon* in the left panel.

3. Click the *Developer* tab check box in the list box at the right to insert a check mark. Click OK to close the Word Options dialog box.

   The DEVELOPER tab displays to the right of the VIEW tab on the ribbon.

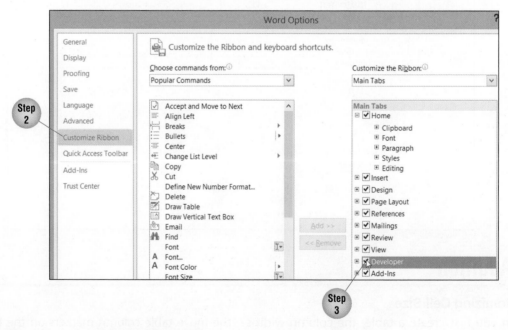

4. Open **CVPPatientForm.docx**.

5. Save CVPPatientForm.docx as a template. Begin by pressing the F12 key to display the Save As dialog box.

6 At the Save As dialog box, click the *Save as type* option box and then click *Word Template (*.dotx)* at the drop-down list.

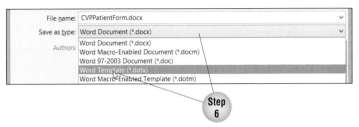

7 Navigate to the WordMedS4 folder on your storage medium, type **UpdateTemplate** in the *File name* text box, and then press Enter.

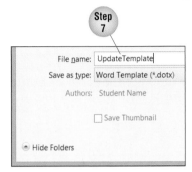

8 Position the mouse pointer to the right of the text *Patient Name:* and then click the left mouse button. This positions the insertion point one space to the right of the colon after *Patient Name:*.

9 Click the DEVELOPER tab and then click the Plain Text Content Control button Aa in the Controls group.

This inserts a plain text content control with the text *Click here to enter text*.

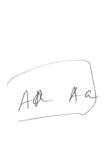

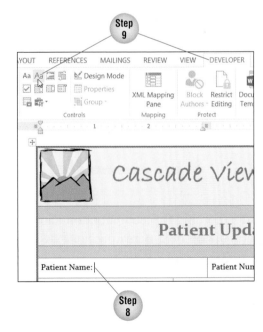

continues

10 Insert plain text content control fields in the remaining cells as shown in Figure W4.7. To insert the check boxes in the *Check the appropriate box identifying with whom the patient lives.* section, click in the desired cell and then click the Check Box Content Control button ☑ in the Controls group.

Data you enter into the form will replace the content control text.

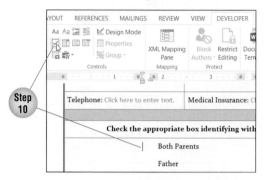

11 Protect the template by clicking the Restrict Editing button 🗎 in the Protect group on the DEVELOPER tab.

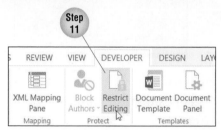

12 At the Restrict Editing task pane, click the *Allow only this type of editing in the document* check box to insert a check mark, click the down-pointing arrow at the right of the option box in the *Editing restrictions* section, and then click *Filling in forms* at the drop-down list.

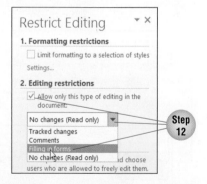

13 Click the Yes, Start Enforcing Protection button and then click OK at the Start Enforcing Protection dialog box. (Creating a password is optional.)

14 Close the Restrict Editing task pane by clicking the Close button that displays in the upper right corner of the task pane.

15 Save, print, and then close **UpdateTemplate.dotx**.

Cascade View Pediatrics

Patient Update

Patient Name: Click here to enter text.	**Patient Number:** Click here to enter text.

Address: Click here to enter text.	**City:** Click here to enter text.	**State:** Click here to enter text.	**Zip:** Click here to enter text.

Telephone: Click here to enter text.	**Medical Insurance:** Click here to enter text.

Check the appropriate box identifying with whom the patient lives.

☐ Both Parents   ☐ Mother

☐ Father   ☐ Other – Specify: Click here to enter text.

Guardian Information	**Guardian Information**
Relationship: Click here to enter text.	**Relationship:** Click here to enter text.
Name: Click here to enter text.	**Name:** Click here to enter text.
Address: Click here to enter text.	**Address:** Click here to enter text.
City: Click here to enter text. **State:** Click here to enter text. **Zip:** Click here to enter text.	**City:** Click here to enter text. **State:** Click here to enter text. **Zip:** Click here to enter text.
Home Telephone: Click here to enter text.	**Home Telephone:** Click here to enter text.

In Brief

Create Form Template
1. Open desired document.
2. Press F12.
3. At Save As dialog box, click *Save as type* option box and then click *Word Template (*.dotx)*.
4. Navigate to desired folder, type template name, and then press Enter.
5. Click DEVELOPER tab.
6. Type document, using buttons on DEVELOPER tab to insert content controls as needed.
7. Click Restrict Editing button.
8. Click *Allow only this type of editing in the document* check box.
9. Click down-pointing arrow at right of option in *Editing restrictions* section and then click *Filling in forms*.
10. Click Yes, Start Enforcing Protection button.
11. Click OK at Start Enforcing Protection dialog box.

In Addition

Planning the Form Layout

When planning the layout of a form, consider the following points:

- Group like items together in the form, as this makes providing complete and accurate information easier for the person filling in the form.
- Place the most important information at the top of the form to increase the likelihood of obtaining it.
- Use fonts, colors, lines, and graphics purposefully and sparingly, as overuse of such design elements tends to clutter a form and make it difficult to read.
- Use white space and lines to separate and clearly identify each section.

Saving a Template to the Custom Office Templates Folder

If you save a document as a template to the Custom Office Templates folder in the Documents folder on your computer, the template will be available at the New backstage area. Create a new document based on the template saved in the Custom Office Templates folder by clicking the FILE tab, clicking the *New* option, clicking the *PERSONAL* option, and then clicking the desired template thumbnail. Templates saved in any other location are not available at the New backstage area.

Activity 4.11

Filling In and Printing a Form Document

After you create, protect, and save a form template, you can use it to create a personalized form document. When you open a protected form template, the insertion point is automatically positioned in the first form field. Enter the appropriate information and then press the Tab key to move the insertion point to the next form field. You can move the insertion point to a previous form field by pressing Shift + Tab. To fill in a check box form field, click the check box. If necessary, click the check box again to remove the X from the form field.

Project

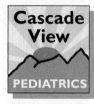

A patient that is a minor child has arrived at the clinic for an appointment. You will enter the updated information for the patient and her parents using the Patient Update form.

1. Create a form with the **UpdateTemplate.dotx** template. To begin, click the File Explorer button on the Taskbar.

2. At the File Explorer window, navigate to the WordMedS4 folder on your storage device and then double-click ***UpdateTemplate.dotx***.

    This opens a new document based on the form template.

3. Word displays the form document with the *Patient Name:* content control selected. Type the name **Jolie Pearson**, as shown below and in Figure W4.8.

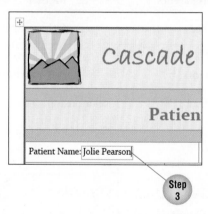

4. Press the Tab key to move to the next content control.

5. Fill in the remaining information as shown in Figure W4.8. Press the Tab key to move the insertion point to the next content control and press Shift + Tab to move the insertion point to the previous content control. To insert an X in a check box, click the check box. If you insert an X by mistake, click the check box again to remove it.

6. When the form is completed, save the document in the WordMedS4 folder on your storage medium and name it **WMedS4-CVPUpdate**.

7. Print and then close **WMedS4-CVPUpdate.docx**.

FIGURE W4.8 Filled-in Form

Cascade View Pediatrics

Patient Update

Patient Name: Jolie Pearson	Patient Number: 210-99

Address: 4512 North Aurora	City: Portland	State: OR	Zip: 97233

Telephone: (503) 555-3847	Medical Insurance: Premiere Group

Check the appropriate box identifying with whom the patient lives.

☒ Both Parents   ☐ Mother

☐ Father   ☐ Other – Specify: Click here to enter text.

Guardian Information	**Guardian Information**
Relationship: Mother	Relationship: Father
Name: Michelle Pearson	Name: Mark Pearson
Address: 4512 North Aurora	Address: 4512 North Aurora
City: Portland State: OR Zip: 97233	City: Portland State: OR Zip: 97233
Home Telephone: (503) 555-3847	Home Telephone: (503) 555-3847

In Brief

Fill In Form
1. Click File Explorer button on Taskbar.
2. Navigate to desired folder and then double-click desired template file.
3. Type text to insert text or click check box to insert check mark.
4. Press Tab key to move to next field or press Shift + Tab to move to previous field.

In Addition

Customizing Plain Text Content Control Properties

To change options for a plain text content control, select the plain text content control and then click the Properties button in the Controls group on the DEVELOPER tab. This displays the Content Control Properties dialog box, shown at the right. At this dialog box, you can apply a title or tag to the content control, lock the content control, and apply formatting options.

Customizing Check Box Content Control Properties

You can customize check box content control options at the Content Control Properties dialog box, shown at the right. Display this dialog box by selecting a check box content control and then clicking the Properties button in the Controls group on the DEVELOPER tab. At the dialog box, you can specify options such as check box symbols and formatting options.

Activity 4.12

Editing a Form Template

You can create a form template and the template text can be edited and saved in the normal manner. However, if you create and protect a form template, the text in the template cannot be changed. If you need to make changes to a template, open the template in the same manner as you would open a normal document in Word. With the template open, unprotect it by clicking the DEVELOPER tab, clicking the Restrict Editing button in the Protect group, and then clicking the Stop Protection button at the Restrict Editing task pane. Make the desired changes to the template and then protect the template again.

Project After using the Patient Update form a couple of times, you realize that you need to add additional fields. You will update the form template to include new content controls.

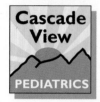

1. Press Ctrl + F12 to display the Open dialog box.

2. At the Open dialog box, navigate to the WordMedS4 folder on your storage medium and then double-click *UpdateTemplate.dotx*.

3. Unprotect the template document by clicking the DEVELOPER tab and then clicking the Restrict Editing button in the Protect group.

4. At the Restrict Editing task pane, click the Stop Protection button that displays toward the bottom.

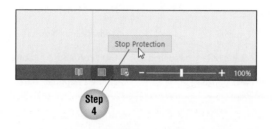

Step 4

5. Insert a new row at the bottom of the table. To do this, click in one of the cells in the bottom row, click the TABLE TOOLS LAYOUT tab, and then click the Insert Below button in the Rows & Columns group.

Step 5

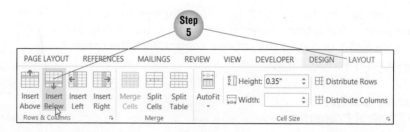

6 Click in the first column of the new row, type **Work Telephone:**, and then press the spacebar.

7 Insert a plain text content control by clicking the DEVELOPER tab and then clicking the Plain Text Content Control button in the Controls group.

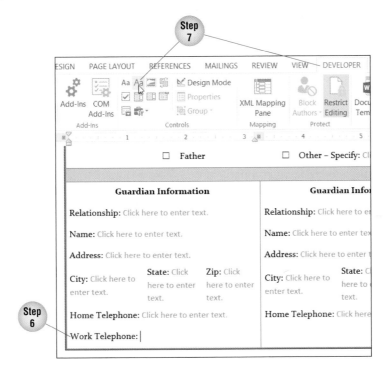

In Brief

Edit Template Document
1. Open template document.
2. Click DEVELOPER tab.
3. Click Restrict Editing button.
4. Click Stop Protection button in Restrict Editing task pane.
5. Make desired changes.
6. Click Yes, Start Enforcing Protection button in task pane.
7. Click OK at Start Enforcing Protection dialog box.

8 Press the Right Arrow key to deselect the content control, press the Tab key to move the insertion point to the new cell in the second column, type **Work Telephone:**, press the spacebar, and then insert a plain text content control.

9 Protect the document by clicking the Yes, Start Enforcing Protection button in the Restrict Editing task pane.

10 Click OK at the Start Enforcing Protection dialog box.

11 Close the Restrict Editing task pane.

12 Save **UpdateTemplate.dotx**.

In Addition

Creating a Form with Legacy Tools

Click the Legacy Tools button in the Controls group on the DEVELOPER tab and a drop-down list displays with a number of fields you can insert in a form, including a text, check box, or drop-down list form field. The Text Form Field button in the Legacy Tools drop-down list is similar to the Plain Text Content Control button. To insert a text form field, position the insertion point in the desired location, click the Legacy Tools button in the Controls group on the DEVELOPER tab, and then click the Text Form Field button. This inserts a gray shaded box in the form. This shaded box is the location where data is entered when a person fills in the form.

Activity 4.13

Creating and Filling In a Form with a Drop-Down List Content Control

Some fields in a form may require the person entering the information to choose from a list of specific options. You can create this type of field by using the Drop-Down List Content Control button in the Controls group on the DEVELOPER tab. After inserting a drop-down list content control, click the Properties button in the Controls group and the Content Control Properties dialog box displays. Use options at this dialog box to type the options you want to include in the list. A drop-down list content control in a form displays as a content control placeholder with a down-pointing arrow at the right side of the box. When entering data in a form, click the down-pointing arrow and then click the desired option at the drop-down list.

Project

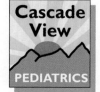

After looking at the Patient Update form, you realize that the field after *Medical Insurance:* should be changed to a drop-down form field since your clinic only accepts medical insurance from three healthcare companies.

1 With **UpdateTemplate.dotx** open, unprotect the template by clicking the DEVELOPER tab and then clicking the Restrict Editing button. At the task pane, click the Stop Protection button.

2 To change the *Medical Insurance:* plain text content control to a drop-down content control, begin by clicking the plain text content control, clicking the content control tab, and then pressing the Delete key.

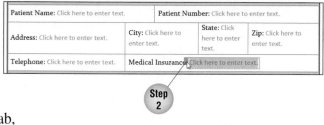

This removes the plain text content control from the cell.

3 Click the Drop-Down List Content Control button in the Controls group on the DEVELOPER tab.

4 Click the Properties button in the Controls group.

This displays the Content Control Properties dialog box.

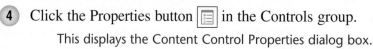

5 At the Content Control Properties dialog box, click the Add button.

6 At the Add Choice dialog box, type **Health Plus America** in the *Display Name* text box and then click OK.

7 Click the Add button, type **Premiere Group** in the *Display Name* text box, and then click OK. Click the Add button, type **Healthwise Cooperative**, and then click OK. Click the Add button, type **Self Insured**, and then click OK.

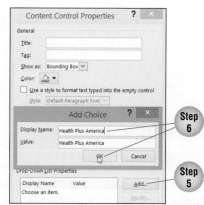

8 Click OK to close the Content Control Properties dialog box.

9 Protect the template by clicking the Yes, Start Enforcing Protection button in the task pane and then clicking OK at the Start Enforcing Protection dialog box.

10. Close the Restrict Editing task pane.

11. Save and then close **UpdateTemplate.dotx**.

12. Click the File Explorer button on the Taskbar, navigate to the WordMedS4 folder on your storage medium, and then double-click *UpdateTemplate.dotx*.

13. Fill in the text and check boxes as shown in Figure W4.9. Press the Tab key to move to the next field or press Shift + Tab to move to the previous field. To fill in the drop-down form field, click the down-pointing arrow at the right of the *Medical Insurance:* option box and then click *Healthwise Cooperative* at the drop-down list.

14. Save the completed form and name it **WMedS4-PatUpdate**.

15. Print and then close **WMedS4-PatUpdate.docx**.

In Brief

Insert Drop-Down Form Field
1. Click DEVELOPER tab.
2. Click Drop-Down List Content Control button.

Display Drop-Down Form Field Properties Dialog Box
1. Select drop-down form field.
2. Click Properties button in Controls group on DEVELOPER tab.

FIGURE W4.9 Filled-in Form

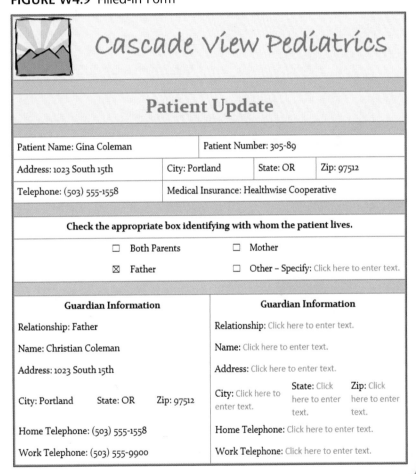

In Addition

Selecting an Option from a Drop-down List

When filling in a drop-down form field, make the field active and then either click the down-pointing arrow at the right side of the form field or press Alt + Down Arrow on the keyboard. At the drop-down list that displays, click the desired choice.

You may also use the Up or Down Arrow keys to navigate to the desired choice and then press the Enter key to select it.

Features Summary

Feature	Ribbon Tab, Group	Button	Option
check box content control	DEVELOPER, Controls		
delete column	TABLE TOOLS LAYOUT, Rows & Columns		*Delete Columns*
delete row	TABLE TOOLS LAYOUT, Rows & Columns		*Delete Rows*
drop-down content control	DEVELOPER, Controls		
Insert Address Block dialog box	MAILINGS, Write & Insert Fields		
insert column	TABLE TOOLS LAYOUT, Rows & Columns	OR	
Insert Greeting Line dialog box	MAILINGS, Write & Insert Fields		
insert merge field	MAILINGS, Write & Insert Fields		
insert row	TABLE TOOLS LAYOUT, Rows & Columns	OR	
Insert Table dialog box	INSERT, Tables		*Insert Table*
plain text content control	DEVELOPER, Controls	Aa	
protect document	DEVELOPER, Protect		
start mail merge	MAILINGS, Start Mail Merge		
table	INSERT, Tables		
Table Properties dialog box	TABLE TOOLS LAYOUT, Table		
table styles	TABLE TOOLS DESIGN, Table Styles		

Knowledge Check

Completion: In the space provided at the right, write in the correct term, symbol, or command.

1. A merge generally involves two documents: the main document and this. _____
2. Use buttons on this tab to merge documents. _____
3. Insert this type of field in a main document at the location where you want to insert variable information during a merge. _____
4. Click this hyperlink in the Mail Merge Recipients dialog box to display the Filter and Sort dialog box with the Sort Records tab selected. _____
5. Create a table by using the Table button on this tab. _____
6. Press this key to move the insertion point to the next cell in a table. _____
7. Press these keys to move the insertion point to the previous cell in a table. _____
8. To insert a row above the current row in a table, click this button in the Rows & Columns group on the TABLE TOOLS LAYOUT tab. _____
9. Center a table between the left and right margins with the *Center* option in the *Alignment* section of this dialog box. _____
10. Apply predesigned table styles with options in the Table Styles group on this tab. _____
11. Use options in this group on the DEVELOPER tab to insert content controls into a form. _____
12. Click the Restrict Editing button and this task pane displays. _____
13. Click this button in the Controls group to insert a content control identifying a location for users to enter text in a form. _____
14. Use this button in the Controls group to insert a field containing a list of options. _____

Skills Review

Review 1 Creating and Merging Letters

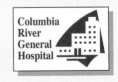
Columbia
River
General
Hospital

1. Use the Mail Merge feature to prepare six letters using the information shown in Figures W4.10 and W4.11 on page 212. When completing the steps, consider the following:
   a. Create a data source using the information shown in Figure W4.10. (Enter the records in this order—*Watanabe, Reeves, Torres, Wickstrom, O'Leary,* and *Fuentes.*) Save the data source document in the WordMedS4 folder on your storage medium and name it **CRGHEdList**.
   b. Type the letter shown in Figure W4.11, using your initials in place of the *xx*. Insert a fill-in field for the *(School)* field. (You determine the prompt message.) ***Hint: Remove the hyperlink from the web address by right-clicking the web address and then clicking*** **Remove Hyperlink** ***at the shortcut menu.***

FIGURE W4.10 Review 1 Data Source

Mr. Paul Watanabe
Division Street Clinic
5330 Division Street
Portland, OR 97255

Mr. Ramon Torres
Youth and Family Services
8904 McLoughlin Boulevard
Oak Grove, OR 97267

Ms. Suzanna O'Leary
Family Counseling Center
100 Center Street
Oak Grove, OR 97268

Ms. Nora Reeves
Community Counseling
1235 North 122nd Avenue
Portland, OR 97230

Dr. Thomas Wickstrom
Columbia Mental Health Center
550 Columbia Street
Portland, OR 97305

Dr. Christina Fuentes
Parenting Services
210 Martin Luther King Way
Portland, OR 97403

FIGURE W4.11 Review 1 Letter

February 1, 2016

«AddressBlock»

«GreetingLine»

The staff in the Education Department at Columbia River General Hospital has prepared parent education classes designed for parents of children between the ages of 5 and 10. Classes focus on a commonsense approach to parenting and provide parents with practical ideas about setting limits and teaching children to make responsible choices. Parents are given ideas and techniques that can be used at home to help children develop decision-making and problem-solving skills.

Qualified family counselors will teach the classes, which will begin Monday, March 7, and end Wednesday, April 6. Classes will be held from 7:00 to 8:30 p.m. at (School). Cost for the classes is based on a sliding-fee scale. For more information on these parenting classes and how parents can register, as well as directions to the school, please call me at (503) 555-2500 or visit us online at www.emcp.net/crgh.

Sincerely,

Laura Latterell
Education Director

xx
CRGHEdLtrs.docx

c. Click the Finish & Merge button and then click *Edit Individual Documents* at the drop-down list.

d. At the Merge to New Document dialog box, make sure *All* is selected and then click the OK button.

e. When merging the letters, type the following in each specific record:

Record 1	**Jefferson Elementary School**
Record 2	**Jefferson Elementary School**
Record 3	**Evergreen Elementary School**
Record 4	**Jefferson Elementary School**
Record 5	**Evergreen Elementary School**
Record 6	**Jefferson Elementary School**

2. Save the merged letters in the normal manner in the WordMedS4 folder on your storage medium and name the document **WMedS4-R-CRGHEdLtrs**.

3. Print and then close **WMedS4-R-CRGHEdLtrs.docx**. (This document will print six letters.)

4. Save the main document in the normal manner in the WordMedS4 folder on your storage medium and name it **WMedS4-R-CRGHEdMainDoc**.

5. Close **WMedS4-R-CRGHEdMainDoc.docx**.

Review 2 Preparing Envelopes

1. Use the Mail Merge feature to prepare envelopes for the letters created in Review 1.

2. Specify **CRGHEdList.mdb** as the data source document.

3. Save the merged envelope document in the WordMedS4 folder on your storage medium and name the document **WMedS4-R-CRGHEdEnvs**.

4. Print and then close **WMedS4-R-CRGHEdEnvs.docx**. (Manual feed may be required when printing.)

5. Close the envelope main document without saving it.

Review 3 Creating Chart Notes Using a Table

1. Open **NSMCLtrhd.docx** and then save it with the name **WMedS4-R-NSMCNotes**. (If necessary, change the zoom to *100%*.)

2. Click the *No Spacing* style, change the font to Constantia, and add 12 points of spacing before paragraphs. ***Hint: Add 12 points of spacing before paragraphs by clicking the Line and Paragraph Spacing button in the Paragraph group on the HOME tab and then clicking* Add Space Before Paragraph *at the drop-down list.***

3. Create a table with 2 columns and 20 rows.

4. Select and then merge each row (individually) as shown in Figure W4.12 on page 214. ***Hint: To merge cells, select the cells and then click the Merge Cells button in the Merge group on the TABLE TOOLS LAYOUT tab.***

5. Type the text in the cells as shown in Figure W4.12.

6. Select the title, *CHART NOTES*, change the font size to 16 points, apply bold formatting, and change the paragraph alignment to center.

7. Apply Gold, Accent 4, Lighter 60% shading to the top row. ***Hint: Do this with the Shading button in the Table Styles group on the TABLE TOOLS DESIGN tab.***

8. Save, print, and then close **WMedS4-R-NSMCNotes.docx**.

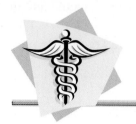

North Shore Medical Clinic
7450 Meridian Street, Suite 150
Portland, OR 97202
(503) 555-2330
www.emcp.net/nsmc

CHART NOTES	
NAME	DOB
DATE	AGE
Reason for visit:	
B/P	PULSE
SHEENT	
Neck	
Lungs	
Cardiovascular	
Abdomen	
Genitourinary	
Musculoskeletal	
Neurologic/Psychiatric	
Lab/X-rays	
Impressions:	
Plan:	

Review 4 Preparing a Form

1. Create the form shown in Figure W4.13 on page 216 as a template. Begin by opening **CRGHSecPayerForm.docx** from the WordMedS4 folder on your storage medium. With the document open, press the F12 key to display the Save As dialog box, change the *Save as type* option to *Word Template (*.dotx),* navigate to the WordMedS4 folder on your storage medium, type **CRGHSPFormTemplate** in the *File name* text box, and then press Enter.

2. Insert the plain text content controls and check box content controls as shown in Figure W4.13. For the *Name of Insurance Company:* cell, insert a drop-down list content control with the following options: *Assure Medical*, *Premiere Group*, *Sound Medical*, *Health Plus*, and *First Choice*.

3. Protect the template document to only allow filling in the form.

4. Save and then close **CRGHSPFormTemplate.dotx**.

5. Create a form document from the **CRGHSPFormTemplate** template. Begin by clicking the File Explorer button on the Taskbar, navigating to the WordMedS4 folder on your storage medium, and then double-clicking ***CRGHSPFormTemplate.dotx***.

6. Insert the following data in the specified fields:

Patient Name:	**Wyatt Johnston**
Patient Number:	**839488**
Address:	**3107 North Cedar Street**
City:	**Portland**
State:	**OR**
Zip:	**97429**
Telephone:	**(503) 555-4775**
Date of Birth:	**05/15/1975**

   Insert a check mark in the *Yes* check box for the first question and insert a check mark in the *No* check box for each of the second through sixth questions.

Name of Insurance Company:	Choose *Health Plus* from the drop-down list.
Telephone Number:	**1-800-555-3995**
Name of Policy Holder:	**Wyatt Johnston**
Policy Number:	**RT-90338**

7. Save the document with the name **WMedS4-R-CRGHPayer**.

8. Print and then close **WMedS4-R-CRGHPayer.docx**.

Columbia River General Hospital

4550 Fremont Street ● Portland, Oregon 97045 ● (503) 555-2000

SECONDARY PAYER FORM

Patient Name: Click here to enter text.		Patient Number: Click here to enter text.	
Address: Click here to enter text.	City: Click here to enter text.	State: Click here to enter text.	Zip: Click here to enter text.
Telephone: Click here to enter text.		Date of Birth: Click here to enter text.	

Please answer the following questions related to your illness or injury:

Yes	No	
☐	☐	Is illness/injury due to an automobile accident?
☐	☐	Is illness/injury due to an accident covered by Workers' Compensation?
☐	☐	Does the Black Lung Program cover this illness?
☐	☐	Are you eligible for coverage under the Veterans Administration?
☐	☐	If under 65, do you have Medicare coverage due to a disability?
☐	☐	Do you have coverage under a spouse's health insurance plan?

Name of Insurance Company: Choose an item.	Telephone Number: Click here to enter text.
Name of Policy Holder: Click here to enter text.	Policy Number: Click here to enter text.

Skills Assessment

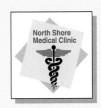

Assessment 1 Creating and Merging Letters

1. Use the Mail Merge feature to create the letter shown in Figure W4.14 on page 218 and merge it with the **NSMCPatientsDS.mdb** data source document with the following specifications:
   a. Browse to the WordMedS4 folder and then double-click *NSMCPatientsDS.mdb*. Display the Mail Merge Recipients dialog box by clicking the Edit Recipient List button and then add the following record:

Title:	**Mrs.**
First Name:	**Lola**
Last Name:	**Solberg**
Address Line 1:	**23100 North Tillicum**
Address Line 2:	(leave blank)
City:	**Portland**
State:	**OR**
ZIP Code:	**97402**
Home Phone:	**(503) 555-3437**
Specialty:	**Obstetrics**

   b. With the Mail Merge Recipients dialog box displayed, identify only those records containing a specialty of *Obstetrics*.
   c. Type the letter shown in Figure W4.14. (Use your initials in place of the *xx*.)
   d. Click the Finish & Merge button and then click *Edit Individual Documents* at the drop-down list.
   e. At the Merge to New Document dialog box, make sure *All* is selected and then click OK.
2. Save the merged letters in the normal manner in the WordMedS4 folder on your storage medium and name the document **WMedS4-A1-NSMCClassLtrs**.
3. Print and then close **WMedS4-A1-NSMCClassLtrs.docx**. (Three letters should print.)
4. Save the main document in the normal manner in the WordMedS4 folder on your storage medium and name the document **WMedS4-A1-NSMCClassMainDoc**.
5. Close **WMedS4-A1-NSMCClassMainDoc.docx**.

October 19, 2016

«AddressBlock»

«GreetingLine»

North Shore Medical Clinic is partnering with the Education Department at Columbia River General Hospital and offering childbirth education classes. A certified nurse practitioner teaches the classes at various times during the year. Participants in the class meet once a week for six weeks.

You can register for the classes directly with Columbia River General Hospital by calling the Education Department at (503) 555-2500 or by contacting us at (503) 555-2330. The fee for the classes is $75 payable directly to Columbia River General Hospital.

Sincerely,

Lee Elliot
Office Manager

xx
NSMCClassLtrs.docx

Assessment 2 Modifying and Formatting a Calendar

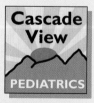

1. Open **CVPCalendar.docx** and then save it with the name **WMedS4-A2-CVPCalendar**.
2. Delete one of the middle rows in the calendar. (Do not delete the first or last row because the table border may get deleted.)
3. Select the entire table and then change the row height to 1.2 inches. *Hint: Do this with the* **Table Row Height** *measurement box in the Cell Size group on the TABLE TOOLS LAYOUT tab.*
4. With the table still selected, change the font to 10-point Candara.
5. Position the insertion point in any cell in the second row and then change the row height to 0.2 inches.
6. Merge the cells in the top row.
7. With the top row selected (one cell), change the font size to 26 points, turn on bold formatting, click the Align Center button in the Alignment group on the TABLE TOOLS LAYOUT tab, apply Gold, Accent 4, Lighter 60% shading, and then type the text shown in the cell in Figure W4.15.

8. Select the second row, change the font size to 11 points, turn on bold formatting, click the Align Center button in the Alignment group on the TABLE TOOLS LAYOUT tab, apply Gold, Accent 4, Lighter 80% shading, and then type the text shown in the second row in Figure W4.15.
9. Type the text in each cell as shown in Figure W4.15.
10. Save, print, and then close **WMedS4-A2-CVPCalendar.docx**.

FIGURE W4.15 Assessment 2

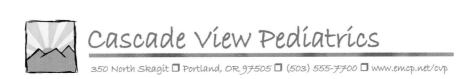

Cascade View Pediatrics

350 North Skagit ☐ Portland, OR 97505 ☐ (503) 555-7700 ☐ www.emcp.net/cvp

Parenting Classes
April 2016

Sunday	Monday	Tuesday	Wednesday	Thursday	Friday	Saturday
					1 Mom & Baby 9:30 to 11:00 a.m.	2
3	4 Basic Parenting 7:00 to 8:30 p.m.	5	6 Basic Parenting 7:00 to 8:30 p.m.	7	8 Mom & Baby 9:30 to 11:00 a.m.	9
10	11 Basic Parenting 7:00 to 8:30 p.m.	12	13 Basic Parenting 7:00 to 8:30 p.m.	14	15 Mom & Baby 9:30 to 11:00 a.m.	16
17	18 Basic Parenting 7:00 to 8:30 p.m.	19	20 Basic Parenting 7:00 to 8:30 p.m.	21	22 Mom & Baby 9:30 to 11:00 a.m.	23
24	25 Basic Parenting 7:00 to 8:30 p.m.	26	27 Basic Parenting 7:00 to 8:30 p.m.	28	29 Mom & Baby 9:30 to 11:00 a.m.	30

Assessment 3 Formatting and Filling in a Medical History Questionnaire

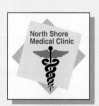

1. Create the form shown in Figure W4.16 as a template. Begin by opening **NSMCMedHistory.docx** from the WordMedS4 folder on your storage medium. With the document open, press the F12 key to display the Save As dialog box, change the *Save as type* option to *Word Template (*.dotx)*, navigate to the WordMedS4 folder on your storage medium, type **NSMCMedHistoryTemplate** in the *File name* text box, and then press Enter.
2. Press Ctrl + End and then create the third table in the medical history document as shown in Figure W4.16. Use the other two tables in the document as a guideline for formatting the third table. After creating the table, insert the content controls in all three tables as shown in the figure.
3. Protect the document.
4. Save and then close **NSMCMedHistoryTemplate.dotx**.
5. Create a form document from **NSMCMedHistoryTemplate.dotx**. Begin by clicking the File Explorer button on the Taskbar, navigating to the WordMedS4 folder on your storage medium, and then double-clicking *NSMCMedHistoryTemplate.dotx*.
6. Fill in the first table with the following information:
   a. Patient's name is Sean Joslin, his patient ID number is 5423, and his insurance is Premiere Group. Insert the current date in the *Date:* content control.
   b. Click the *Yes* check box after the *Prior operations?* question and then type **Appendectomy, 2008** in the *Specify:* content control.
   c. Click the *No* check box for the next two questions.
   d. Click the *Yes* check box after the *Current medications?* question and then type **Prilosec, Tylenol** in the *List:* content control.
7. Fill in the second table with the following information:
   a. In the *Mother* column, click the check boxes for *Asthma* and *Eczema/dermatitis*.
   b. In the *Father* column, click the check box for *High blood pressure*.
   c. In the *Relative* column, click the check boxes for *Arthritis*, *Cancer*, *Heart disease*, and *High blood pressure*.
8. Fill in the third table with the following information:
   a. Click the *Yes* check box after the *Currently employed?* question and then type **Firefighter** in the *Occupation:* content control.
   b. Click the *No* check box for the next three questions.
   c. Click the *Yes* check box after the *Married?* question.
9. Save the document with the name **WMedS4-A3-MedHistory**.
10. Print and then close **WMedS4-A3-MedHistory.docx**.

Assessment 4 Converting a Table to Text

1. Use Word's Help feature to learn how to convert a table to text.
2. Open **Table.docx** and save it with the name **WMedS4-A4-Table**.
3. Convert the table to text, separating text with tabs.
4. Save, print, and then close **WMedS4-A4-Table.docx**.

HELP

FIGURE W4.16 Assessment 3

MEDICAL HISTORY QUESTIONNAIRE

Patient Name: Click here to enter text.	Patient ID#: Click here to enter text.
Insurance: Click here to enter text.	Date: Click here to enter text.

PAST MEDICAL HISTORY

	Yes	No	
Prior operations?	☐	☐	Specify: Click here to enter text.
Prior major illness?	☐	☐	Specify: Click here to enter text.
Allergies to medications?	☐	☐	List: Click here to enter text.
Current medications?	☐	☐	List: Click here to enter text.

FAMILY HISTORY

	Mother	Father	Relative
Allergies	☐	☐	☐
Arthritis	☐	☐	☐
Asthma	☐	☐	☐
Cancer	☐	☐	☐
Diabetes	☐	☐	☐
Eczema/dermatitis	☐	☐	☐
Heart disease	☐	☐	☐
High blood pressure	☐	☐	☐
Lung disease	☐	☐	☐
Other: Click here to enter text.	☐	☐	☐

SOCIAL HISTORY

	Yes	No	
Currently employed?	☐	☐	Occupation: Click here to enter text.
Pregnant?	☐	☐	
Smoke tobacco?	☐	☐	Daily quantity: Click here to enter text.
Drink alcohol?	☐	☐	Daily quantity: Click here to enter text.
Married?	☐	☐	

Assessment 5 Locating Information and Writing a Memo

1. Two doctors from the clinic are traveling to Chicago for a medical conference. Lee Elliott has asked you to find information on round-trip airfare from Portland to Chicago. For the departure date, use the first Monday of the next month and for the return date, use the first Saturday after the departure date. Use an Internet travel company (such as Expedia or Travelocity) to search for flights. The doctors want to leave sometime between 9:00 a.m. and noon and return sometime between noon and 3:00 p.m.
2. Open **NSMCMemoForm.docx** and then, using the flight information you found, write a memo to Lee Elliott that includes a table containing information such as airline names, flight numbers, times, and cost. Format and modify the table so the information is attractive and easy to read.
3. Save the completed memo and name it **WMedS4-A5-Conference**.
4. Print and then close **WMedS4-A5-Conference.docx**.

Marquee Challenge

Challenge 1 Preparing a Treadmill Exercise Test Form

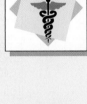

1. Open **NSMCLtrhd.docx** and then save it with the name **WMedS4-C1-Treadmill**.
2. Change the spacing after paragraphs to 0 points.
3. Create the document shown in Figure W4.17.
4. Save, print, and then close **WMedS4-C1-Treadmill.docx**.

Challenge 2 Preparing a Pre-operative Questions Form

1. Open **NSMCPreOpQuestions.docx** from the WordMedS4 folder on your storage medium and then save it as a template with the name **NSMCPreOpQuestionsTemplate**. *Hint: Do this at the Save As dialog box.*
2. Insert data in the table, format the table, and insert text content controls and check box content controls so your form appears the same as shown in Figure W4.18 on page 224.
3. Protect the template document and only allow filling in the form.
4. Save and then close **NSMCPreOpQuestionsTemplate.dotx**.
5. Create a form document from **NSMCPreOpQuestionsTemplate.dotx**. You determine the information to insert in the form.
6. Save the document with the name **WMedS4-C2-PreOp**.
7. Print and then close **WMedS4-C2-PreOp.docx**.

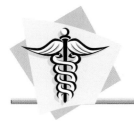

North Shore Medical Clinic
7450 Meridian Street, Suite 150
Portland, OR 97202
(503) 555-2330
www.emcp.net/nsmc

TREADMILL EXERCISE TEST

EXERCISE					
Stage (mph – grade)	Blood Pressure	Heart Rate	Premature Beats	ST mm	ST slope
AT REST					
Stage 1/2 (1.7 mph – 5%)					
Stage I (1.7 mph – 10%)					
Stage II (2.5 mph – 12%)					
Stage III (3.4 mph – 14%)					
Stage IV (4.2 mph – 16%)					
Stage V (5.0 mph – 18%)					
Stage VI (5.5 mph – 22%)					
Stage VII (6.0 mph – 22%)					

RECOVERY					
RECOVERY	Blood Pressure	Heart Rate	Premature Beats	ST mm	ST slope
IMMEDIATE					
1 Minute					
3 Minutes					
5 Minutes					
7 Minutes					

FIGURE W4.18 Challenge 2

PRE-OPERATIVE QUESTIONS

Patient Name: Click here to enter text.		Patient ID#: Click here to enter text.	
Birth Date: Click here to enter text.		Surgery Date: Click here to enter text.	

Do you now have or have you ever had:

	Yes	No	
Anesthesia	☐	☐	When? Click here to enter text.
Difficulty with anesthesia	☐	☐	What? Click here to enter text.
A relative who has difficulty with anesthesia	☐	☐	What? Click here to enter text.
Asthma, bronchitis, or other lung problems	☐	☐	
Abnormal chest x-ray	☐	☐	
Hypertension, chest pain, irregular heart beat	☐	☐	What? Click here to enter text.
Heart attack, heart murmur, abnormal EKG	☐	☐	What? Click here to enter text.
Bleeding or clotting problems	☐	☐	
Convulsions or seizures	☐	☐	
Stroke, muscle weakness, numbness, dizziness	☐	☐	
Hepatitis or jaundice	☐	☐	
Diabetes	☐	☐	
Kidney problems or blood in your urine	☐	☐	
Cortisone pills or injections	☐	☐	
Taking aspirin, ibuprofen, or other blood thinner	☐	☐	
Taking prescription drugs	☐	☐	List: Click here to enter text.
Smoke tobacco	☐	☐	

Using
EXCEL
in the
Medical Office

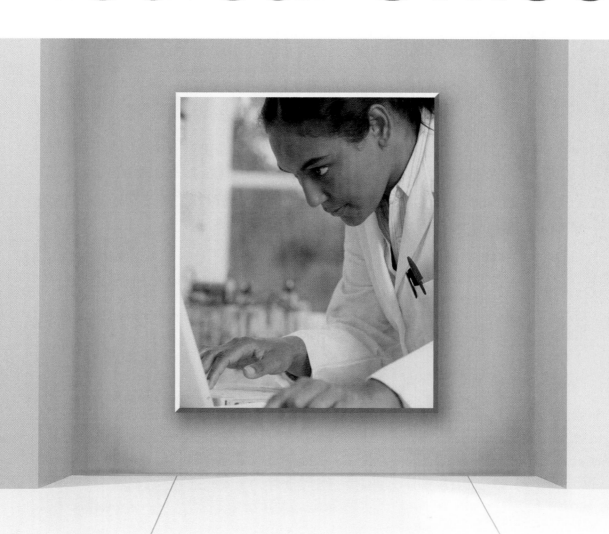

Introducing
EXCEL 2013

Microsoft Excel 2013 is a popular choice among individuals and companies for presenting and analyzing data. Excel organizes information in columns and rows in a document called a worksheet. Once a worksheet has been created, you can perform analyses of hypothetical situations such as "What if medical supplies increase in price by 4%?" Changing a value in a worksheet causes Excel to automatically recalculate any other values dependent on the number you changed. In an instant, your question is answered.

In Section 1, you will create new worksheets by entering labels, values, and formulas. To improve your efficiency, you will learn to use tools such as the fill handle and special techniques for performing common tasks such as copying. Section 2 presents editing and formatting you can use to improve a worksheet's appearance and correct errors. Section 3 introduces function formulas; visual elements such as charts, clip art, and drawing objects; page layout and print options; and data management features for working with lists.

In each of the three Excel sections, you will prepare medical worksheets for two clinics and a hospital as described below.

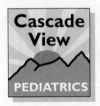

Cascade View Pediatrics is a full-service pediatric clinic that provides comprehensive primary pediatric care to infants, children, and adolescents.

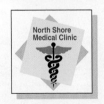

North Shore Medical Clinic is an internal medicine clinic dedicated to providing exceptional care to all patients. The physicians in the clinic specialize in a number of fields including internal medicine, family practice, cardiology, and dermatology.

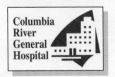

Columbia River General Hospital is an independent, not-for-profit hospital with the mission of providing high-quality, comprehensive care to patients and improving the health of members of the community.

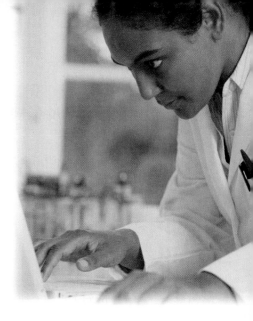

Excel SECTION 1
Analyzing Data Using Excel

Skills

- Start Excel and identify features in the Excel window
- Save a workbook using Save and Save As
- Enter labels and values
- Use the fill handle to enter a series
- Enter formulas
- Create a formula using Sum
- Copy a formula
- Test a worksheet for accuracy
- Apply the Accounting format to values
- Right-align labels
- Sort a selection
- Use the Help feature
- Center a label across multiple columns
- Change the page orientation to landscape
- Preview and print a worksheet
- Display cell formulas in a worksheet
- Navigate a large worksheet using the mouse and the keyboard
- Jump to a specific cell using Go To
- Create a new workbook using a template

Student Resources

Before beginning the activities in Excel Section 1, copy to your storage medium the ExcelMedS1 folder from the Student Resources CD. This folder contains the data files you need to complete the projects in this Excel section.

Projects Overview

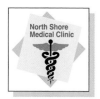

Create a payroll worksheet, browse a supplies inventory and standard exam room cost report, create an invoice, create a purchase order for medical supplies, and create an invoice for in-service training.

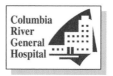

Edit an executive management salary report, calculate funds needed for a professional development budget, and prepare a surgery cost report.

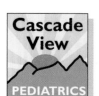

Complete an estimated travel expenses worksheet and calculate costs and registration fees for a medical seminar.

Activity 1.1

Completing the Excel Worksheet Cycle

In Excel, information is created in a ***worksheet*** and saved in a file called a ***workbook***. A workbook can contain several worksheets. A worksheet contains horizontal and vertical lines drawn in a grid to create columns and rows. Data is entered into a ***cell***, which is the intersection of a column with a row. Columns are lettered A to Z, AA to AZ, BA to BZ, and so on. The last column in a worksheet is labeled *XFD*. Rows are numbered 1, 2, 3, and so on. A column letter and a row number identify each cell. For example, A1 is the cell address for the intersection of column A with row 1. Each worksheet in Excel contains 16,384 columns and 1,048,576 rows. By default, an Excel workbook contains one worksheet, labeled *Sheet1*. Additional worksheets can be inserted as needed.

Project

You have been asked to update the Executive Management Salary Report for the Columbia River General Hospital by adding and editing data. As you update the data, you will view the impact of the new data on cells used to calculate salary and benefit costs.

Columbia
River
General
Hospital

1. At the Windows Start screen, click the Excel 2013 tile.

2. At the Excel 2013 opening screen, click the *Blank workbook* template.

3. At the Excel screen, identify the various features by comparing your screen with the one shown in Figure E1.1. If necessary, maximize the Excel window. Depending on your screen resolution, what you see may vary slightly from what is shown in the figure. Refer to Table E1.1 for a description of the screen features.

4. Click the FILE tab and then click the *Open* option at the backstage area.

   The backstage area organizes file management tasks into options such as *Open*, *Save*, *Save As*, and *Print*.

FIGURE E1.1 Excel Worksheet Screen

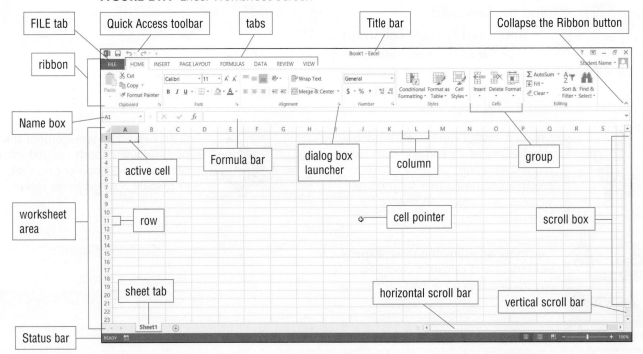

GST
= D3* $C$13   (F4)   Price of GST Per Unit

= select cell → select GST → F4 → Enter

TABLE E1.1 Excel Screen Features and Descriptions

Feature	Description
active cell	location in the worksheet that will display typed data or be affected by any commands applied
cell pointer	used to select cells by clicking or dragging the mouse
Collapse the Ribbon button	when clicked, removes the ribbon from the screen; when double-clicked, redisplays the ribbon
dialog box or task pane launcher	when clicked, opens a dialog box or task pane with more options for that group
FILE tab	when clicked, displays backstage area that contains options for working with and managing files
Formula bar	displays the contents stored in the active cell
Name box	displays the address or name assigned to the active cell
New sheet button	when clicked, inserts a new worksheet in the workbook
Quick Access toolbar	contains buttons for commonly used commands, making it possible to execute them with a single mouse click
ribbon	area containing the tabs with options and buttons divided into groups
sheet tab	when clicked, makes the worksheet active; tab name can be edited or assigned a color
Status bar	displays current mode, action messages, view buttons, and Zoom slider bar
tabs	contain commands and buttons organized into groups
Title bar	displays workbook name followed by program name
vertical and horizontal scroll bars	used to view parts of the worksheet beyond the current screen
worksheet area	contains cells used to create the worksheet

select Row
↓
insert
↓
sheet rows

click between 2 Rows

select → wrap text

select → sort A-Z

write
↓
Then drag to Autofill

select → sheet
↓
Review
↓
New comment

5   At the Open backstage area, click the desired location in the middle panel (contains the four location options). For example, click the *OneDrive* option preceded by your name if you are opening a workbook from your OneDrive or click the *Computer* option if you are opening a workbook from your computer's hard drive or a USB Flash drive.

= C3 / number
(Price for 1 unit)

Home → insert
↓
sheet columns

6   Click the Browse button.

> Press Ctrl + F12 to display the Open dialog box without displaying the Open backstage area.

Step 7

Total Price

7   At the Open dialog box, navigate to the ExcelMedS1 folder on your storage medium.

= Price of GST
+
Price for 1 unit

> To change to a different drive, click the drive letter in the *This PC* section of the Navigation pane. (You may need to scroll down the Navigation pane to see the *This PC* section.) Change to a different folder by double-clicking the folder name in the Content pane.

Page Layout
↓
Orientation
↓
Landscape
↓
Page setup

8   Double-click *CRGHExecutiveSalaries.xlsx* in the Content page of the Open dialog box.

> This workbook contains one worksheet with the salary and benefits report for the executive management team at Columbia River General Hospital. Notice some of the cells are empty. You will enter these values in Steps 11 through 14.

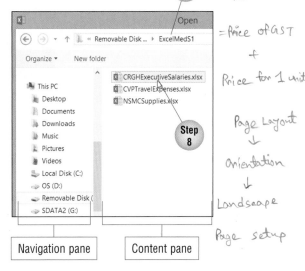

Navigation pane   Content pane

continues

Activity 1.1   229

9 Click the FILE tab and then click the *Save As* option.

10 At the Save As backstage area, click the current folder (the end of the current folder path name should end in *ExcelMedS1*) that displays below the *Current Folder* heading.

> Use the *Save As* option when you want to create a copy of a workbook with a different name. Use the *Save* option to save the workbook with the current name.

11 At the Save As dialog box, with ExcelMedS1 the active folder on your storage medium, press the Home key, type **EMedS1-** at the beginning of the current file name in the *File name* text box, and then press Enter or click the Save button.

> Press the F12 function key to display the Save As dialog box without displaying the Save As backstage area. Excel workbooks have the file extension *.xlsx* at the end of their names. When naming a file, do not change or delete this file extension, because this file extension tells the operating system to open the file in Microsoft Excel. If you change or delete the extension, the operating system will not know which program is associated with the data and will not be able to open the file.

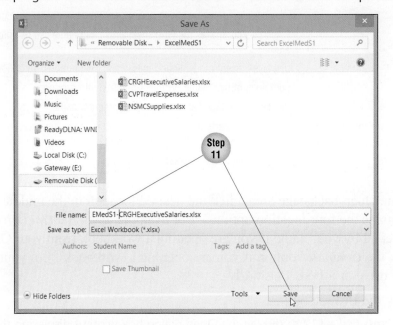

12 Move the cell pointer to the intersection of column F and row 8 (cell F8) and then click to make cell F8 the active cell.

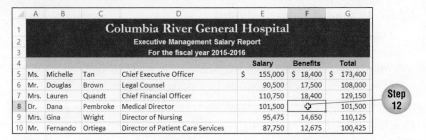

13 Type 16400 and then press Enter.

> You do not need to type a comma in the thousands place. The column is formatted to insert the comma automatically. (You will learn about this formatting in Section 2.) Notice that the entry in cell G8 has changed. This is because the formula in cell G8 was dependent on cell F8. As soon as you entered a value in cell F8, any other dependent cells were automatically updated. Can you identify other cells that changed as a result of the new value in cell F8?

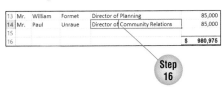

14 Click cell E14 to make it active and then type 85000.

15 Click cell F14 to make it active, type 9275, and then press Enter.

16 Double-click cell D14. Using the Right Arrow or Left Arrow keys, position the blinking insertion point immediately right of the comma, press the Backspace key to delete the comma, press the spacebar to insert a space, type of, and then press Enter.

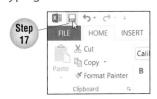

> Doing this fixes an inconsistency in the directors' titles in column D. Double-clicking a cell opens the cell for editing. A blinking insertion point will appear inside the cell. Edit the entry by using the arrow keys to move the insertion point, pressing the Backspace key or the Delete key to remove text, and then typing new text.

17 Click the Save button 🖫 on the Quick Access toolbar.

18 Click the FILE tab, click the *Print* option, and then click the Print button.

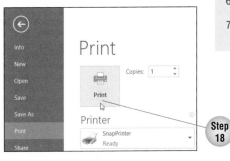

> You can save steps to print a workbook by adding a Quick Print button to the Quick Access toolbar. To add the button, click the Customize Quick Access Toolbar button that displays at the right side of the toolbar and then click *Quick Print* at the drop-down list. The worksheet's page layout options have been set to print the worksheet in landscape orientation, centered horizontally between the left and right margins. You will learn how to change these options in a later activity.

19 Click the FILE tab and then click the *Close* option to close the workbook. Click the FILE tab and click the *Close* option to close the blank workbook.

> When no workbooks are currently open, Excel displays a blank gray screen.

In Brief

Open Workbook
1. Click FILE tab.
2. Click *Open*.
3. Click desired location in middle panel.
4. Click Browse button.
5. At Open dialog box, navigate to desired folder.
6. Double-click workbook name.

Save Workbook
1. Click Save button on Quick Access toolbar.
2. At Save As backstage area, click desired location in middle panel.
3. Click Browse button.
4. At Save As dialog box, navigate to desired folder.
5. Type document name.
6. Click Save button or press Enter.

Save Workbook with New Name
1. Click FILE tab.
2. Click *Save As* option.
3. At Save As backstage area, click desired location in middle panel.
4. Click Browse button.
5. At Save As dialog box, navigate to desired folder.
6. Type document name.
7. Click Save button or press Enter.

In Addition

Using AutoComplete

As you start to type a new entry in a cell, the AutoComplete feature in Excel will attempt to complete it for you. If the first few letters that you type match another entry in the column, Excel automatically fills in the remaining text. Press Tab, Enter, or one of the arrow keys to accept the suggested text, or continue typing the correct text.

You can turn off AutoComplete at the Excel Options dialog box. Do this by clicking the FILE tab and then clicking *Options*. Click *Advanced* in the left panel, click the *Enable AutoComplete for cell values* check box to remove the check mark, and then click OK.

Activity 1.2

Entering Labels and Values; Using Fill Options

A *label* is an entry in a cell that helps the reader relate to the values in the corresponding column or row. Labels are generally entered first when creating a new worksheet since they define the layout of the data in the columns and rows. By default, Excel aligns labels at the left edge of the column. A *value* is a number, formula, or function that can be used to perform calculations within the worksheet. By default, Excel aligns values at the right edge of the column. Take a few moments to plan or sketch out the layout of a new worksheet before entering labels and values. Determine the calculations you will need to execute, as well as how best to display the data so that it will be easily understood and interpreted.

Project You need to create a new payroll worksheet for the hourly paid staff at the North Shore Medical Clinic. Begin by entering labels and values.

1 At the blank Excel screen, click the FILE tab, click the *New* option, and then click the *Blank workbook* template at the New backstage area.

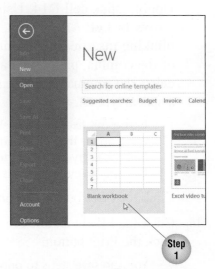

> You can also open a new blank workbook by using the keyboard shortcut Ctrl + N. You can also insert a New button on the Quick Access toolbar. To insert the button, click the Customize Quick Access Toolbar button that displays at the right side of the toolbar and then click *New* at the drop-down list.

2 With cell A1 active, type **Payroll** as the title for the new worksheet.

> When you type a new entry in a cell, the entry appears in the Formula bar as well as within the active cell in the worksheet area. To end a cell entry, press Enter, move to another cell in the worksheet, or click the Enter button on the Formula bar.

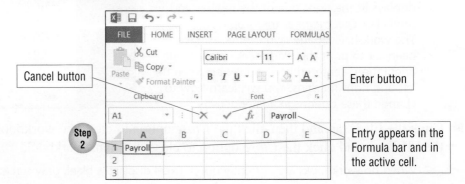

3 Press Enter.

4 With A2 the active cell, type **Week Ended: January 31, 2016** and then press Enter.

> Notice that the entry in cell A2 is overflowing into columns B and C. You can allow a label to spill over into adjacent columns as long as you do not plan to enter other data in the overflow cells. In a later section, you will learn how to adjust column widths to prevent overflow.

5 Enter the remaining labels as shown below by making the appropriate cell active, typing the label, and then pressing Enter or clicking another cell. (Do not complete the labels for the days of the week beyond *Sun*, as this will be done in Steps 6–8.)

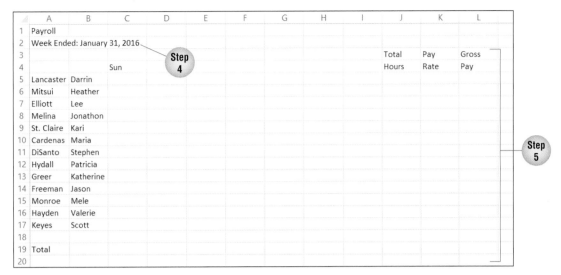

6 Click in cell C4 to make it active.

A thick green border surrounds the active cell. A small green square, known as the ***fill handle***, displays in the bottom right corner of the active cell. The fill handle is used to populate adjacent cells with the same or consecutive data. The entries that are automatically inserted in the adjacent cells are dependent on the contents of the active cell. You will use the fill handle in cell C4 to automatically enter the remaining days of the week in cells D4 through I4.

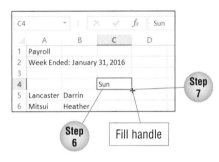

Fill handle

7 Using the mouse, point to the fill handle in cell C4. The cell pointer changes from a large white cross ⊹ to a thin black cross ✚.

8 Hold down the left mouse button, drag the pointer to cell I4, and then release the left mouse button.

The entries *Mon* through *Sat* appear in cells D4 through I4. As you drag the pointer to the right, a green border surrounds the selected cells and a ScreenTip appears below the pointer indicating the label or value that will be inserted. When you release the left mouse button, the cells remain selected and the Auto Fill Options button appears. Clicking the Auto Fill Options button causes a drop-down list to appear with various alternative actions for filling data in the cells.

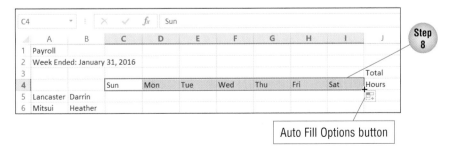

Auto Fill Options button

continues

9 Click cell C5 to make it active.

10 Type **8** and then press the Right Arrow key.

11 Type **5** in cell D5 and then press the Right Arrow key.

12 Type the following values in the cells indicated:

E5: **6**

F5: **8**

G5: **5**

H5: **0**

I5: **8**

13 Make cell F5 the active cell.

14 Using the mouse, point to the fill handle in cell F5, drag the pointer down to cell F17, and then release the mouse button.

> This time the active cell contained a value. The value *8* is copied down to the adjacent cells.

	A	B	C	D	E	F	G
1	Payroll						
2	Week Ended: January 31, 2016						
3							
4			Sun	Mon	Tue	Wed	Thu
5	Lancaster	Darrin	8	5	6	8	5
6	Mitsui	Heather				8	
7	Elliott	Lee				8	
8	Melina	Jonathon				8	
9	St. Claire	Kari				8	
10	Cardenas	Maria				8	
11	DiSanto	Stephen				8	
12	Hydall	Patricia				8	
13	Greer	Katherine				8	
14	Freeman	Jason				8	
15	Monroe	Mele				8	
16	Hayden	Valerie				8	
17	Keyes	Scott				8	
18							
19	Total						
20							

Step 14

15 Enter the remaining values for employee hours as shown below. Use the fill handle where there are duplicate values in adjacent cells to enter the data as efficiently as possible.

	A	B	C	D	E	F	G	H	I
1					Payroll				
2					Week Ended: January 31, 2016				
3									
4			Sun	Mon	Tue	Wed	Thu	Fri	Sat
5	Lancaster	Darrin	8	5	6	8	5	0	8
6	Mitsui	Heather	0	8	6	8	7	5	0
7	Elliott	Lee	8	8	0	8	7	7	0
8	Melina	Jonathon	8	8	0	8	7	8	0
9	St. Claire	Kari	0	8	0	8	8	7	0
10	Cardenas	Maria	0	0	0	8	8	7	8
11	DiSanto	Stephen	8	0	0	8	8	7	8
12	Hydall	Patricia	8	0	0	8	8	7	8
13	Greer	Katherine	8	6	8	8	0	0	8
14	Freeman	Jason	0	5	8	8	6	0	8
15	Monroe	Mele	5	6	8	8	0	8	0
16	Hayden	Valerie	6	4	8	8	0	8	0
17	Keyes	Scott	7	6	8	8	0	8	0
18									

Step 15

16 Make cell K5 the active cell, type **10.25**, and then press Enter.

17 Position the cell pointer over cell K5, hold down the left mouse button, drag down to cell K17, and then release the mouse button.

> A group of two or more adjacent cells is referred to as a *range*. Select a range of cells when you want to perform an action on more than one cell at once.

18 With the HOME tab active, click the Fill button [↓] in the Editing group and then click *Down* at the drop-down list.

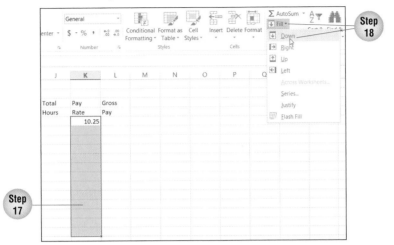

19 Click in any cell in the worksheet to deselect the range of cells in column K.

20 Click the Save button on the Quick Access toolbar.

21 At the Save As backstage area, click the desired location in the middle panel (*OneDrive* or *Computer*) and then click the *ExcelMedS1* folder that displays below the *Recent Folders* heading.

22 At the Save As dialog box with ExcelMedS1 the active folder, type **EMedS1-NSMCPayJan31** in the *File name* text box and then press Enter.

In Addition

Using the Fill Handle

The fill handle is versatile and can be used to enter a series of values, dates, times, or other labels as a pattern. The pattern is established based on the cells you select before dragging the fill handle. In the worksheet shown below, the cells in columns C through J were all populated using the fill handle. In each row, the first two cells in columns A and B were selected and then the fill handle was dragged right to column J. Notice the variety of patterns used to extend a series.

Use the Auto Fill Options button drop-down list to control how the series is entered. After dragging the fill handle, the Auto Fill Options button is displayed at the end of the series. Pointing at the button causes it to expand and display a down-pointing arrow. Click the down-pointing arrow and then select the desired fill action at the drop-down list. By default, *Fill Series* is selected.

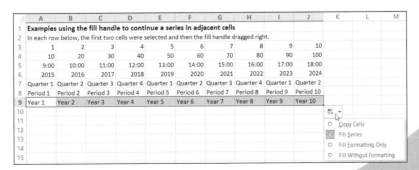

Activity 1.3

Performing Calculations Using Formulas

A *formula* is entered into a cell to perform mathematical calculations in a worksheet. All formulas in Excel begin with the equals sign (=). After the equals sign, the addresses of the cells involved in the formula are entered between mathematical operators. The mathematical operators are + (addition), – (subtraction), * (multiplication), / (division), and ^ (exponentiation). An example of a valid formula is =A3*B3, which means that the value in A3 is multiplied by the value in B3 and the result is placed in the formula cell. By including the cell address in the formula rather than the actual value displayed in the cell, you can utilize the powerful recalculation feature in Excel. If you change the contents of a cell that is part of one or more formulas, the formula automatically recalculates so that all values in the worksheet are current.

Project

North Shore Medical Clinic

To calculate total hours and gross pay for the first two medical office assistants listed in the payroll worksheet for the North Shore Medical Clinic, you will use two methods to enter formulas.

1. With **EMedS1-NSMCPayJan31.xlsx** open, make cell J5 the active cell.

   Begin a formula by making active the cell in which you want the result to be placed.

2. Type **=C5+D5+E5+F5+G5+H5+I5** and then press Enter.

   The values in cells C5 through I5 are added and the result, *40*, is displayed in cell J5. You can type cell column letters in a formula in uppercase or lowercase letters. If you type lowercase column letters in a formula, Excel will convert the letters to uppercase when you press Enter.

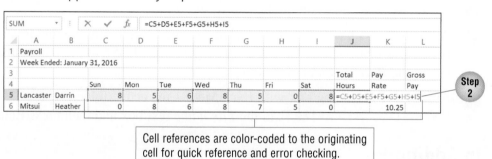

Cell references are color-coded to the originating cell for quick reference and error checking.

3. Press the Up Arrow key to make cell J5 the active cell.

   Notice that the result of the formula is displayed in the worksheet area and the formula used to calculate the result is shown in the Formula bar.

4. Make cell J6 the active cell, type the formula **=C6+D6+E6+F6+G6+H6+I6**, and then press Enter.

   Seem like too much typing? A more efficient way to add a series of cells to a formula will be introduced in the next activity.

5. Make cell L5 active.

   To calculate gross pay, you need to multiply the total hours by the pay rate. In Steps 6–10, you will enter this formula using the pointing method.

6. Type an equals sign (=).

7. Click in cell J5.

   A moving dashed border (called a *marquee*) displays around cell J5, indicating that it is the cell included in the formula, and the cell address is added to the formula cell (J5) with a blinking insertion point after the reference. Notice that the word POINT displays at the left side of the Status bar, which indicates that you are using the pointing method to create a formula.

8 Type an asterisk (*), which is the multiplication operator.

> The marquee surrounding cell J5 disappears. Cell J5 is color-coded with the same color used for the J5 cell reference within the formula cell.

9 Click in cell K5. A marquee displays around the cell and the cell address is added to the formula in cell L5. Both the cell and the reference display in the same color.

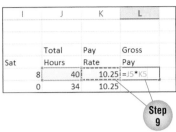

Step 9

Step 10

10 Click the Enter button ✓ on the Formula bar.

> The result, *410*, is displayed in cell L5. In Activity 1.6 you will learn how to display two decimal places for cells containing dollar values.

11 To calculate the gross pay for Heather Mitsui, type the formula **=J6*K6** in cell L6 and then press Enter.

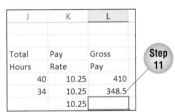

Step 11

12 Click the Save button on the Quick Access toolbar.

In Brief

Enter Formula
1. Activate formula cell.
2. Type =.
3. Type first cell address.
4. Type operator symbol.
5. Type second cell address.
6. Continue Steps 3–5 until finished.
7. Press Enter or click Enter button.

Enter Formula Using Pointing Method
1. Activate formula cell.
2. Type =.
3. Click first cell.
4. Type operator symbol.
5. Click second cell.
6. Repeat Steps 3–5 until finished.
7. Press Enter or click Enter button.

In Addition

Order of Operations

If you include several operators in a formula, Excel calculates the result using the following order of operations: negations (e.g., –1) first, then percents (%), then exponentiations (^), then multiplication and division (* and /), and finally addition and subtraction (+ and –). If a formula contains more than one operator at the same level of precedence—for example, both an addition and a subtraction operation—Excel calculates the equation from left to right. To change the order of operations, include parentheses around the part of the formula you want calculated first.

Formula	Calculation
=B5*C5/D5	Both operators are at the same level of precedence—Excel would multiply the value in B5 times the value in C5 and then divide the result by the value in D5.
=B5+B6+B7*C10	Multiplication takes precedence over addition, so Excel would first multiply the value in B7 times the value in C10. Excel would then take the value in B5, add to it the value in B6, and then add the result of the multiplication.
=(B5+B6+B7)*C10	Because of the parentheses, Excel would first add the values in B5 through B7, then multiply this sum times the value in C10.

Activity 1.4

Using the SUM Function

In the previous activity, the formulas used to calculate the hours worked by the first two employees were lengthy. A more efficient way to calculate the total hours is to use one of Excel's built-in functions, called SUM. A *function* is a preprogrammed formula. The structure of a formula utilizing a function begins with the equals sign (=), followed by the name of the function, and then the *argument*, which is the term given to the values identified within parentheses. For example, to calculate the total hours for Darrin Lancaster in cell J5, you would enter =*SUM(C5:I5)*. In this example, the argument C5:I5 contains the starting cell and the ending cell separated by a colon (:), which indicates a range, or a rectangular-shaped block of cells, to be summed. Since the SUM function is used frequently, an AutoSum button is available on the HOME tab.

Project

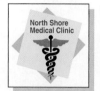

Lee Elliott, North Shore Medical Clinic's office manager, wants you to use a more efficient method of payroll calculation, so you will use the SUM function to calculate the hours worked.

1. With **EMedS1-NSMCPayJan31.xlsx** open, make cell J5 the active cell and then press the Delete key.

   This deletes the formula in the cell. Although there was nothing wrong with the formula already entered in cell J5, you are deleting it so that the formulas in the completed worksheet will be consistent.

2. Click the AutoSum button Σ in the Editing group on the HOME tab. (Make sure to click the button rather than the button arrow.) A marquee surrounds cells C5 through I5 and a ScreenTip appears below the formula cell indicating the correct format for the SUM function. Excel enters the formula =*SUM(C5:I5)* in cell J5.

   The suggested range C5:I5 is selected within the formula so that you can highlight a different range with the mouse if the suggested range is not correct.

Step 2

SUM		▾	:	✕	✓	f_x	=SUM(C5:I5)					
	A	B	C	D	E	F	G	H	I	J	K	L	M
1	Payroll												
2	Week Ended: January 31, 2016												
3										Total	Pay	Gross	
4			Sun	Mon	Tue	Wed	Thu	Fri	Sat	Hours	Rate	Pay	
5	Lancaster	Darrin	8	5	6	8	5	0	8	=SUM(C5:I5)		0	
6	Mitsui	Heather	0	8	6	8	7	5	0	SUM(**number1**, [number2], …)		5	
7	Elliott	Lee	8	8	0	8	7	7	0		10.25		
8	Melina	Jonathon	8	8	0	8	7	8	0		10.25		

3. Press Enter.

   Since the range suggested by Excel is correct, finish the formula by pressing Enter or by clicking the Enter button on the Formula bar.

4. With cell J6 the active cell, press the Delete key to delete the existing formula.

5. Click the AutoSum button. When Excel displays the formula =*SUM(C6:I6)*, click the Enter button in the Formula bar.

6. With cell J7 the active cell, click the AutoSum button.

   This time, the range of cells Excel is suggesting to add (J5:J6) is the wrong range. When you click the AutoSum button, Excel looks for multiple values in the cells immediately above the active cell. In this case, there are multiple values in the cells immediately above J7 so Excel inserts J5:J6 as the range in the SUM formula. You need to correct the range of cells that you want to add.

7 Position the cell pointer over cell C7, hold down the left mouse button, drag the pointer to the right to cell I7, and then release the mouse button.

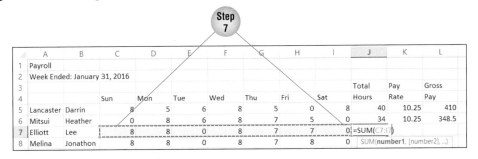

Step 7

	A	B	C	D	E	F	G	H	I	J	K	L
1	Payroll											
2	Week Ended: January 31, 2016											
3										Total	Pay	Gross
4			Sun	Mon	Tue	Wed	Thu	Fri	Sat	Hours	Rate	Pay
5	Lancaster	Darrin	8	5	6	8	5	0	8	40	10.25	410
6	Mitsui	Heather	0	8	6	8	7	5	0	34	10.25	348.5
7	Elliott	Lee	8	8	0	8	7	7	0	=SUM(C7:I7)		
8	Melina	Jonathon	8	8	0	8	7	8	0	SUM(**number1**, [number2], ...)		

8 Press Enter.

> Now that you have seen how the AutoSum button operates, you already know that the suggested range for the next employee's total hours will be incorrect. In Step 9, you will select the range of cells *first* to avoid the incorrect suggestion.

9 Position the cell pointer over cell C8, hold down the left mouse button, drag the pointer to cell J8, and then release the mouse button.

> Notice that you are including J8, the cell that will display the result, in the range of cells.

10 Click the AutoSum button.

> The result, *39*, appears in cell J8.

	A	B	C	D	E	F	G	H	I	J
1	Payroll									
2	Week Ended: January 31, 2016									
3									Total	Pay
4			Sun	Mon	Tue	Wed	Thu	Fri	Sat	Hours	Rate
5	Lancaster	Darrin	8	5	6	8	5	0	8	40
6	Mitsui	Heather	0	8	6	8	7	5	0	34
7	Elliott	Lee	8	8	0	8	7	7	0	38
8	Melina	Jonathon	8	8	0	8	7	8	0	39
9	St. Claire	Kari	0	8	0	8	8	7	0	

Steps 9-10

11 Click cell J8 and look in the Formula bar at the formula the SUM function created: *=SUM(C8:I8)*.

> Since Excel created the correct SUM formula from a range of selected cells, you decide to try calculating total hours for more than one employee in one step using the method employed in Steps 9 and 10 but with an expanded range.

12 Position the cell pointer over cell C9, hold down the left mouse button, drag the pointer down and to the right to cell J17, and then release the mouse button.

13 Click the AutoSum button.

14 Starting with J9 and ending with J17, click each of the cells to confirm that the correct formulas appear in the Formula bar.

	C	D	E	F	G	H	I	J
	Sun	Mon	Tue	Wed	Thu	Fri	Sat	Total Hours
	8	5	6	8	5	0	8	40
	0	8	6	8	7	5	0	34
	8	8	0	8	7	7	0	38
	8	8	0	8	7	8	0	39
	0	8	0	8	8	7	0	31
	0	0	0	8	8	7	8	31
	8	0	0	8	8	7	8	39
	8	0	0	8	8	7	8	39
	8	6	8	8	0	0	8	38
	0	5	8	8	6	0	8	35
	5	6	8	8	0	8	0	35
	6	4	8	8	0	8	0	34
	7	6	8	8	0	8	0	37

Steps 12-13

15 Click the Save button on the Quick Access toolbar.

Enter SUM Function
1. Make result cell active.
2. Click AutoSum button.
3. Press Enter or drag to select correct range and then press Enter.

OR

1. Drag to select range of cells to be summed, including result cell.
2. Click AutoSum button.

Activity 1.5

Copying Formulas

Many times you may create a worksheet in which several formulas are basically the same. For example, in the payroll worksheet, the formula to total the hours is =SUM(C5:I5) for Darrin Lancaster, =SUM(C6:I6) for Heather Mitsui, and so on. The only differences between the two formulas are the row numbers. Whenever formulas are this similar, you can use the Copy and Paste feature to copy the formula from one cell to another. The cell from which the original formula is copied is called the *source*, and the cell into which the formula is pasted is called the *destination*. When the formula is pasted, Excel automatically changes column letters or row numbers to reflect the destination location. By default, Excel assumes *relative addressing*—cell addresses update relative to the destination.

Project

To simplify your completion of the payroll worksheet for the North Shore Medical Clinic, you will copy formulas using two methods: Copy and Paste and the fill handle.

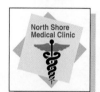

1. With **EMedS1-NSMCPayJan31.xlsx** open, make cell L6 active.

   This cell contains the formula =J6*K6 to calculate the gross pay for Heather Mitsui. You will copy this formula to the remaining cells in column L to complete the *Gross Pay* column.

2. Click the Copy button in the Clipboard group on the HOME tab. (Make sure to click the button rather than the button arrow.)

   A marquee surrounds the active cell, indicating that the source contents have been copied to the Clipboard, which is a temporary storage location. The content being copied is the formula =J6*K6 — not the value 348.5.

3. Select the range L7:L17. To do this, position the cell pointer over cell L7, hold down the left mouse button, drag the pointer down to cell L17, and then release the mouse button.

4. Click the Paste button in the Clipboard group. (Do not click the button arrow.)

   Excel pastes the formula into the selected cells and displays the results. The Paste Options button appears. Clicking this button will display a drop-down list with various alternatives for pasting the data. The marquee remains around the source cell and the destination cells remain highlighted. The marquee disappears as soon as you start another activity or press the Esc key.

5. Press the Esc key to remove the marquee and the Paste Options button, click cell L7, and then look at the entry in the Formula bar: =J7*K7.

   The row number in the source formula was increased by one to reflect the destination.

6. Use the Down Arrow key to check the remaining formulas in column L.

7. Make cell C19 active.

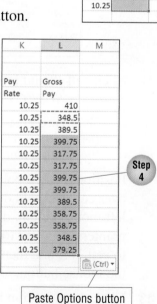

Paste Options button

8 Click the AutoSum button and then click the Enter button in the Formula bar.

> The SUM function inserts the formula =SUM(C5:C18). Next, you will copy the formula using the fill handle.

9 Drag the fill handle in cell C19 right to cell L19.

> When the active cell contains a formula, dragging the fill handle causes Excel to copy the formula and change the cell references relative to each destination.

In Brief
Copy Formula
1. Make source cell active.
2. Click Copy button.
3. Select destination cell(s).
4. Click Paste button.

	A	B	C	D	E	F	G	H	I	J	K	L
1	Payroll											
2	Week Ended: January 31, 2016											
3										Total	Pay	Gross
4			Sun	Mon	Tue	Wed	Thu	Fri	Sat	Hours	Rate	Pay
5	Lancaster	Darrin	8	5	6	8	5	0	8	40	10.25	410
6	Mitsui	Heather	0	8	6	8	7	5	0	34	10.25	348.5
7	Elliott	Lee	8	8	0	8	7	7	0	38	10.25	389.5
8	Melina	Jonathon	8	8	0	8	7	8	0	39	10.25	399.75
9	St. Claire	Kari	0	8	0	8	8	7	0	31	10.25	317.75
10	Cardenas	Maria	0	0	0	8	8	7	8	31	10.25	317.75
11	DiSanto	Stephen	8	0	0	8	8	7	8	39	10.25	399.75
12	Hydall	Patricia	8	0	0	8	8	7	8	39	10.25	399.75
13	Greer	Katherine	8	6	8	8	0	0	8	38	10.25	389.5
14	Freeman	Jason	0	5	8	8	6	0	8	35	10.25	358.75
15	Monroe	Mele	5	6	8	8	0	8	0	35	10.25	358.75
16	Hayden	Valerie	6	4	8	8	0	8	0	34	10.25	348.5
17	Keyes	Scott	7	6	8	8	0	8	0	37	10.25	379.25
18												
19	Total		66	64	52	104	64	72	48	470	133.25	4817.5
20												

Step 9

Need Help?

If the results do not appear in D15 through L15, you probably dragged the cell pointer instead of the fill handle. Click cell C15 and try again, making sure you drag using the thin black cross.

10 Make cell K19 the active cell and then press the Delete key.

> The sum of the *Pay Rate* column is not useful information.

11 Make D19 the active cell and then look at the entry in the Formula bar: =SUM(D5:D18).

> The column letters in the source formula were changed to reflect the destination.

12 Use the Right Arrow key to check the formulas in the remaining columns.

13 Click the Save button on the Quick Access toolbar.

In Addition

Understanding Copy and Paste versus Fill

What is the difference between Copy and Paste and the fill handle? When you use Copy, the contents of the source cell(s) are placed in the Clipboard. The data will remain in the Clipboard and can be pasted several times in the current worksheet or into an open document in another program.

Use Copy and Paste when the formula is to be inserted more than once into nonadjacent cells. Use the fill handle when the formula is only being copied to adjacent cells.

Activity 1.6

Testing a Worksheet; Improving Worksheet Appearance; Sorting

When you have finished building a worksheet, verifying the accuracy of the formulas you entered is a good idea. The worksheet could contain formulas that are correct in structure but not mathematically correct for the situation. For example, the wrong range may be included in a SUM formula, or parentheses missing from a multioperator formula may cause an incorrect result. Various methods can be employed to verify a worksheet's accuracy. One method is to create a proof formula in a cell beside or below the worksheet that will verify the totals. For example, in the payroll worksheet, the *Total Hours* column can be verified by creating a formula that adds all of the hours for all of the employees.

Data in Excel can be rearranged by sorting rows in ascending order or descending order. You can select a single column or define a custom sort to specify multiple columns that determine the sort order.

Project

To confirm the accuracy of your calculations in the payroll worksheet, you will enter proof formulas. You will then use two formatting options to improve the worksheet's appearance. Finally, you will sort the worksheet in ascending order by last name.

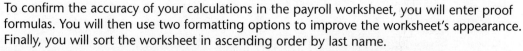

North Shore Medical Clinic

1. With **EMedS1-NSMCPayJan31.xlsx** open, make cell A21 the active cell.

2. Type **Hours**, press Alt + Enter, type **Proof**, and then press Enter.

Alt + Enter is the command to insert a line break in a cell. This command is used when you want multiple lines within the same cell. The height of the row automatically expands to accommodate the multiple lines.

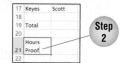

Step 2

3. Make cell B21 the active cell.

4. Click in the Formula bar, type **=SUM(C5:I17)**, and then click the Enter button or press Enter. (Alternatively, click the AutoSum button and then drag the pointer across the range of cells C5:I17.)

Excel displays the result, *470,* which verifies that the total hours amount in cell J19 is correct. Can you think of another formula that would have accomplished the same objective? *Hint: Think of the direction you added to arrive at the total hours in cell J19.*

Step 4

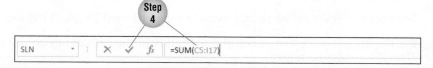

Need Help?

Didn't get 470? One of the cell entries is incorrect. Check your worksheet against the data provided in previous activities to see if the difference between 470 and your result is equal to a cell entry that you missed or mistyped.

5 Make cell A22 the active cell.

6 Type **Gross**, press Alt + Enter, type **Pay Proof**, and then press Enter.

7 Make cell B22 the active cell.

> Since all of the employees are paid at the same rate, you can verify the *Gross Pay* column by multiplying the total hours by the pay rate.

8 Type **=J19*K5** and then press the Right Arrow key.

> The result, *4817.5*, confirms that the value in cell L19 is correct. The importance of testing a worksheet cannot be emphasized enough. Worksheets often contain important financial or statistical data that can form the basis for strategic business decisions.

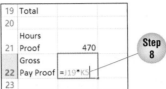

9 Look at the completed worksheet shown below. Notice that some of the values in column L show no decimals while others show 1 or 2 decimal places. Also notice that the labels do not align directly over the values below them.

Labels do not align directly over values.

	A	B	C	D	E	F	G	H	I	J	K	L
1	Payroll											
2	Week Ended: January 31, 2016											
3										Total	Pay	Gross
4			Sun	Mon	Tue	Wed	Thu	Fri	Sat	Hours	Rate	Pay
5	Lancaster	Darrin	8	5	6	8	5	0	8	40	10.25	410
6	Mitsui	Heather	0	8	6	8	7	5	0	34	10.25	348.5
7	Elliott	Lee	8	8	0	8	7	7	0	38	10.25	389.5
8	Melina	Jonathon	8	8	0	8	7	8	0	39	10.25	399.75
9	St. Claire	Kari	0	8	0	8	8	7	0	31	10.25	317.75
10	Cardenas	Maria	0	0	0	8	8	7	8	31	10.25	317.75
11	DiSanto	Stephen	8	0	0	8	8	7	8	39	10.25	399.75
12	Hydall	Patricia	8	0	0	8	8	7	8	39	10.25	399.75
13	Greer	Katherine	8	6	8	8	0	0	8	38	10.25	389.5
14	Freeman	Jason	0	5	8	8	6	0	8	35	10.25	358.75
15	Monroe	Mele	5	6	8	8	0	8	0	35	10.25	358.75
16	Hayden	Valerie	6	4	8	8	0	8	0	34	10.25	348.5
17	Keyes	Scott	7	6	8	8	0	8	0	37	10.25	379.25
18												
19	Total		66	64	52	104	64	72	48	470		4817.5
20												
21	Hours Proof	470										
22	Gross Pay Proof	4817.5										
23												

Decimal places are not consistent.

continues

10 Select the range of cells L5:L19.

These final steps in building a worksheet are meant to improve the appearance of cells. In column L, Excel uses up to 15 decimal places for precision when calculating values. Since the *Gross Pay* column represents a sum of money, you will format these cells using the Accounting format.

11 Click the Accounting Number Format button $\boxed{\$}$ in the Number group on the HOME tab.

The Accounting format adds a dollar sign, a comma in the thousands place, and two decimal places to each value in the selection.

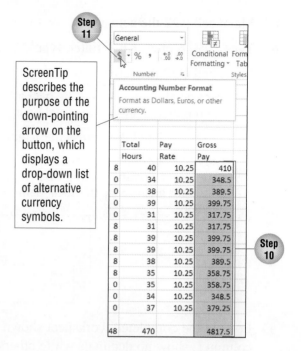

Step 11

ScreenTip describes the purpose of the down-pointing arrow on the button, which displays a drop-down list of alternative currency symbols.

Step 10

Accounting Number Format
Format as Dollars, Euros, or other currency.

Total Hours	Pay Rate	Gross Pay
8	40	10.25	410
0	34	10.25	348.5
0	38	10.25	389.5
0	39	10.25	399.75
0	31	10.25	317.75
8	31	10.25	317.75
8	39	10.25	399.75
8	39	10.25	399.75
8	38	10.25	389.5
8	35	10.25	358.75
0	35	10.25	358.75
0	34	10.25	348.5
0	37	10.25	379.25
48	470		4817.5

12 Make cell B22 the active cell and then click the Accounting Number Format button.

13 Select the range of cells C3:L4.

As previously mentioned, labels are aligned at the left edge of a column while values are aligned at the right edge. In the next step, you will align the labels at the right edge of the column so they appear directly over the corresponding values.

14 Click the Align Right button $\boxed{\equiv}$ in the Alignment group on the HOME tab.

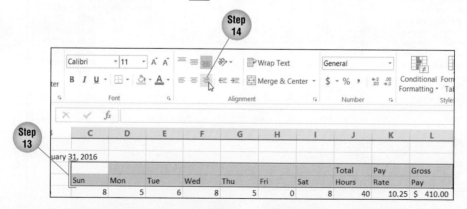

Step 14

Step 13

15 Click in any cell to deselect the range.

In the next steps, you will sort the names in the payroll worksheet so that they are in alphabetical order by last name.

16 Select the range of cells A5:L17.

You are selecting the range before performing the sort since you do not want to include the cells above and below the list of names in the sort.

17 Click the Sort & Filter button in the Editing group on the HOME tab.

18 Click *Sort A to Z* at the drop-down list.

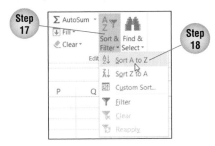

Step 17

Step 18

19 Click in any cell to deselect the range. Compare your sorted worksheet to the one shown below.

	A	B	C	D	E	F	G	H	I	J	K	L
1	Payroll											
2	Week Ended: January 31, 2016											
3										Total	Pay	Gross
4			Sun	Mon	Tue	Wed	Thu	Fri	Sat	Hours	Rate	Pay
5	Cardenas	Maria	0	0	0	8	8	7	8	31	10.25	$ 317.75
6	DiSanto	Stephen	8	0	0	8	8	7	8	39	10.25	$ 399.75
7	Elliott	Lee	8	8	0	8	7	7	0	38	10.25	$ 389.50
8	Freeman	Jason	0	5	8	8	6	0	8	35	10.25	$ 358.75
9	Greer	Katherine	8	6	8	8	0	0	8	38	10.25	$ 389.50
10	Hayden	Valerie	6	4	8	8	0	8	0	34	10.25	$ 348.50
11	Hydall	Patricia	8	0	0	8	8	7	8	39	10.25	$ 399.75
12	Keyes	Scott	7	6	8	8	0	8	0	37	10.25	$ 379.25
13	Lancaster	Darrin	8	5	6	8	5	0	8	40	10.25	$ 410.00
14	Melina	Jonathon	8	8	0	8	7	8	0	39	10.25	$ 399.75
15	Mitsui	Heather	0	8	6	8	7	5	0	34	10.25	$ 348.50
16	Monroe	Mele	5	6	8	8	0	8	0	35	10.25	$ 358.75
17	St. Claire	Kari	0	8	0	8	8	7	0	31	10.25	$ 317.75
18												
19	Total		66	64	52	104	64	72	48	470		$4,817.50
20												
21	Hours Proof	470										
22	Gross Pay Proof	$4,817.50										

employees sorted in ascending alphabetical order by last name

20 Click the Save button on the Quick Access toolbar.

In Addition

Rotating Text in Cells

The Alignment group on the HOME tab contains an Orientation button, which can be used to rotate text within cells. Text can be rotated counterclockwise, clockwise, changed to vertical alignment, rotated up vertically, or rotated down vertically. Often, text set in narrow columns is angled to improve the label appearance. In the image shown at the right, the cells containing the days of the week in the payroll worksheet are angled down counterclockwise.

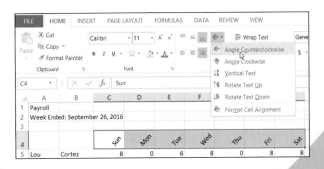

Activity 1.7

Using Help

An extensive online Help resource is available that contains information on Excel features and commands. Click the Microsoft Excel Help button located near the upper right corner of the screen to display the Excel Help window. By default, the Help feature searches for an Internet connection. If you are not connected to the Internet, an offline message displays in the Excel Help window. Make sure you are connected to the Internet to complete the steps in the activity. Another way to access Help resources is to point to a button on a tab and then press the F1 function key.

Project

Lee Elliott reviewed the payroll worksheet you created. Lee thinks the first two title rows would look better if they were centered over the columns in the worksheet. You will use the Help feature to look up the steps to do this.

1 With **EMedS1-NSMCPayJan31.xlsx** open, make cell A1 the active cell.

To center the title rows above the columns in the worksheet, you decide to browse the buttons in the Alignment group on the HOME tab. The Merge & Center button seems appropriate but you are not sure of the steps to work with this feature.

2 Point to the Merge & Center button in the Alignment group on the HOME tab and read the information that displays in the ScreenTip.

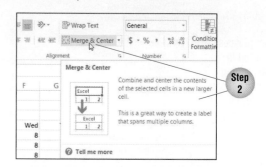

3 With the pointer still resting on the Merge & Center button, press the F1 function key and then read the information on merging cells that displays in the Excel Help window. Make sure you scroll down the window and read all of the information provided by Excel Help.

4 Close the Excel Help window by clicking the Close button in the upper right corner of the window.

5 Select the range of cells A1:L1 and then click the Merge & Center button in the Alignment group on the HOME tab.

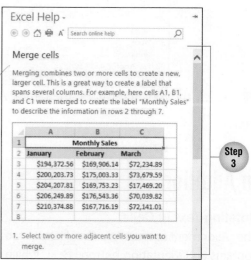

Cell A1 is merged across columns A through L and the text *Payroll* is automatically centered within the merged cell.

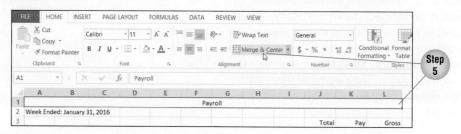

6 Select the range of cells A2:L2 and then click the Merge & Center button.

The two titles in the payroll worksheet are now centered over the cells below them.

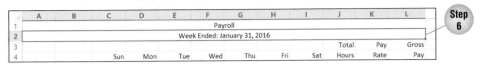

In Brief

Use Help
1. Click Microsoft Excel Help button.
2. Type search text.
3. Click Search online help button.
4. Click desired hyperlink.

7 Click the Microsoft Excel Help button [?] located near the upper right corner of the screen.

You can also access Help resources by typing a search phrase and browsing related topics in the Help window.

8 Click in the search text box, type **preview worksheet**, and then click the Search online help button or press Enter.

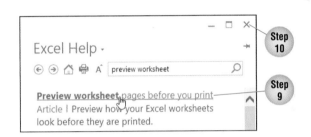

9 Click the <u>Preview worksheet pages before you print</u> hyperlink and then read the information that displays in the window.

Since Microsoft Office Online is updated frequently, your search results list may vary. The hyperlink may have a slightly different title or position within the list.

10 Close the Excel Help window.

11 Click the Save button on the Quick Access toolbar.

In Addition

Using Excel Help Window Buttons

The Excel Help window contains five buttons that display to the left of the search box. Use the Back and Forward buttons to navigate in the window. Click the Home button to return to the Excel Help window opening screen. If you want to print information on a topic or feature, click the Print button and then click the Print button at the Print dialog box. You can make the text in the Excel Help window larger by clicking the Use Large Text button. In addition to these five buttons, the Excel Help window contains a Pin Help button located near the upper right corner of the window. Click this button and the Excel Help window remains on the screen, even as you work in a worksheet. Click the button again to remove (unpin) the window from the screen.

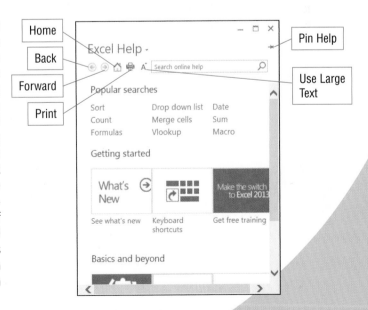

Activity 1.8

Previewing; Changing Page Orientation; Printing a Workbook

Many times a worksheet is printed to create a paper copy, or **hard copy**, that can be filed or attached to a report. Large, complex worksheets are often easier to proofread and reference in hard copy. Display the Print backstage area to preview the worksheet and modify print options. To display the Print backstage area, click the FILE tab and then click the *Print* option. At the Print backstage area, a preview of how the worksheet will look when printed displays at the right side.

The center of the Print backstage area is divided into three sections: *Print, Printer,* and *Settings*. Use the galleries in each category to modify print options. For example, to change the page orientation of a worksheet, click the third button from the top in the *Settings* section (contains the text *Portrait Orientation*). Click *Landscape Orientation* at the drop-down list. Once you have selected all of the desired printing options, click the Print button in the *Print* section to print the worksheet.

Project

The payroll worksheet Is finished. You want to preview the worksheet and then print a copy for the office manager.

1. With **EMedS1-NSMCPayJan31.xlsx** open, make cell A24 the active cell and then type the student information your instructor has directed you to include on printouts. For example, type your first and last names and then press Enter.

   Make sure you have checked with your instructor as to whether you should include other identifying information such as your program or class number.

2. Click the FILE tab and then click the *Print* option to display the worksheet in the Print backstage area as shown in Figure E1.2.

FIGURE E1.2 Print Backstage Area

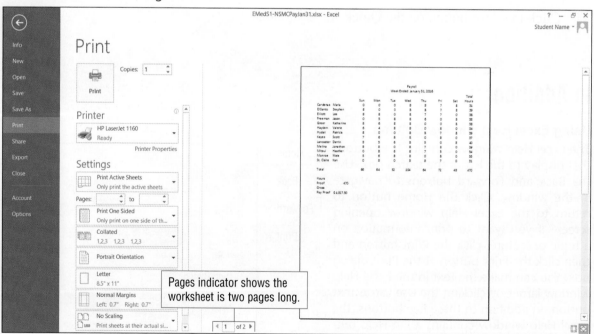

3 The right side of the backstage area displays the first page of the worksheet as it will look when printed with the current print options. The pages indicator at the bottom left of the preview shows that you are viewing page 1 of 2 pages. Click the Next Page button ▶ at the right of the indicator to display page 2.

4 The second page of the printout appears, showing the columns that could not fit on page 1.

5 Click the orientation gallery (currently displays *Portrait Orientation*) in the *Settings* category of the Print backstage area.

> One way to fit the printout on one page is to change the orientation from portrait to landscape. In *portrait* orientation, the content is printed on paper that is taller than it is wide. In *landscape* orientation, the content is rotated to print on paper that is wider than it is tall.

6 Click *Landscape Orientation* at the drop-down list.

> The preview updates to show the worksheet in landscape orientation. Notice that all of the columns now fit on one page.

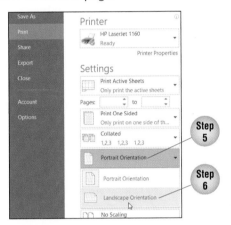

7 Click the Print button.

> The Print backstage area closes and the worksheet prints on the default printer. The default settings in the Print backstage area are to print one copy of all pages in the active worksheet. You will learn how to further adjust page layout and print settings in a later section.

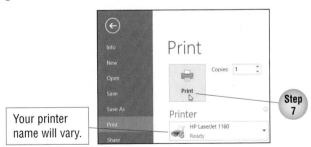

Your printer name will vary.

8 At the worksheet, scroll to the right until you see the vertical dashed line between columns located to the right of the *Gross Pay* column.

> The dashed vertical line represents a page break. Page breaks display in a worksheet after you have previewed or printed it. A worksheet containing more rows than can fit on one page will display a horizontal dashed line below the last row that can fit on the page. The dashed lines do not print.

9 Click the Save button on the Quick Access toolbar.

In Brief

Preview Worksheet
1. Click FILE tab.
2. Click *Print* option.

Change to Landscape Orientation
1. Click FILE tab.
2. Click *Print* option.
3. Click orientation gallery.
4. Click *Landscape Orientation*.

Activity 1.9

Displaying Formulas; Navigating a Worksheet

Sometimes you may want to print a worksheet with the formulas, rather than the formula results, displayed in the cells. Printing a second copy of a worksheet with the cell formulas displayed is a good idea when the worksheet contains complicated formulas that would take you a long time to recreate. To display cell formulas, click the FORMULAS tab and then click the Show Formulas button in the Formula Auditing group. You can also display formulas with the keyboard shortcut Ctrl + `. Displaying formulas in worksheet cells causes the cells to expand, which means you

may need to scroll to the right or scroll down to locate certain data or cells. To scroll with the mouse, use the horizontal and vertical scroll bars. Scrolling using the scroll bars does not change which cell is currently active. You can also scroll using the arrow keys or other keyboard commands. Scrolling using the keyboard changes which cell is currently active. To navigate to a specific cell in a worksheet, use the Go To feature. Display the Go To dialog box by clicking the Find & Select button in the Editing group on the HOME tab and then clicking *Go To* at the drop-down list.

Project

You will print a second copy of the payroll worksheet with the cell formulas displayed and then practice navigating the worksheet using the scroll bars and keyboard shortcuts.

1 With **EMedS1-NSMCPayJan31.xlsx** open, click the FORMULAS tab.

2 Click the Show Formulas button in the Formula Auditing group.

> The cells in the worksheet are automatically expanded and cells that contain formulas now display the formula rather than the formula results.

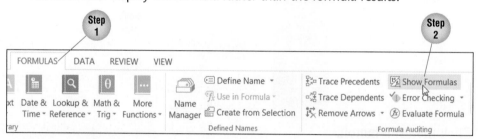

3 Click the FILE tab and then click the *Print* option.

4 At the Print backstage area, click the Print button.

> The worksheet will print on two pages in the expanded cell formulas view. In a later section you will learn how to adjust column widths and scale a worksheet to reduce the number of pages on which it prints.

5 Position the mouse pointer on the right scroll arrow at the right edge of the horizontal scroll bar and then click the left mouse button a few times to scroll to the right edge of the worksheet.

6 Position the mouse pointer on the horizontal scroll box, hold down the left mouse button, drag the scroll box to the left edge of the horizontal scroll bar, and then release the mouse button.

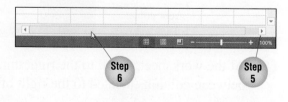

> The width or height of the scroll box indicates the proportional amount of the used cells in the worksheet that are visible in the current window. The position of the scroll box within the scroll bar indicates the relative location of the visible cells within the remainder of the worksheet.

7 Press Ctrl + Home to make cell A1 the active cell.

8 Press the Page Down key once.

> Each time you press the Page Down key, you move the active cell down one screen.

9 Press the Page Up key once.

> Each time you press the Page Up key, you move the active cell up one screen.

10 Click the Find & Select button 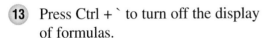 in the Editing group on the HOME tab and then click *Go To* at the drop-down list.

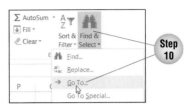

Step 10

11 At the Go To dialog box, type **L15** in the *Reference* text box and then click OK or press Enter.

> Notice that using Go To changed the active cell to cell L15 and made the cell visible on the screen.

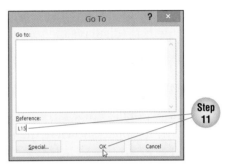

12 Use the Up, Down, Left, and Right Arrow keys to practice moving around the worksheet.

> Holding down a directional arrow key causes the screen to scroll very quickly. Table E1.2 provides more keyboard shortcuts you can use to navigate in a worksheet.

Step 11

13 Press Ctrl + ` to turn off the display of formulas.

> The ` symbol is the grave symbol. On the keyboard, it is usually located immediately to the left of the 1 key.

14 Click the Save button on the Quick Access toolbar.

15 Click the FILE tab and then click the *Close* option at the backstage area.

In Brief
Go to Specific Cell
1. Click Find & Select button.
2. Click *Go To*.
3. Type cell address.
4. Click OK.

TABLE E1.2 Keyboard Navigation Shortcuts

Press	To move to
Arrow keys	one cell up, down, left, or right
Ctrl + Home	A1
Ctrl + End	last cell in worksheet
Home	beginning of row
Page Down	down one screen
Page Up	up one screen
Alt + Page Down	one screen to the right
Alt + Page Up	one screen to the left

In Addition

Displaying Formulas at the Excel Options Dialog Box

In addition to the Show Formulas button on the FORMULAS tab and the keyboard shortcut, you can also display formulas at the Excel Options dialog box. Display this dialog box by clicking the FILE tab and then clicking *Options*. At the Excel Options dialog box, click *Advanced* in the left panel, click the *Show formulas in cells instead of their calculated results* check box in the *Display options for this worksheet* section to insert a check mark, and then click OK.

Activity 1.10

Creating a Workbook from a Template

Excel includes worksheets that are formatted for specific purposes such as creating budgets, sales invoices, inventories, timecards, and financial statements. These preformatted worksheets are called *templates*. Templates can be customized and saved with a new name to reflect individual company data. Templates are available at the New backstage area and can be downloaded from Office.com.

Project

Darrin Lancaster has asked you to complete an invoice for a recent exam. You decide to use a template to do this since the template has formulas already entered.

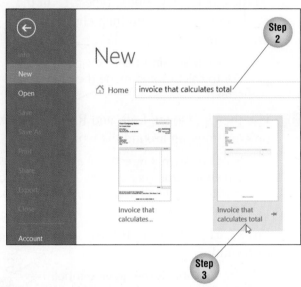

1. Click the FILE tab and then click the *New* option.

2. At the New backstage area, search for invoice templates by clicking in the search text box (displays the text *Search for online templates*), typing **invoice that calculates total**, and then pressing Enter.

3. Double-click the invoice template shown at the right.

4. Review the template, observing the type of information required and the way data is arranged on the page. Save the workbook in the ExcelMedS1 folder with the name **EMedS1-NSMCInvoice**.

5. Click in cell A2 (displays the text *Your Company Name*), type **North Shore Medical Clinic**, and then press Enter.

6. Type **7450 Meridian Street, Suite 150** and then press Enter.

7. Type **Portland, OR 97202** and then press Enter.

8. Type **(503) 555-2330** and then press Enter.

9. Type **dlancaster@emcp.net** and then press Enter four times.

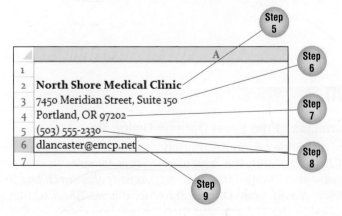

10 With cell A10 the active cell (displays the text *Name*), type **AJ Estman** and then press Enter.

11 Press the Delete key to remove the text in cell A11 and then press Enter.

12 Type **430 Island Drive** and then press Enter.

13 Type **Portland, OR 97204** and then press Enter.

14 Type **(503) 555-1578** and then press Enter.

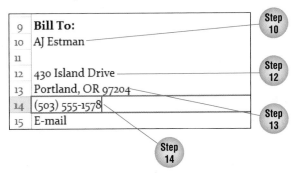

15 Press the Delete key to remove the text in cell A15.

16 Enter the following data in the specified cells:
    A19:   **Annual Physical Exam**
    B19:   **143.81**
    A20:   **Lab Analysis: Blood, Urine**
    B20:   **109.45**

Notice how the total amount is automatically calculated in cell B21 because the template included a formula.

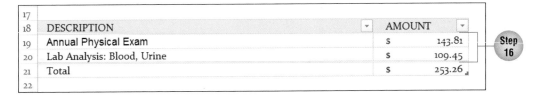

17 Save, print and then close **EMedS1-NSMCInvoice.xlsx**.

In Addition

Pinning a Template

If you use a template on a regular basis, consider pinning the template to the New backstage area. To do this, hover your mouse over the template and then click the gray left-pointing stick pin (*Pin this item to the list*.) that displays to the right of the template name. To unpin the template, click the down-pointing stick pin (*Unpin this item from the list*).

Features Summary

Feature	Ribbon Tab, Group	Button	Quick Access Toolbar	FILE Tab Option	Keyboard Shortcut
Accounting format	HOME, Number	$			
align right	HOME, Alignment	≡		*Options*	
close a workbook				*Close*	Ctrl + F4
copy	HOME, Clipboard	🗐			Ctrl + C
fill down	HOME, Editing	⬇, *Down*			Ctrl + D
fill left	HOME, Editing	⬇, *Left*			
fill right	HOME, Editing	⬇, *Right*			Ctrl + R
fill up	HOME, Editing	⬇, *Up*			
Go To	HOME, Editing	🔍			Ctrl + G
Help		?			F1
insert line break					Alt + Enter
merge and center	HOME, Alignment	⬌			
new workbook				*New*	Ctrl + N
Open backstage area				*Open*	Ctrl + O
Open dialog box					Ctrl + F12
paste	HOME, Clipboard	📋			Ctrl + V
Print backstage area				*Print*	Ctrl + P or Ctrl + F2
save			💾	*Save*	Ctrl + S
save with a new name				*Save As*	F12
show formulas	FORMULAS, Formula Auditing	🔢			Ctrl + `
sort	HOME, Editing	A/Z▼			
SUM function	HOME, Editing	Σ			Alt + =

Knowledge Check

Completion: In the space provided at the right, write in the correct term, command, formula, or option.

1. This area of the Excel screen contains options and buttons divided into tabs and groups.   _____

2. This area displays the formula stored within the cell (not the result).   _____

3. The cell pointer changes to this when pointing to the small green square in the bottom right corner of the active cell.   _____

4. You would enter this formula to divide the contents of cell C6 by the contents of cell C12.   _____

5. This is the term for the method used to create a formula by typing the equals sign and operator symbols and clicking to insert the cell references.   _____

6. This term is used to refer to the values identified within parentheses in the SUM function.   _____

7. The AutoSum button is located in this group on the HOME tab.   _____

8. Do this action if Excel suggests the wrong range after you click the AutoSum button.   _____

9. This button appears after copied cells are pasted into the destination.   _____

10. This is the term for the formulas entered beside or below a worksheet to verify the worksheet's accuracy.   _____

11. This format adds a dollar sign, a comma in the thousands place, and two decimal places to each value in the selected range.   _____

12. Click the Sort & Filter button in the Editing group on the HOME tab and then click this option at the drop-down list to sort a list in ascending order.   _____

13. This keyboard shortcut will display the Excel Help window when you are pointing to a button.   _____

14. Display this backstage area to change the page orientation.   _____

15. Open this dialog box to type the address of a cell that you want to make active.   _____

Skills Review

Note: If you submit your work in hard copy, check with your instructor before completing these reviews to find out if you need to print two copies of each worksheet with one of the copies showing the cell formulas instead of the calculated results.

Review 1 Entering Labels and Values; Formatting Cells

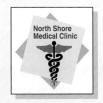

North Shore
Medical Clinic

1. Create a new workbook using the Blank workbook template.
2. Enter the labels and data shown in Figure E1.3. Use the fill handle whenever possible to facilitate data entry. Do not format the cells.
3. Select the range of cells G12:G20 and then apply the Accounting format.
4. Deselect the range and then save the workbook with the name **EMedS1-R-NSMCPOtoMedCare**.

FIGURE E1.3 Review 1 Worksheet

	A	B	C	D	E	F	G
1	North Shore Medical Clinic						
2	Purchase Order						
3							
4	Vendor:						
5	Medcare Medical Supplies			Telephone		Fax	
6	1913 NE 7th Avenue			(503) 555-4589		(800) 555-6315	
7	Portland, OR 97212-3906						
8							
9							
10							
11	Item				Order Qty	Unit	Price
12	Disposable shoe cover				1	per 300	38.15
13	Disposable bouffant cap				1	per 100	7.91
14	Disposable examination table paper				8	per roll	9.1
15	Disposable patient gown				8	per doz.	8.25
16	Disposable patient slippers				8	per doz.	4.35
17	Disposable skin staple remover				8	per doz.	35.9
18	Dispoasable skin stapler				8	per doz.	42.55
19	Disposable thermometer tips				8	per 100	5.13
20	Disposable earloop mask				8	per 50	6.48
21							

Review 2 Entering and Copying Formulas; Using AutoSum

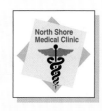

1. With **EMedS1-R-NSMCPOtoMedCare.xlsx** open, enter the following labels and create the following formulas by typing them into the Formula bar or the cell, using the pointing method, or clicking the AutoSum button:
   a. In cell H11, type the label **Line Total**.
   b. In cell H12, multiply the order quantity by the price by entering **=E12*G12**.
   c. Use the fill handle to copy the formula to cells H13:H20.
   d. In cell F22, type the label **Subtotal**.
   e. In cell H22, use a Sum function to add the range of cells H12:H20.
   f. In cell F23, type the label **Shipping**.
   g. In cell H23, type the value **25**.
   h. In cell F24, type the label **Order Total**.
   i. In cell H24, calculate the purchase order total by entering **=H22+H23**.
2. Apply the Accounting format to cell H23.
3. Save **EMedS1-R-NSMCPOtoMedCare.xlsx**.

Review 3 Improving the Appearance of the Worksheet; Previewing and Printing

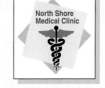

1. With **EMedS1-R-NSMCPOtoMedCare.xlsx** open, select cells A1:H1 and then click the Merge & Center button.
2. Merge and center cells A2:H2.
3. Select the range of cells E11:H11 and then apply center alignment.
4. Select the range of cells E12:E20 and then apply center alignment.
5. Make cell A9 the active cell, type the following label, and then press Enter: **Terms: 1%/10, net 30 days. No substitutions.**
6. Display the worksheet in the Print backstage area. Preview and then print the worksheet.
7. Save **EMedS1-R-NSMCPOtoMedCare.xlsx**.

Review 4 Using Help

1. With **EMedS1-R-NSMCPOtoMedCare.xlsx** open, display the Excel Help window, type **How do I add a background color?** in the search box, and then press Enter.
2. Scroll down the search results list and then click the <u>Apply or remove a cell shading format</u> hyperlink.
3. Read the information displayed in the Excel Help window about filling cells with solid colors.
4. Close the Excel Help window.
5. Select the range of cells A11:H11 and then apply the Blue, Accent 5, Lighter 60% fill color using the Fill color button in the Font group, as you learned in Help.
6. Select the range of cells A1:A2 and then apply the Blue, Accent 5, Lighter 40% fill color.
7. Deselect cells A1:A2.
8. Save, print, and then close **EMedS1-R-NSMCPOtoMedCare.xlsx**.

Skills Assessment

Note: If you submit your work in hard copy, check with your instructor before completing these assessments to find out if you need to print two copies of each worksheet with one of the copies showing the cell formulas instead of the calculated results.

Assessment 1 Adding Values and Formulas to a Worksheet

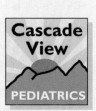

1. Open **CVPTravelExpenses.xlsx**.
2. Save the workbook with the name **EMedS1-A1-CVPTravelExpenses**.
3. You have been asked by Sydney Larsen, office manager at Cascade View Pediatrics, to calculate the estimated travel expenses for the American Academy of Pediatrics members who will be attending the International Pediatric Medical Conference in Toronto, Ontario, Canada, May 22–26. Sydney has already received quotes for airfare, hotel, and airport transfers. This information is summarized below.
   - Return airfare from Portland to Toronto is $566.00 per person.
   - Sydney has negotiated a hotel rate of $536.75 per room for the duration, with two persons per room.
   - Airport Transfer Limousine Service charges a flat rate of $75.00 in Toronto and $55.00 in Portland for all travelers.
   - All of the above prices include taxes and fees and are quoted in U.S. dollars.
   - Members attending the conference include:
        Dr. Raphaël Severin
        Dr. Joseph Yarborough
        Dr. Beth Delaney
        Deanna Reynolds, Child Development Specialist
4. Cascade View Pediatrics reimburses all traveling employees for food expenses at the rate of $70.00 per day.
5. Enter the appropriate values and formulas to complete the worksheet.
6. Make any formatting changes you think would improve the appearance of the worksheet.
7. Save, print, and then close **EMedS1-A1-CVPTravelExpenses.xlsx**.

Assessment 2 Creating a New Workbook for a Seminar

1. Sydney Larsen, office manager of Cascade View Pediatrics, has asked you to prepare a cost estimate for a seminar on ADHD treatment strategies that Dr. Beth Delaney is hosting for the local chapter of the American Academy of Pediatrics. Using the following information, create a worksheet that will calculate the total seminar costs and the registration fee that needs to be charged to each member in order to cover these costs.
   a. Create a new workbook using the Blank workbook template and then create a worksheet to summarize the seminar costs for 75 members using the following prices:
      - Rental fee for the meeting room at the Hilton Portland & Executive Tower is $50.00.
      - Rental fee for the audio-visual equipment Dr. Delaney needs for her presentation is $45.00 for the day.
      - Handouts, name badges, and other materials have been estimated at $23.95 (for all supplies).
      - Morning coffee and refreshments are quoted at $2.17 per person.
      - Lunch is quoted at $7.90 per person.

b. Calculate the total cost.

c. In a separate row below the total cost, calculate the cost per member.

2. Make any formatting changes you think would improve the appearance of the worksheet.

3. Save the workbook and name it **EMedS1-A2-CVPADHDSeminar**.

4. Print and then close **EMedS1-A2-CVPADHDSeminar.xlsx**.

Assessment 3 Creating a New Workbook to Estimate Funds Needed

Columbia
River
General
Hospital

1. Laura Latterell, education director at Columbia River General Hospital, has asked you to prepare an estimate of the funds needed in the professional development budget for 2016. Professional development funding includes in-service sessions, continuing education course fees, and conference registration fees. All other related costs such as travel expenses are funded directly from each medical professional's department budget. Create a new workbook to calculate the total 2016 professional development budget. Include a subtotal for each category of funded professional development.

2. A survey of the department managers has provided the following information:
   • There are in-service training requests for 15 sessions throughout the year. Sessions are run by consultants Laura hires at the rate of $60.00 per session.
   • There are the following requests for continuing education courses:

       18 requests for doctors at $350.00 per course
       30 requests for nurses at $295.00 per course
       12 requests for respiratory therapists at $185.00 per course
       14 requests for anesthesiologists at $192.00 per course
       11 requests for radiologists at $195.00 per course
       10 requests for physical therapists at $160.00 per course
       10 requests for management staff at $150.00 per course
       10 requests for support staff at $135.00 per course

3. The hospital buys block registrations for the following conferences:

American Medical Association national annual conference	$6,500.00
American Academy of Nursing annual conference	$5,750.00
International Respiratory Congress	$4,100.00
Radiological Society of North America annual meeting	$2,250.00
American Society of Anesthesiologists annual conference	$3,700.00
American Physical Therapy Association annual conference	$1,775.00
American Hospital Association annual meeting	$1,950.00

4. Make any formatting changes you think would improve the appearance of the workbook.

5. Save the workbook with the name **EMedS1-A3-CRGHPDBudget**.

6. Print and then close **EMedS1-A3-CRGHPDBudget.xlsx**.

Assessment 4 Experimenting with Hiding Zero Values

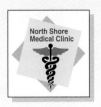

1. Open **NSMCSupplies.xlsx**.
2. Save the workbook with the name **EMedS1-A4-NSMCSupplies**.
3. Open the Excel Options dialog box and then click *Advanced* in the left pane. Scroll down to the section titled *Display options for this worksheet*.
4. Click the *Show a zero in cells that have zero value* check box to remove the check mark and then click OK. Notice that all cells in the worksheet that had a zero value now display as blank cells.
5. At the Print backstage area, change the page orientation to landscape.
6. Print page 1 of the worksheet.
7. Save and then close **EMedS1-A4-NSMCSupplies.xlsx**.

Assessment 5 Creating a School Budget

1. Create a worksheet to calculate the estimated total cost of completing your diploma or certificate. You determine the items that need to be included in the worksheet. You might include tuition fees, textbooks, supplies, accommodation costs, transportation, telephone, food, and entertainment. Use the Internet to find reasonable cost estimates if you do not want to use your own personal data. Arrange the labels and values by quarter, semester, or academic year according to your preference. Make sure to include a cell that shows the total cost of your education.
2. Save the worksheet with the name **EMedS1-A5-SchoolBudget**.
3. Apply alignment and formatting options as necessary to improve the appearance of the worksheet.
4. If necessary, change the page orientation to landscape and then print the worksheet.
5. Save and then close **EMedS1-A5-SchoolBudget.xlsx**.

Marquee Challenge

Challenge 1   Preparing a Surgery Average Cost Report

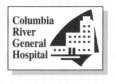

1. At a blank workbook, enter the data shown in Figure E1.4.
2. Use the following information to complete the worksheet:
   a. Total average cost in column K is the sum of items starting with column F (*Ward*) and ending with column J (*Pharmacy*).
   b. Total cost of all cases in column L is column K (*Total Avg Cost*) times column D (*Cases*).
3. Apply the Accounting format to the values in columns K and L.
4. Add a grand total for all cases at the bottom of column L. Label the value appropriately.
5. Save the workbook with the name **EMedS1-C1-CRGHAvgCostAnalysis**.
6. At the Print backstage area, change the page orientation to landscape and then print the worksheet.
7. Close **EMedS1-C1-CRGHAvgCostAnalysis.xlsx**.

Challenge 2   Completing an Invoice

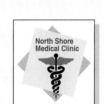

1. Use a template to create the worksheet shown in Figure E1.5 on page 262. At the New backstage area, click in the *Search for online templates* text box and then type **invoice with tax**.
2. Double-click the *Service invoice with tax calculation* template.
3. Enter the information and data shown in Figure E1.5, letting the formulas calculate the amount, subtotal, sales tax, and total.
4. Save the workbook with the name **EMedS1-C2-NSMCInvToCRGH**.
5. Print and then close **EMedS1-C2-NSMCInvToCRGH.xlsx**.

FIGURE E1.4 Challenge 1

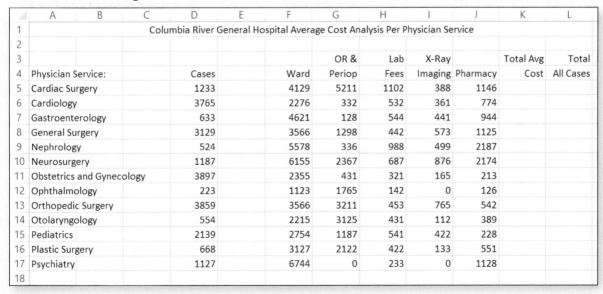

	A	B	C	D	E	F	G	H	I	J	K	L
1	Columbia River General Hospital Average Cost Analysis Per Physician Service											
2												
3							OR &	Lab	X-Ray		Total Avg	Total
4	Physician Service:			Cases		Ward	Periop	Fees	Imaging	Pharmacy	Cost	All Cases
5	Cardiac Surgery			1233		4129	5211	1102	388	1146		
6	Cardiology			3765		2276	332	532	361	774		
7	Gastroenterology			633		4621	128	544	441	944		
8	General Surgery			3129		3566	1298	442	573	1125		
9	Nephrology			524		5578	336	988	499	2187		
10	Neurosurgery			1187		6155	2367	687	876	2174		
11	Obstetrics and Gynecology			3897		2355	431	321	165	213		
12	Ophthalmology			223		1123	1765	142	0	126		
13	Orthopedic Surgery			3859		3566	3211	453	765	542		
14	Otolaryngology			554		2215	3125	431	112	389		
15	Pediatrics			2139		2754	1187	541	422	228		
16	Plastic Surgery			668		3127	2122	422	133	551		
17	Psychiatry			1127		6744	0	233	0	1128		
18												

North Shore Medical Clinic

INVOICE

7450 Meridian Street, Suite 150
Portland, OR 97202
Phone (503) 555-2330   Fax (503) 555-2335

DATE: (use current date)
INVOICE # A-128

BILL TO:
Laura Latteral, Education Director
Columbia River General Hospital
4550 Fremont Street
Portland, OR 97045
(503) 555-2000 ext. 2347

FOR: Educational Services

DESCRIPTION	HOURS	RATE	AMOUNT
In-Service Training Session	2.00	$60.00	$ 120.00
		SUBTOTAL	$ 120.00
		TAX RATE	10.00%
		SALES TAX	12.00
		OTHER	
		TOTAL	$ 132.00

Make all checks payable to North Shore Medical Clinic
Total due in 15 days. Overdue accounts subject to a service charge of 1% per month.

THANK YOU FOR YOUR BUSINESS!

Excel SECTION 2
Editing and Formatting Worksheets

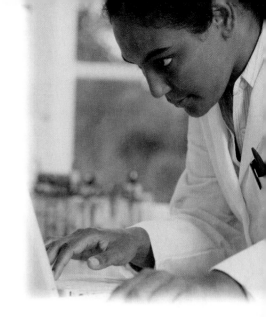

Skills

- Insert, move, and resize clip art and pictures
- Edit the content of cells
- Clear cells and cell formatting
- Use proofing tools
- Insert and delete columns and rows
- Move and copy cells
- Use the Paste Options button to link cells
- Adjust column widths and row heights
- Change the font, size, style, and color of cell contents
- Apply numeric formats and adjust the number of decimal places
- Use Undo
- Change cell alignment and indentation
- Insert and edit comments
- Add borders and shading
- Use Format Painter
- Apply cell styles
- Apply a theme
- Find and replace cell entries and formats
- Freeze and unfreeze panes
- Change the zoom percentage
- Create formulas with absolute addresses

Student Resources

Before beginning the activities in Excel Section 2, copy to your storage medium the ExcelMedS2 folder from the Student Resources CD. This folder contains the data files you need to complete the projects in this Excel section.

Projects Overview

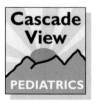

Edit and format a revenue summary report.

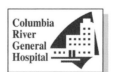

Edit and format a laboratory requisitions billing report, edit and format research data for a medical conference presentation, research and create a workbook on healthcare costs, create a staffing worksheet for the neurology department, and create a radiology requisition form.

Activity 2.1

Inserting, Moving, and Resizing Clip Art and Pictures

Microsoft Office includes a gallery of media images you can insert in a document, such as clip art, photographs, and illustrations. Use the Online Pictures button on the INSERT tab to search for and insert images from Office.com. Once an image has been inserted, it can be moved, resized, or deleted. Format an image with options at the PICTURE TOOLS FORMAT tab. A company logo, digital picture, or any other image file you have saved on your hard drive can also be inserted into a worksheet using the Pictures button in the Illustrations group on the INSERT tab.

Project

Sydney Larsen, office manager of Cascade View Pediatrics, has started a January revenue summary report for Dr. Joseph Yarborough. Sydney would like you to enhance the report's appearance before she submits it. You decide to add two images to the worksheet.

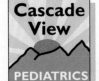

1. Open **CVPRevYarborough.xlsx**. *Note: This worksheet contains intentional spelling errors that will be corrected in the next activity.*

2. Save the workbook in the ExcelMedS2 folder with the name **EMedS2-CVPRevYarborough**.

3. Make cell A38 the active cell.

4. Click the INSERT tab and then click the Online Pictures button ![icon] in the Illustrations group.

    This displays the Insert Pictures window with search boxes.

5. Click in the *Office.com Clip Art* text box, type **stethoscope**, and then press Enter.

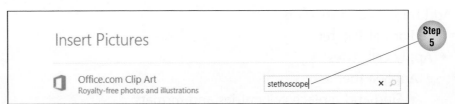

6. Scroll through the images in the Insert Pictures window until you see the clip art image shown below. Double-click the image to insert it in the worksheet.

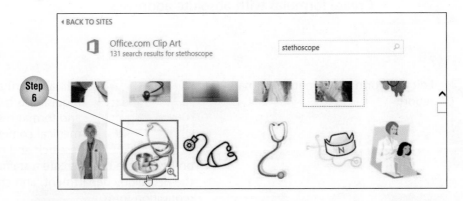

Need Help?

Select an alternative image if the clip art shown is not available.

7 Position the mouse pointer on the white sizing handle in the bottom right corner of the image, hold down the left mouse button, and then drag up and to the left until the image fits within rows 38 to 42.

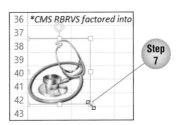

8 Move the mouse pointer over the image until the move icon (four-headed arrow) appears attached to the pointer, hold down the left mouse button, and then drag the image to the right until it is aligned in the center of column E.

9 Make cell A1 the active cell, click the INSERT tab, and then click the Pictures button in the Illustrations group.

10 At the Insert Picture dialog box, navigate to the ExcelMedS2 folder on your storage medium and then double-click ***CVPLogo.png***.

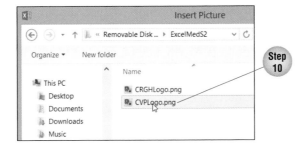

11 Click in the *Shape Height* measurement box in the Size group on the PICTURE TOOLS FORMAT tab, type **0.8**, and then press Enter.

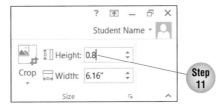

12 Click in any cell to deselect the logo image.

13 Save **EMedS2-CVPRevYarborough.xlsx**.

In Addition

Using the PICTURE TOOLS FORMAT Tab

When a clip art image or picture is selected, the contextual PICTURE TOOLS FORMAT tab becomes available. Customize the image using picture tools or picture styles. Use the Crop button to remove unwanted areas of the image. You can also set a specific height or width measurement for the image. Buttons in the Arrange group allow you to control the alignment, rotation, and order of the image within the worksheet.

Activity 2.2

Editing and Clearing Cells; Using Proofing Tools

The contents of a cell can be edited directly within the cell or in the Formula bar. Clearing a cell can involve removing the cell contents, format, or both. The Spelling feature is a useful tool to assist with correcting typing errors within a worksheet. After completing a spelling check, you will still need to proofread the worksheet since the spelling checker will not highlight all errors and cannot check the accuracy of values. Other proofing tools available in Excel include a Research feature to search for external information, a Thesaurus to find a word with a similar meaning, and a Translate tool to translate a selected word into a different language.

Project

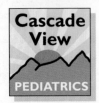

Sydney's report for Dr. Yarborough contains some typographical errors. It also needs updating after Sydney reviewed the day sheets from the medical accounting program. Sydney has asked you to correct the errors and finish the report.

1 With **EMedS2-CVPRevYarborough.xlsx** open, double-click in cell E15.

> When you double-click in a cell, a blinking insertion point appears inside it and the word *EDIT* appears in the Status bar. The position of the insertion point within the cell varies depending on the location of the cell pointer when Edit mode is activated.

2 Press the Right Arrow or Left Arrow key as needed to move the insertion point between the *4* and *5* and then press the Delete key.

3 Type **3** and then press Enter.

4 Make cell E30 the active cell.

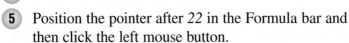

Step 3

5 Position the pointer after *22* in the Formula bar and then click the left mouse button.

> The cell pointer changes to an I-beam pointer $\boxed{\text{I}}$ when it hovers over the Formula bar.

6 Press Backspace to delete *2*, type **4**, and then click the Enter button on the Formula bar.

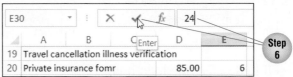

Step 6

7 Make cell A16 the active cell and then press Delete.

> Pressing the Delete key or the Backspace key clears only the contents of the cell; formatting applied to the cell remains in effect.

8 Select the range of cells F7:F8. Click the Clear button $\boxed{\text{✐}}$ in the Editing group on the HOME tab and then click *Clear All* at the drop-down list.

> Clicking *Clear All* removes everything from a cell, including formatting.

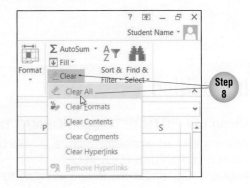

Step 8

9 Press Ctrl + Home to make cell A1 the active cell.

10 Click the REVIEW tab and then click the Spelling button.

The spelling checker starts at the active cell. Words within the worksheet that are not found in the built-in dictionary are highlighted as potential errors. Use buttons in the Spelling dialog box to skip the word (Ignore Once or Ignore All), replace the word with the highlighted word in the *Suggestions* list box (Change), or add the word to the dictionary (Add to Dictionary) if it is spelled correctly.

11 Click the Change button in the Spelling dialog box to instruct Excel to replace *assesment* with *assessment*.

Excel stops at the next row and flags the same spelling error. A quick glance down the worksheet reveals this word is frequently misspelled throughout the worksheet.

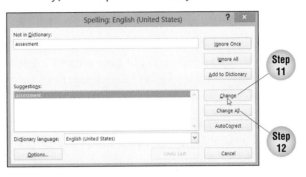

12 Click the Change All button in the Spelling dialog box to replace all occurrences of *assesment* with *assessment*.

13 Click the Change All button to replace *fomr* with *form*. If the spelling checker stops at *RBRVS* in cell A36, click the Ignore Once button.

14 Click OK at the message informing you that the spelling check is complete.

15 Make cell A29 the active cell.

16 Click the Thesaurus button in the Proofing group on the REVIEW tab.

When you click the Thesaurus button, the Thesaurus task pane displays at the right side of the screen. Use the Thesaurus task pane to replace a word in the worksheet with another word of similar meaning.

17 Point to the word *Replication* in the list box in the Thesaurus task pane, click the down-pointing arrow that appears, and then click *Insert* at the drop-down list.

The word *Photocopying* is replaced with *Replication* in cell A29.

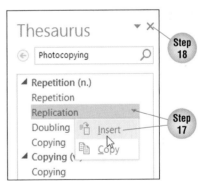

18 Click the Close button in the upper right corner of the Thesaurus task pane.

19 Save **EMedS2-CVPRevYarborough.xlsx**.

In Brief

Edit Cell
1. Double-click in cell.
2. Insert and/or delete text.
3. Press Enter or click another cell.

Clear Cell
1. Click cell.
2. Click Clear button on HOME tab.
3. Click *Clear All, Clear Formats, Clear Contents,* or *Clear Comments.*

Check Spelling
1. Click REVIEW tab.
2. Click Spelling button.
3. Click Ignore Once, Ignore All, Change, or Add to Dictionary as required.
4. Click OK when spelling check is complete.

In Addition

Using the Research Task Pane

Use the Research task pane to search for information online without leaving the worksheet. For example, you can conduct a general Internet search or look up information in online encyclopedias or on business reference sites. Display the Research task pane by clicking the Research button in the Proofing group on the REVIEW tab. Choose the online source by clicking the down-pointing arrow at the right of the option box located below the *Search for* text box.

Activity 2.3

Inserting and Deleting Columns and Rows

Insert rows or columns using options at the Insert button drop-down list in the Cells group on the HOME tab or at the shortcut menu that displays when you right-click a selected area of the worksheet. Rows are inserted above the active cell or row and existing rows are shifted down. Columns are inserted to the left of the active cell or column and existing columns are shifted right. When rows or columns are deleted, data automatically shifts up or to the left to fill the space and references in formulas are updated to reflect this.

Project

Sydney has provided you with new data to insert into the worksheet. To improve the layout of the report, you decide to insert blank rows before each fee category and remove the blank row that was created when you deleted *Hospital physicals* in the last activity.

Cascade View
PEDIATRICS

1. With **EMedS2-CVPRevYarborough.xlsx** open, position the pointer (displays as a right-pointing black arrow) over row indicator 18, hold down the left mouse button, drag the mouse down over row indicator 19, and then release the mouse.

   This selects rows 18 and 19.

2. Click the HOME tab, click the Insert button arrow in the Cells group, and then click *Insert Sheet Rows* at the drop-down list.

   Two blank rows are inserted above row 18. All rows below the inserted rows are shifted down.

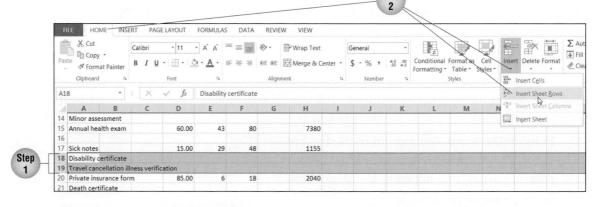

3. Click in cell A18, type **Hearing assessment**, and then press Enter.

4. Type **Speech assessment** in cell A19 and then press Enter.

5. Type the data for hearing and speech assessment as follows:

   | D18: **26.50** | E18: **4** | F18: **2** |
   | D19: **31.50** | E19: **7** | F19: **5** |

6. Enter formulas to calculate the totals for hearing and speech assessment as follows:

   H18: =(E18+F18)*D18
   H19: =(E19+F19)*D19

Steps 3-6

	A	D	E	F	H
16					
17	Sick notes	15.00	29	48	1155
18	Hearing assessment	26.50	4	2	159
19	Speech assessment	31.50	7	5	378
20	Disability certificate				
21	Travel cancellation illness verification				

7 Position the pointer over row indicator 16 and then click the left mouse button to select the entire row.

8 Click the Delete button arrow ⊟ in the Cells group and then click *Delete Sheet Rows* at the drop-down list.

> The contents of row 16 are removed from the worksheet.

9 Select row 11. Hold down the Ctrl key, select rows 24 and 29, and then release the mouse button and the Ctrl key.

> Holding down the Ctrl key allows you to select multiple rows or columns that are not adjacent.

10 Position the pointer within any of the three selected rows, right-click to display the shortcut menu and Mini toolbar, and then click *Insert* at the shortcut menu.

11 Position the pointer over column indicator G and then right-click.

> Right-clicking the column indicator selects the column and displays the shortcut menu and Mini toolbar at the same time.

12 At the shortcut menu, click *Delete*.

> The contents of the columns to the right of the deleted column are shifted left to fill in the space.

13 Click in any cell in the worksheet to deselect the column.

14 Save **EMedS2-CVPRevYarborough.xlsx**.

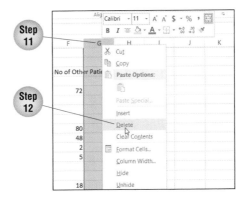

In Brief

Insert Rows or Columns
1. Select number of rows or columns to add.
2. Click Insert button arrow.
3. Click Insert Sheet Rows or Insert Sheet Columns.

Delete Rows or Columns
1. Select rows or columns to be deleted.
2. Click Delete button arrow.
3. Click Delete Sheet Rows or Delete Sheet Columns.

In Addition

Inserting and Deleting Cells

In this activity, you inserted and deleted entire rows and columns, but you can also insert new blank cells or delete a range of cells within the worksheet area. To insert new blank cells, select the amount of cells you need to add at the desired location of the additional cells, and then click the Insert button in the Cells group, or click the Insert button arrow and then click *Insert Cells* at the drop-down list to display the dialog box shown at the right. Using the dialog box, you can choose to shift existing cells right or down. Click the Delete button in the Cells group to delete a selected range of cells and cause the cells below the deleted range to shift up. Click the Delete button arrow and then click *Delete Cells* to open the Delete dialog box. The Delete dialog box contains options similar to those available at the Insert dialog box.

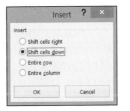

Activity 2.4

Moving and Copying Cells

You learned how to use copy and paste to replicate formulas in the payroll worksheet for the North Shore Medical Clinic. In this activity, you will practice using copy and paste and cut and paste to copy or move the contents of a cell or range of cells to another location in the worksheet. The selected cells being cut or copied are called the *source*. The cell or range of cells receiving the source data is called the *destination*. If data already exists in the destination cells, Excel replaces the contents. Cells cut or copied to the Clipboard can be pasted more than once in the active workbook, another workbook, or another Office application.

Project

Continue to work on the report by moving, copying, and linking cell contents. To do this, you will use buttons in the Clipboard group on the HOME tab and a method called *drag and drop*.

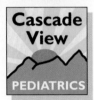

1. With **EMedS2-CVPRevYarborough.xlsx** open, make cell A40 the active cell.

2. Click the Cut button ✂ in the Clipboard group on the HOME tab.

   A marquee surrounds the source after you use the Cut or Copy commands, indicating the cell contents have been placed in the Clipboard.

3. Make cell A9 the active cell and then click the Paste button in the Clipboard group. (Do not click the Paste button arrow, as this displays a drop-down list of options.)

   The text is moved from cell A40 to cell A9. In the next step, you will move the contents of a cell using a method called *drag and drop*.

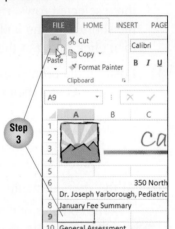

Step 3

4. Make cell A10 the active cell.

5. Point to any one of the four borders surrounding the selected cell.

   When you point to a border, the pointer changes from the thick white cross to a white arrow with the move icon (four-headed arrow) attached to it.

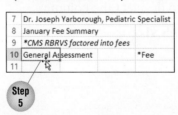

Step 5

6. Hold down the left mouse button, drag the cell down one row to cell A11, and then release the mouse button.

   A green border appears as you drag, indicating where the cell contents will be placed when you release the mouse button. The destination cell or range also displays in a ScreenTip below the green border.

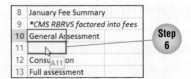

Step 6

7. Make cell D34 the active cell.

   Dr. Yarborough charges the same fee for telephone prescription renewals and sick notes, so Sydney wants you to link the sick notes fee to the telephone prescription renewal fee. That way, if the fee changes, you will only need to type the new fee in one of the two cells, but they will both be updated.

8. Click the Copy button in the Clipboard group.

9 Make cell D17 the active cell, click the Paste button arrow in the Clipboard group, and then click the Paste Link button in the *Other Paste Options* section of the Paste button drop-down gallery.

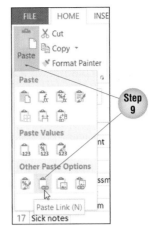

> The existing data in cell D17 is replaced with the value copied from cell D34 and the source and destination cells are now linked. Linking the cells means that any change made to the source cell (D34) will automatically be applied to the destination cell (D17). A Paste Options button appears next to the destination cell (D17). Click the button to access the Paste Options drop-down gallery if you want to choose another paste option. See the In Addition section at the bottom of this page for more information on the Paste drop-down gallery.

10 Press Esc to remove the marquee from cell D34.

11 Make cell D34 the active cell, edit the value to read *16.50*, and then press Enter.

> Notice that the value in cell D17 is automatically changed to *16.50*.

12 Select the range of cells E27:G27.

13 Point to any one of the four borders surrounding the selected range until the pointer displays as a white arrow with the move icon attached to it, hold down the Ctrl key, and then drag the mouse to the range of cells E28:G28. Release the mouse button and then release the Ctrl key.

> Holding down the Ctrl key while dragging copies cells.

In Brief

Move or Copy Cells
1. Select source cells.
2. Click Cut or Copy button.
3. Select starting destination cell.
4. Click Paste button.

Copy and Link Cells
1. Select source cells.
2. Click Copy button.
3. Select destination cell.
4. Click Paste button arrow.
5. Click Paste Link button.

	A	B	C	D
11	General Assessment			
12	Consultation			94.50
13	Full assessment			
14	Intermediate assessment			
15	Minor assessment			
16	Annual health exam			60.00
17	Sick notes			16.50
18	Hearing assessment			26.50
19	Speech assessment			31.50
20	Disability certificate			
21	Travel cancellation illness verification			
22	Private insurance form			85.00
23	Death certificate			
24	Life insurance certificate			
25				
26	Specific Assessment			
27	Day care assessment			55.00
28	Day care form			
29	Camp physical assessment			40.00
30	Camp form			
31				
32	Other Charges			
33	Replication			
34	Telephone prescription renewal			16.50

> The contents of cell D17 change automatically since the cell is linked to cell D34.

	A	B	C	E	F	G
26	Specific Assessment					
27	Day care assessment	55.00		34	0	1870
28	Day care form					
29	Camp physical assessment	40.00		10		1720

E28:G28 — Step 13

14 Make cell D28 the active cell, type **30.00**, and then press Enter.

15 Save **EMedS2-CVPRevYarborough.xlsx**.

In Addition

Using the Paste Drop-down Gallery

The Paste drop-down gallery (shown at the right) can be accessed via the Paste button arrow in the Clipboard group, the Paste Options button that appears after an entry has been pasted into a cell, or the shortcut menu that appears when you right-click a cell. The drop-down list is divided into three sections: *Paste*, *Paste Values*, and *Other Paste Options*. Each section includes buttons for various paste options. Hover the mouse over a button to view a ScreenTip that describes the button's purpose as well as a pre-view of the paste option applied to the cell in the worksheet. The Paste drop-down gallery is context sensitive, meaning that the buttons that appear are dependent on the type of content that has been cop-ied and the location in which the content is being pasted.

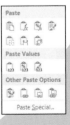

Activity 2.5

Adjusting Column Width and Row Height; Using AutoFit

By default, columns in Excel are all the same width (8.11 characters, or 80 pixels) and rows are all the same height (14.40 points, or 24 pixels). While Excel automatically adjusts the heights of rows to accommodate the text within the cells, it does not automatically adjust column widths. In some cases you do not have to increase the width when the text is too wide for the column, since labels "spill over" into the next cell to the right, but if the next cell to the right contains data, some of the content will be hidden. In this case, you will want to manually increase the width of the column to show all of the content. You can also manually increase the height of rows to add more space between them. This can help to improve readability or draw attention to a series of cells. There are a few ways to adjust column width and row height, including AutoFit. When using AutoFit, Excel automatically adjusts the width or height based on the longest or tallest entry.

Project

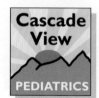

To improve the readability of the report, you will adjust the widths of columns in which the entire heading is not currently visible and increase the height of the row containing the column headings.

1. With **EMedS2-CVPRevYarborough.xlsx** open, make any cell in column E the active cell.

2. Click the Format button in the Cells group on the HOME tab and then click *Column Width* at the drop-down list.

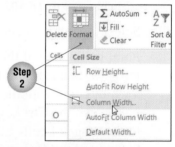

3. At the Column Width dialog box, type **20** and then click OK or press Enter.

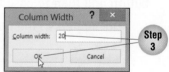

   In the next step, you will use the mouse to adjust the width of column F.

4. Position the mouse pointer on the boundary line between columns F and G in the column indicator row until the pointer changes to a left-and-right-pointing arrow with a vertical line in the middle ⟷.

5. Hold down the left mouse button, drag the boundary line to the right until *Width: 17.00 (160 pixels)* displays in the ScreenTip, and then release the mouse button. ***Note: The pixel value that displays in parentheses may vary depending on your monitor's settings. Use the point values given in this book to complete activities.***

   As you drag the boundary line to the right or left, a dotted line appears in the worksheet area indicating the new width of the column. If, after decreasing a column's width, cells that previously had numbers in them now display as a series of pound symbols (######), the column is too narrow. Excel displays pound symbols instead of displaying only a part of a numeric value so that you do not confuse the partially displayed value with the actual full value. Widen the column to redisplay the numbers.

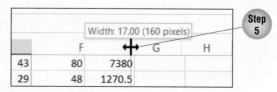

6 Make cell A21 the active cell, click the Format button in the Cells group, and then click *AutoFit Column Width* at the drop-down list.

> The *AutoFit Column Width* option adjusts the width of the column to accommodate the content in the active cell. You can also double-click a column's boundary line to AutoFit the width to accommodate the longest entry.

7 By using either the Column Width dialog box or dragging the column boundary, increase the width of column D to *10 (97 pixels)*.

> After reviewing the worksheet, you decide the two columns with dollar values should be the same width. In the next steps, you will learn how to change the width of multiple columns in one operation.

8 Click column indicator D, hold down the Ctrl key, and then click column indicator G.

9 Position the mouse pointer on either one of the two columns' right boundary lines until the pointer becomes a left-and-right-pointing arrow with a vertical line in the middle.

> Any change made to the width of one column will be applied to both of the selected columns.

10 Drag the boundary line to the right until *Width: 15.00 (142 pixels)* displays in the ScreenTip and then release the mouse button.

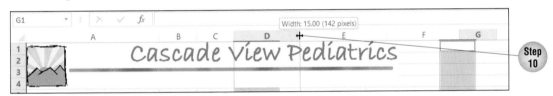

11 Click in any cell to deselect the columns.

> Do not be concerned that the columns appear too wide — you will improve the layout as you work through the next several activities.

12 Position the mouse pointer on the boundary line between rows 10 and 11 until the pointer becomes an up-and-down-pointing arrow with a horizontal line in the middle.

13 Drag the boundary line down until *Height: 21.00 (35 pixels)* displays in the ScreenTip and then release the mouse button.

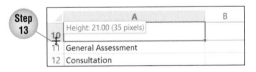

14 Save **EMedS2-CVPRevYarborough.xlsx**.

In Addition

Using the Row Height Dialog Box

Using the Row Height dialog box (shown at the right) to adjust row height works similarly to using the Column Width dialog box to adjust the width of a column. Click any cell within the row, click the Format button in the Cells group on the HOME tab, and then click *Row Height* at the drop-down list. Type the desired height and then press Enter or click OK.

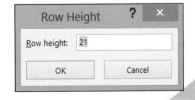

In Brief

Increase or Decrease Column Width
1. Select column(s).
2. Click Format button in Cells group.
3. Click *Column Width*.
4. Type desired width.
5. Click OK.

Increase or Decrease Row Height
1. Select row(s).
2. Click Format button in Cells group.
3. Click *Row Height*.
4. Type desired height.
5. Click OK.

Adjust Width or Height Using Mouse
Drag boundary to right of column or below row, or double-click boundary to AutoFit.

Activity 2.6

In Excel, the *font* is the typeface used to display data in electronic and print formats. The default font in Excel is Calibri, but many other fonts are available. The size of the font is measured in units called *points*. A point is approximately 1/72 of an inch, measured vertically. The default font size in Excel is 11 points. The larger the point size, the larger the type. Each font's style can be changed to **bold**, *italic*, or ***bold italic***. By default, cell entries display in black with a white background. Changing the color of the font and/or the color of the background (called *fill*) can add interest or emphasis to the text.

Project

To visually enhance Dr. Yarborough's revenue report, you will change the font and font size and apply formatting such as bold and color.

1. With **EMedS2-CVPRevYarborough.xlsx** open, make cell A6 the active cell.

2. Click the Font button arrow in the Font group on the HOME tab, scroll down the list of fonts in the drop-down gallery, and then point to *Book Antiqua*. Notice that Excel applies the font to the active cell so that you can preview the result. This feature is called *live preview*. Click *Book Antiqua* to apply the font to cell A6.

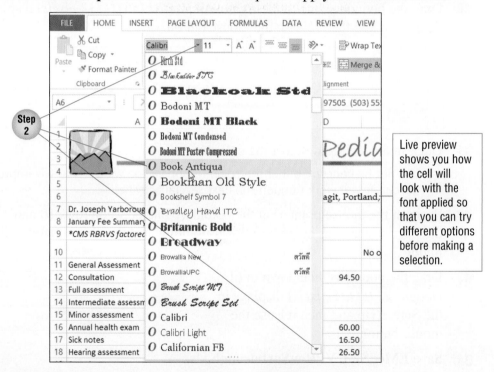

Live preview shows you how the cell will look with the font applied so that you can try different options before making a selection.

3. With cell A6 still the active cell, click the Font Size button arrow in the Font group and then click *14* at the drop-down list.

   The row height is automatically increased to accommodate the larger font size.

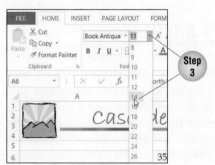

4 With cell A6 still the active cell, click the Font Color button [A ▾] arrow in the Font group and then click *Aqua, Accent 5, Darker 50%* (ninth column, sixth row) in the *Theme Colors* section of the color gallery.

5 With cell A6 still selected, click the Fill Color button [🎨 ▾] arrow in the Font group and then click *Aqua, Accent 5, Lighter 80%* (ninth column, second row) in the *Theme Colors* section of the color gallery.

> *Fill* is the color of the background in the cell. Changing the fill color is sometimes referred to as applying *shading* to a cell.

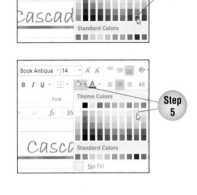

Step 4

Step 5

<!-- In Brief sidebar -->
In Brief

Change Font
1. Select cells.
2. Click Font button arrow.
3. Click desired font.
4. Deselect cells.

Change Font Size
1. Select cells.
2. Click Font Size button arrow.
3. Click desired size.
4. Deselect cells.

Change Font Style
1. Select cells.
2. Click desired font style button.
3. Deselect cells.

6 Click the Bold button [B] in the Font group.

7 Select the range of cells A7:I7 and then click the Merge & Center button in the Alignment group.

8 With cell A7 the active cell, change the font size to 12 points, and then change the font color to *Dark Red* (first color from the left in the *Standard Colors* section).

9 Select the range of cells A8:I8 and apply the same formatting you applied in Steps 7 and 8.

> Since Dark Red is the color you most recently selected from the Font Color button drop-down gallery, you can apply it to cells A8:I8 simply by clicking the Font Color button. You do not need to display the drop-down gallery.

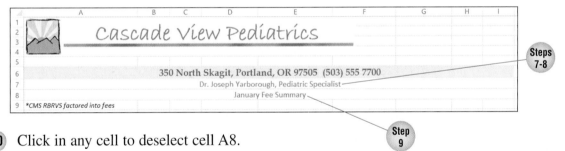

Steps 7-8

Step 9

10 Click in any cell to deselect cell A8.

11 Save **EMedS2-CVPRevYarborough.xlsx**.

In Addition

Using the Format Cells Dialog Box

You can use the Format Cells dialog box with the Font tab selected (shown at the right) to change the font, font size, font style, and color of text. This dialog box also offers additional options such as more Underline styles (*Single, Double, Single Accounting*, and *Double Accounting*) and special effects options (*Strikethrough, Superscript*, and *Subscript*). To display this dialog box, select the cells you want to change and then click the Font group dialog box launcher.

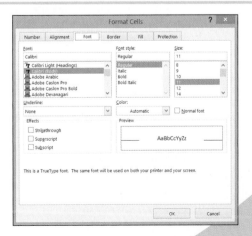

Formatting Numeric Cells;
Adjusting Decimal Places; Using Undo

When creating the payroll worksheet for the North Shore Medical Clinic, you learned how to format numeric cells with the Accounting format, which adds a dollar symbol ($), comma in the thousands place, and two decimal places, and displays negative values in brackets. Other numeric formats in Excel include Comma, Percent, and Currency. By default, cells are initially set to the General format which has no specific numeric style. The number of decimal places in a selected range of cells can be increased or decreased using the Increase Decimal and Decrease Decimal buttons in the Number group on the HOME tab.

Use the Undo button on the Quick Access toolbar to reverse the last action. Excel stores up to 100 actions that can be undone, redone, or repeated. However, it is important to note that some actions (such as Save) cannot be reversed with Undo.

Project

Continue improving the visual appearance of the revenue summary report by applying format options to the numeric cells.

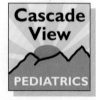

1. With **EMedS2-CVPRevYarborough.xlsx** open, select cell D12, hold down the Ctrl key, and then select cell G12.

2. Click the Accounting Number Format button in the Number group on the HOME tab.

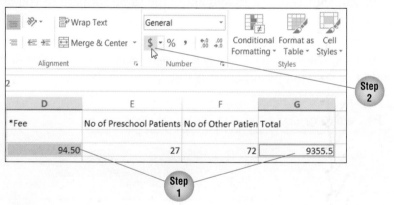

3. Click in any cell to deselect the cells.

4. Select the range of cells G16:G34.

5. Click the Comma Style button in the Number group.

> The Comma format applies the same formatting as the Accounting format, except it does not apply the dollar (or alternative currency) symbol.

6. Click in any cell to deselect the cells and review the numeric values in the worksheet. Only one numeric cell remains that could be improved by applying a format option: cell G38.

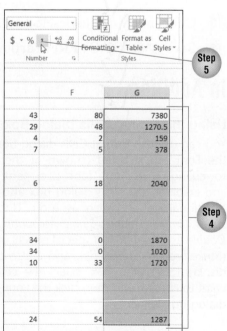

7 Make cell G38 the active cell.

8 Click the Accounting Number Format button in the Number group.

9 Select the range of cells E12:F34 and then click the Increase Decimal button in the Number group twice.

> One decimal place is added to the cells in the selected range each time you click the Increase Decimal button.

10 With the range E12:F34 still selected, click the Decrease Decimal button in the Number group.

> One decimal place is removed from the cells in the selected range when you click the Decrease Decimal button.

11 Click the Undo button on the Quick Access toolbar.

> Excel adds back one decimal place in the range of cells E12:F34.

12 Click the Undo button two times to return the cells to their original state and then click in any cell to deselect the range.

13 Save **EMedS2-CVPRevYarborough.xlsx**.

In Brief

Change Numeric Format
1. Select cells.
2. Click desired format button in Number group.
3. Deselect cells.

Undo Action
Click Undo button on Quick Access toolbar or press Ctrl + Z.

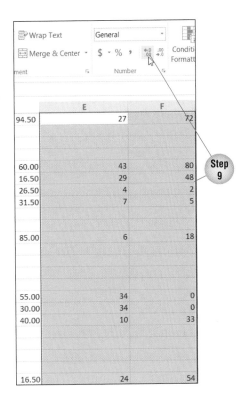

In Addition

Exploring Additional Number Format Options

Click the Number Format button arrow in the Number group on the HOME tab to display a drop-down list (shown at the right) with additional numeric formats including date, time, fraction, and scientific options. Click *More Number Formats* at the bottom of the list to open the Format Cells dialog box with the Number tab selected. Using this dialog box, you can access further customization options for a format, such as displaying negative values in red or creating your own custom format code.

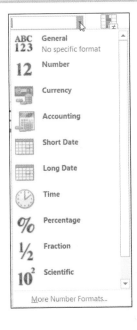

Activity 2.8

Changing the Alignment and Indentation of Cells; Inserting Comments

Data in a cell can be left-aligned, right-aligned, or centered within the column. Use the Increase Indent and Decrease Indent buttons to adjust how far text is indented from the left edge of the cell. The indent is increased or decreased by approximately one character each time one of the buttons is clicked. Using buttons in the top row of the Alignment group on the HOME tab you can change vertical alignment, rotate text, or wrap text within a cell.

A *comment* is a note that can be attached to a cell. A red triangle in the upper right corner of the cell alerts the reader that a comment exists. Hover the mouse pointer over the cell to display the comment in a pop-up box.

Project

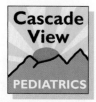

Continue improving the visual appearance of the revenue summary report by editing cells, removing columns, adjusting column widths, aligning cells, and indenting labels. You will also add two comments in cells asking Sydney to verify values before the report is submitted to Dr. Yarborough.

1. With **EMedS2-CVPRevYarborough.xlsx** open, select cell E10 and then edit the contents to read *Preschool Patients*. Select cell F10 and then edit the contents to read *Other Patients*.

2. Select the range of cells E10:F10, click the Format button in the Cells group on the HOME tab, and then click *AutoFit Column Width* at the drop-down list.

3. Delete columns B and C from the worksheet. Refer to Activity 2.3 if you need assistance with this step.

4. Delete columns F and G from the worksheet.

    Although no data existed in any cells within columns F and G, this step corrected the extended merge and centering applied to rows 6–8.

5. Select the range of cells B10:E10.

6. Click the Center button ≡ in the Alignment group on the HOME tab.

    Other buttons in the Alignment group include the Align Left button ≡, which aligns entries at the left edge of the cell, and the Align Right button ≡, which aligns entries at the right edge of the cell.

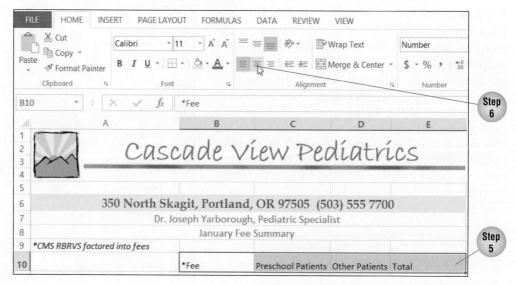

7 Select the range of cells A12:A24.

8 Click the Increase Indent button 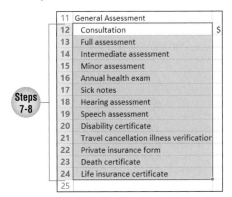 in the Alignment group.

Each time you the click the Increase Indent button, the contents of the selected cells are indented by approximately one character. If you click the Increase Indent button too many times, click the Decrease Indent button ⬅ to return the text to the previous indent position.

11	General Assessment
12	Consultation $
13	Full assessment
14	Intermediate assessment
15	Minor assessment
16	Annual health exam
17	Sick notes
18	Hearing assessment
19	Speech assessment
20	Disability certificate
21	Travel cancellation illness verification
22	Private insurance form
23	Death certificate
24	Life insurance certificate
25	

Steps 7-8

9 Select the range of cells A27:A30 and then click the Increase Indent button.

10 Select the range of cells A33:A36 and then click the Increase Indent button.

11 Select the range of cells B10:E10. Hold down the Ctrl key and then click cells A11, A26, A32, and A38.

Use the Ctrl key to select multiple ranges or cells to which you want to apply a formatting option.

	A	B	C	D	E
10		*Fee	Preschool Patients	Other Patients	Total
11	General Assessment				
12	Consultation	$ 94.50	27	72	$ 9,355.50
13	Full assessment				
14	Intermediate assessment				
15	Minor assessment				
16	Annual health exam	60.00	43	80	7,380.00
17	Sick notes	16.50	29	48	1,270.50
18	Hearing assessment	26.50	4	2	159.00
19	Speech assessment	31.50	7	5	378.00
20	Disability certificate				
21	Travel cancellation illness verification				
22	Private insurance form	85.00	6	18	2,040.00
23	Death certificate				
24	Life insurance certificate				
25					
26	Specific Assessment				
27	Day care assessment	55.00	34	0	1,870.00
28	Day care form	30.00	34	0	1,020.00
29	Camp physical assessment	40.00	10	33	1,720.00
30	Camp form				
31					
32	Other Charges				
33	Repetition				
34	Telephone prescription renewal	16.50	24	54	1,287.00
35	Missed appointments				
36	Missed annual physical				
37					
38	Total				$ 26,480.00
39					

Step 11

12 Click the Bold button in the Font group.

13 Click in any cell to deselect the cells.

continues

14 Select the range of cells B10:E10.

In Activity 2.5, you increased the height of row 10 to 21 points. The Alignment group contains buttons that allow you to control the alignment of the text between the top and bottom borders of the row. In the next step, you will center the text vertically within the cells.

15 Click the Middle Align button ≡ in the Alignment group.

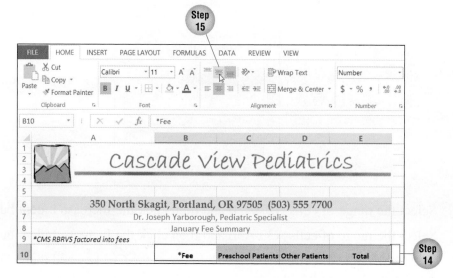

16 Deselect the range.

17 Make cell C30 the active cell.

You want to insert a comment to Sydney Larsen asking her to confirm that there were no charges for camp forms in January.

18 Click the REVIEW tab and then click the New Comment button in the Comments group.

A yellow comment box displays anchored to the active cell. The comment box contains the user's name in bold text at the top and a blinking insertion point. In worksheets accessed by multiple users, the user's name is important because it informs the reader of the name of the person who made the comment.

19 Type **Sydney, please confirm no camp forms were issued in January. Thanks.**

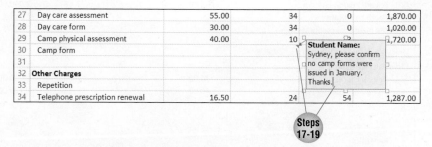

20 Click in any cell outside the comment box.

The comment box closes and a red triangle appears in the upper right corner of cell C30, indicating that a comment exists for the cell.

21 Right-click cell B28 and then click *Insert Comment* at the shortcut menu.

22 Type **Check fee. This is the same rate as last year.**

23 Click in any cell outside the comment box.

24 Hover the cell pointer over cell B28.

> When you hover the cell pointer over a cell that contains a comment, the comment appears in a pop-up box.

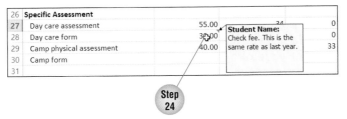

Step
24

25 Right-click cell B28 and then click *Edit Comment* at the shortcut menu.

26 Add the following sentence to the end of the existing comment text:

> **Should this be the same fee as Dr. Severin's?**

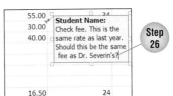

Step
26

27 Click in any cell outside the comment box.

28 Make cell A9 the active cell and then click the Next button ⬚ in the Comments group on the REVIEW tab.

> Excel displays the comment associated with cell B28.

29 Click the Next button in the Comments group.

> Excel displays the comment associated with cell C30.

30 Click the Next button and then click Cancel at the message indicating that Excel has reached the end of the workbook. This instructs Excel not to continue the review at the beginning of the workbook.

> The Comments group also contains a Previous button ⬚ that can be used to view the comment box prior to the active comment.

31 Click in any cell to close the comment associated with cell C30.

32 Save **EMedS2-CVPRevYarborough.xlsx**.

In Brief

Change Horizontal or Vertical Alignment
1. Select cells.
2. Click desired alignment button.
3. Deselect cells.

Indent Text within Cells
1. Select cells.
2. Click Increase Indent button.
3. Deselect cells.

Insert Comment
1. Make desired cell active.
2. Click REVIEW tab.
3. Click New Comment button.
4. Type comment text.
5. Click outside comment box.

In Addition

Printing Comments

By default, comments do not print with a worksheet. To print a worksheet with the comment boxes, you need to specify a *Comments* option at the Page Setup dialog box. Click the PAGE LAYOUT tab, click the Page Setup dialog box launcher at the bottom right of the Page Setup group, click the Sheet tab, and then click the down-pointing arrow at the right of the *Comments* option box in the *Print* section (shown at the right). You can choose to print the comment text at the end of the sheet or as displayed on the sheet.

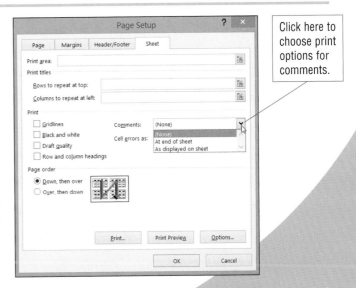

Click here to choose print options for comments.

Activity 2.9

Adding Borders and Shading; Copying Formats with Format Painter

Borders in various styles and colors can be applied to display and print in selected cells within a worksheet. Borders can be added to the top, left, bottom, or right edge of a cell. Use borders to underscore headings or totals or to emphasize cells containing important data. Format Painter copies formatting among cells. Use this feature to quickly and easily apply multiple formatting options from one cell to another.

Project As you get closer to completing the report, you will spend time improving the appearance of the worksheet by adding borders and shading.

1. With **EMedS2-CVPRevYarborough.xlsx** open, select the range of cells A10:E10.

2. Click the Bottom Border button arrow in the Font group on the HOME tab.

   A drop-down list of border style options displays.

3. Click *Top and Bottom Border* at the drop-down list.

4. Click in any cell to deselect the range and view the border.

5. Make cell A11 the active cell, click the Top and Bottom Border button arrow (previously the Bottom Border button), and then click *Outside Borders* at the drop-down list.

6. Make cell A26 the active cell and then click the Outside Borders button (not the button arrow).

   Since the Borders button displays the most recently selected border style, you can apply the Outside Borders option to the active cell without displaying the drop-down list.

7. Make cell A32 the active cell, click the Outside Borders button, and then deselect the cell.

8. Make cell E38 the active cell, click the Outside Borders button arrow, and then click *Top and Double Bottom Border* at the drop-down list.

9. Select the range of cells A17:E17, click the Fill Color button arrow, and then click the *More Colors* option.

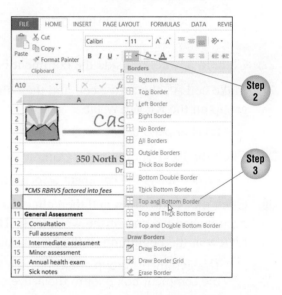

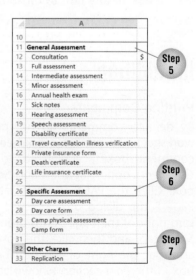

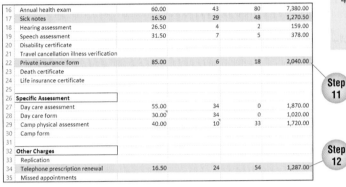

10 At the Colors dialog box with the Standard tab selected, click the light orange color option shown at the right and then click OK.

Step 10

11 With the range A17:E17 still selected, double-click the Format Painter button in the Clipboard group.

> A marquee surrounds the source cell and a paintbrush icon displays attached to the cell pointer. This icon means that the formats have been copied from the source cell(s) and can be applied to multiple cells or ranges. Clicking the Format Painter button once allows you to copy formatting to the next cell or range that you click. The feature automatically turns off after this. Double-clicking the Format Painter button toggles the feature on until you turn it off by clicking the Format Painter button once.

In Brief

Add Borders
1. Select cells.
2. Click Borders button arrow in Font group.
3. Click desired border style.
4. Deselect cells.

Copy Formats
1. Make source cell active.
2. Click or double-click Format Painter button in Clipboard group.
3. Click destination cell(s).
4. If necessary, click Format Painter button to turn off feature.

12 Select the range of cells A22:E22. Notice that the shading is copied to the range and the paintbrush icon remains attached to the cell pointer.

13 Select the range of cells A34:E34.

14 Click the Format Painter button to turn off the feature.

15 Click in any cell to deselect the range.

16 Save **EMedS2-CVPRevYarborough.xlsx**.

16	Annual health exam	60.00	43	80	7,380.00
17	Sick notes	16.50	29	48	1,270.50
18	Hearing assessment	26.50	4	2	159.00
19	Speech assessment	31.50	7	5	378.00
20	Disability certificate				
21	Travel cancellation illness verification				
22	Private insurance form	85.00	6	18	2,040.00
23	Death certificate				
24	Life insurance certificate				
25					
26	**Specific Assessment**				
27	Day care assessment	55.00	34	0	1,870.00
28	Day care form	30.00	34	0	1,020.00
29	Camp physical assessment	40.00	10	33	1,720.00
30	Camp form				
31					
32	**Other Charges**				
33	Replication				
34	Telephone prescription renewal	16.50	24	54	1,287.00
35	Missed appointments				

Step 11

Step 12

In Addition

Creating a Custom Border

If none of the borders available in the drop-down list suit your needs, you can create a custom border. Click the *More Borders* option at the bottom of the Borders button drop-down list to open the Format Cells dialog box with the Border tab selected (as shown below). At this dialog box, you can change to a different line style by clicking another line option in the *Style* list box, and/or change the line color by clicking the down-pointing arrow at the

right of the *Color* option box and then choosing the desired color at the drop-down list. Next, specify where to apply the border by clicking one of the buttons in the *Presets* section, by clicking one or more of the Border buttons along the perimeter of the preview box, or by clicking inside the preview box at the edge of the cell along which you want the border to appear. When you are finished creating the border, click OK.

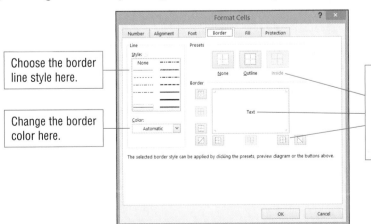

Choose the border line style here.

Change the border color here.

Specify where the border should appear by clicking a button in the *Presets* section, a border button, or inside the preview box along the edge at which you want the border to appear.

Activity 2.10

Applying Cell Styles and Themes

A cell style is a group of predefined formatting options that can be applied with one click. Styles are an efficient way to consistently apply formatting, creating a professional worksheet appearance. Excel provides several cell styles that you can apply or modify, or you can choose to create your own cell style.

A *theme* is a set of formatting choices that includes colors, heading and body text fonts, and lines and fill effects. Excel provides a variety of themes you can use to format a worksheet. The default theme in a new Excel worksheet is Office.

Project

To further finalize the revenue summary report, you will apply cell styles and a theme.

Cascade View
PEDIATRICS

1. With **EMedS2-CVPRevYarborough.xlsx** open, select the range of cells A7:A8.

   You decide to change the formatting of this range to one of the predefined cell styles provided by Excel.

2. Click the Cell Styles button 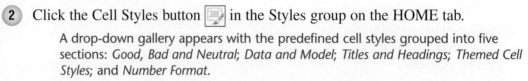 in the Styles group on the HOME tab.

   A drop-down gallery appears with the predefined cell styles grouped into five sections: *Good, Bad and Neutral*; *Data and Model*; *Titles and Headings*; *Themed Cell Styles*; and *Number Format*.

3. Move the mouse over several of the cell style options in the drop-down gallery. Live preview shows you how each style would look when applied to the two title rows.

4. Click the *Heading 4* style in the *Titles and Headings* section.

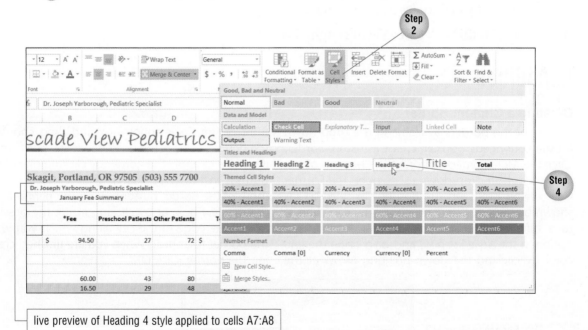

live preview of Heading 4 style applied to cells A7:A8

5 Make cell A11 the active cell, click the Cell Styles button in the Styles group, and then click the *Accent5* style in the *Themed Cell Styles* section.

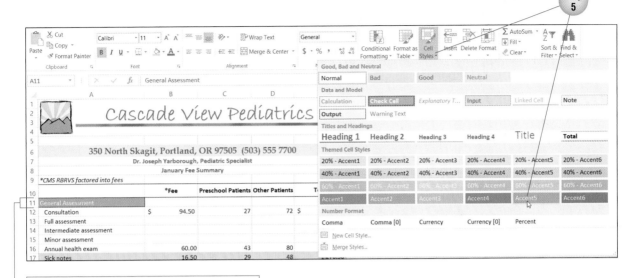

live preview of Accent5 style applied to cell A11

6 Apply the Accent5 style to cells A26 and A32.

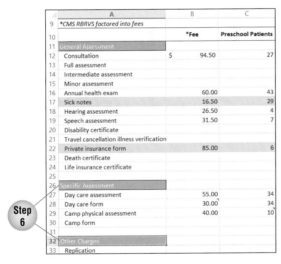

Step 6

7 Deselect the cell(s).

In the next steps you will apply a theme to the worksheet. Changing the theme will cause the fonts, colors, and effects in the cells to change. As with styles, you will be able to view a live preview of the changes before you choose a theme.

continues

(8) Click the PAGE LAYOUT tab.

(9) Click the Themes button 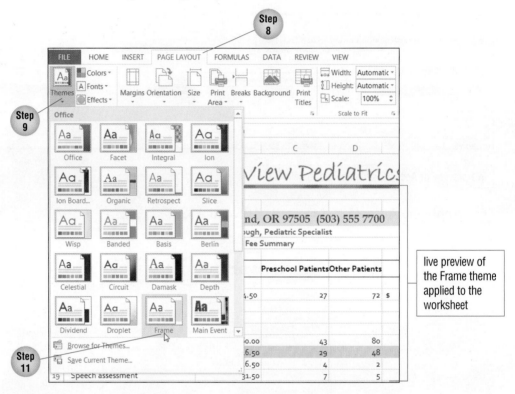 in the Themes group.

(10) Move the mouse over several of the themes in the drop-down gallery and observe the changes that take place in the worksheet.

> Applying a theme affects the entire worksheet. You do not select a cell or range of cells before you apply a theme.

(11) Click *Frame* at the drop-down gallery.

(12) Click the Colors button 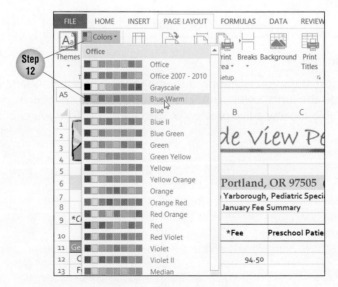 in the Themes group and then click *Blue Warm* at the drop-down gallery.

13 Click the Fonts button 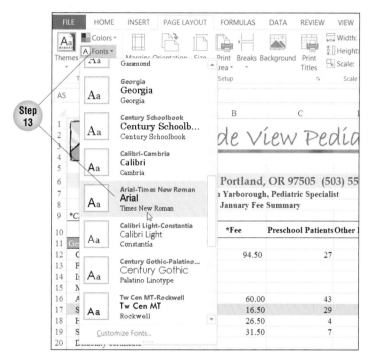 in the Themes group, scroll down the drop-down gallery, and then click *Arial-Times New Roman*.

In Brief

Apply Cell Style
1. Select cells.
2. Click Cell Styles button.
3. Click desired style in drop-down gallery.

Apply Theme
1. Click PAGE LAYOUT tab.
2. Click Themes button.
3. Click desired theme in drop-down gallery.

Need Help?

Applied the wrong theme? Since themes are applied to the entire worksheet, simply go back to the Themes button drop-down gallery and select the correct theme. The existing theme will be replaced.

14 Save **EMedS2-CVPRevYarborough.xlsx**.

In Addition

Creating a New Cell Style

You can create your own cell style by clicking the *New Cell Style* option at the bottom of the Cell Styles drop-down gallery. First, select a cell in the current worksheet and apply all of the formatting to the cell that you want to save in the style. Second, with the cell active, click the Cell Styles button in the Styles group on the HOME tab and then click *New Cell Style* at the drop-down gallery. At the Style dialog box, shown at the right, type a name for the style in the *Style name* text box and then click OK. The new style will appear at the top of the Cell Styles drop-down gallery in a new section titled *Custom*. Custom styles are saved in the workbook in which they are created. You will not see the new style when you open a new workbook; however, you can copy styles from one workbook to another.

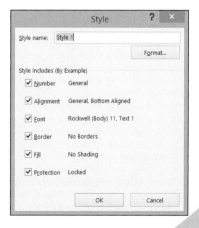

Activity 2.11

Using Find and Replace

Use the Find feature to search for specific content within a worksheet. The Find feature will locate every instance of the text you specify. Use the Replace feature to search for a label, value, or format and automatically replace it with another label, value, or format. The Find and Replace feature ensures that all occurrences of the specified text or formatting are found and/or replaced.

Project

To double-check your work on the revenue summary report, you decide to search the worksheet to make sure you included all of the forms. Sydney Larsen has also reviewed the report and requested that you change all occurrences of *assessment* to *evaluation*.

1 With **EMedS2-CVPRevYarborough.xlsx** open, press Ctrl + Home to make cell A1 the active cell.

2 Click the HOME tab.

3 Click the Find & Select button 🔍 in the Editing group and then click *Find* at the drop-down list.

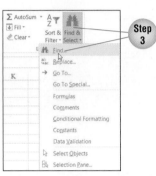

4 Type **form** in the *Find what* text box and then click the Find Next button.

Cell A22, which contains the first occurrence of the word *form*, becomes active.

Need Help?

Can't see the active cell? The Find and Replace dialog box may be obscuring your view. Click in the Title bar and then drag the box to another area of the screen so that you can see the active cell.

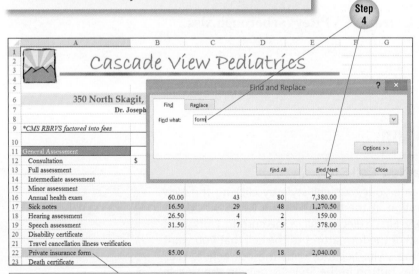

The Find feature moves to the next occurrence of the text each time you click the Find Next button.

5 Click the Find Next button.

The cell containing *Day care form* (cell A28) becomes active.

6 Click the Find Next button.

The cell containing *Camp form* (cell A30) becomes active.

7 Click the Find Next button.

> Excel returns to the first occurrence of *form*, located in cell A22. Although in this small worksheet you could easily have reviewed the form entries by scanning column A, in a large worksheet with many rows and columns, using the Find feature is an efficient way to locate specific text. Using the Find feature also ensures that you do not miss any instances of the text or formatting for which you are searching.

8 Click the Close button to close the Find and Replace dialog box.

9 Click the Find & Select button in the Editing group and then click *Replace* at the drop-down list.

10 Select *form* in the *Find what* text box and then type **assessment**.

11 Press Tab to move the insertion point to the *Replace with* text box and then type **evaluation**.

12 Click the Replace All button.

> Excel searches through the entire worksheet and automatically changes all occurrences of *assessment* to *evaluation*.

13 Click OK at the message informing you that Excel has completed the search and made nine replacements.

14 Click the Close button to close the Find and Replace dialog box.

15 Review the labels in column A of the worksheet and note the replacements that were made.

16 Click the PAGE LAYOUT tab. Click the Width button arrow ⊞ (currently displays *Automatic*) in the Scale to Fit group and then click *1 page* at the drop-down list.

17 Save and then print **EMedS2-CVPRevYarborough.xlsx**.

In Brief

Find Label or Value
1. Click Find & Select button in Editing group.
2. Click *Find*.
3. Type label or value in *Find what* text box.
4. Click Find Next.

Replace Label or Value
1. Click Find & Select button.
2. Click *Replace*.
3. Type label or value in *Find what* text box.
4. Type replacement label or value in *Replace with* text box.
5. Click Find Next or Replace All.

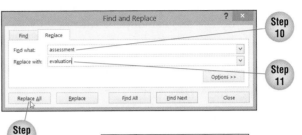

Step 10

Step 11

Step 12

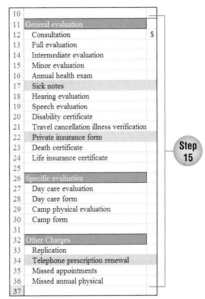

Step 15

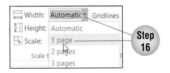

Step 16

In Addition

Replacing Formatting

You can use the Replace feature to find formatting and then replace or remove it. For example, you could find all occurrences of bold and blue font color and replace them with bold and green font color. At the Find and Replace dialog box with the Replace tab selected, click the Options button to display Format buttons to the right of the *Find what* and *Replace with* text boxes (shown at the right). Use these buttons to specify the desired formatting options. The Preview box (which initially displays the text *No Format Set*) displays the formats that will be found and/or replaced.

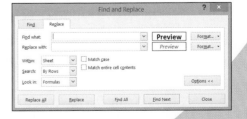

Activity 2.12

Freezing Panes; Changing the Zoom

When you scroll down or to the right to view parts of a worksheet that do not fit in the current window, some column or row headings may scroll off the screen, making it difficult to interpret text or values. You can use the Freeze Panes option to make sure rows and columns remain fixed when scrolling.

Magnify or reduce the worksheet display by dragging the Zoom slider bar button, clicking the Zoom In or Zoom Out buttons, or specifying a zoom percentage at the Zoom dialog box. Changing the on-screen zoom does not affect printing since worksheets print at 100% unless scaling options are changed.

Project

You will freeze row headings in the report to make sure data is easily understood even when scrolling. You will also experiment with various zoom settings to make more cells visible within the current window.

Cascade View PEDIATRICS

1. With **EMedS2-CVPRevYarborough.xlsx** open, make cell A11 the active cell.

2. Click the VIEW tab.

3. Click the Freeze Panes button in the Window group.

4. Click *Freeze Panes* at the drop-down list.

   All rows above the active cell are frozen. A horizontal black line appears, indicating which rows will remain fixed when scrolling, as shown in Figure E2.1.

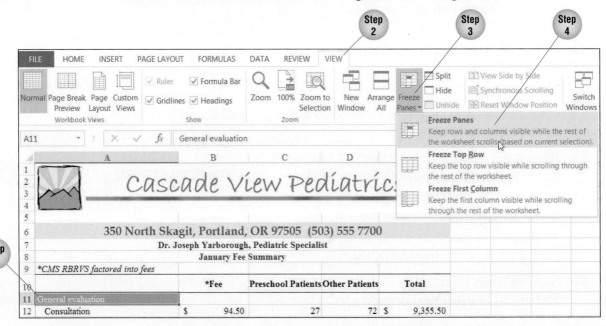

5. Press the Page Down key a few times to scroll down the worksheet.

   Notice that rows 1 through 10 do not scroll off the screen.

6. Press Ctrl + Home. Notice that cell A11 becomes the active cell since cell A1 is frozen.

7. Click the Freeze Panes button in the Window group and then click *Unfreeze Panes* at the drop-down list.

   The *Freeze Panes* option changes to *Unfreeze Panes* when rows or columns have been frozen.

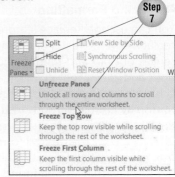

FIGURE E2.1 Worksheet with Rows 1–10 Frozen

	A	B	C	D	E
1					
2			*Cascade View Pediatrics*		
3					
4					
5					
6		350 North Skagit, Portland, OR 97505 (503) 555 7700			
7		Dr. Joseph Yarborough, Pediatric Specialist			
8		January Fee Summary			
9	*CMS RBRVS factored into fees*				
10		*Fee	Preschool Patients	Other Patients	Total
27	Day care evaluation	55.00	34	0	1,870.00
28	Day care form	30.00	34	0	1,020.00
29	Camp physical evaluation	40.00	10	33	1,720.00
30	Camp form				
31					
32	Other Charges				
33	Replication				
34	Telephone prescription renewal	16.50	24	54	1,287.00
35	Missed appointments				
36	Missed annual physical				

Rows 1 to 10 remain fixed in place as you scroll down.

A horizontal black line indicates that the rows above are frozen.

8 Click and drag the button on the Zoom slider bar (located at the right side of the Status bar, above the time on the Taskbar) and watch the cells grow and shrink as you drag right and left.

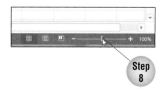

Step 8

9 Drag the Zoom slider button to the halfway mark on the slider bar to redisplay the worksheet at 100%.

10 Click *100%* at the right side of the slider bar to open the Zoom dialog box.

11 Click the *75%* option and then click OK.

12 Click the Zoom In button at the right side of the Zoom slider bar (displays as a plus symbol).

13 Continue to click the Zoom In button until the zoom percentage returns to 100%.

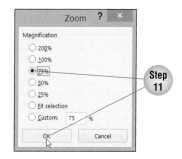

Step 11

When the zoom is set to 100%, clicking the Zoom In or Zoom Out buttons at either side of the slider bar magnifies or shrinks the display of the worksheet by 10%.

14 Save **EMedS2-CVPRevYarborough.xlsx**.

In Addition

Using the Zoom Group on the VIEW Tab

The VIEW tab contains a Zoom group with three buttons to change zoom settings, as shown at the right. Click the Zoom button to display the Zoom dialog box. This is the same dialog box that you displayed in Step 10. Click the 100% button to return the zoom to 100%. Select a range of cells and then click the Zoom to Selection button to zoom so that the selected range fills the worksheet area.

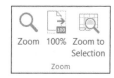

Activity 2.13

Creating Formulas with Absolute Addressing

In previous activities, when you copied and pasted formulas in worksheets, the cell addresses in the destination cells changed automatically *relative* to the destination row or column. The formulas in these worksheets used **relative addressing**. While relative addressing is helpful in many cases, sometimes you need a cell address to remain fixed when it is copied to another location in the worksheet.

To do this, the formulas must include **absolute addressing** for those cell addresses that you do not want to change. Make a cell address absolute by typing a dollar symbol ($) in front of the column letter and/or row number that you want to stay the same. You can also use the F4 function key to cycle through relative, absolute, or mixed variations of the address in which either the row is absolute and the column is relative or vice versa.

Project

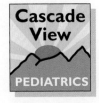

Dr. Yarborough would like to increase his monthly revenue by approximately $1,500. He has asked you to add columns to the report to determine the percentage by which he needs to increase his fees to achieve this goal.

1 With **EMedS2-CVPRevYarborough.xlsx** open, make cell F10 the active cell and then type **New Fee**.

2 Make cell G10 the active cell and then type **New Total**.

3 Make cell F9 the active cell, type **5%**, and then press Enter.

> Placing the percent increase in its own cell will allow you to easily try out different percentages until you find the one that will achieve the $1,500 increase in revenue. In the next steps you will create and copy formulas that will calculate revenue based on a 5% increase in fees.

4 Make cell F12 the active cell, type **=(B12*F9**, press F4, type **)+B12**, and then press Enter.

> You will be copying this formula to the remaining rows, so you need to make sure that the reference to cell F9 stays the same when the formula is duplicated. Pressing F4 causes Excel to insert dollar symbols in front of the row letter and column number immediately left of the insertion point—F9 becomes $F$9, an absolute address.

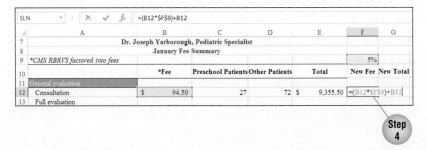

5 Make cell G12 the active cell, type **=(C12+D12)*F12**, and then press Enter.

> The formula to calculate the total revenue does not require an absolute reference. When copying this formula, you want the row numbers to change relative to the destination cells.

6 Make cell F16 the active cell, type **=(B16*$F$9)+B16**, and then press Enter.

> You can type the dollar symbols into the formula rather than inserting them by pressing F4.

	B	C	D	E	F	G
	Joseph Yarborough, Pediatric Specialist					
	January Fee Summary					
					5%	
	*Fee	Preschool Patients	Other Patients	Total	New Fee	New Total
	$ 94.50	27	72 $	9,355.50	$ 99.23	$9,823.28
	60.00	43	80	7,380.00	=(B16*$F$9)+B16	
	16.50	29	48	1,270.50		

Step 6

7 Make cell F16 the active cell and then click the Copy button in the Clipboard group on the HOME tab.

8 Select the range of cells F17:F19, hold down the Ctrl key, and then select cells F22, F27:F29, and F34.

9 Click the Paste button in the Clipboard group. (Make sure to click the button and not the button arrow.)

10 Press the Esc key to remove the marquee from cell F12.

11 Click cell F17 and then look at the Formula bar to see the formula that was pasted into the cell: *=(B17*$F$9)+B17*.

> Notice that the cell address containing the percent value (F9) did not change, while the cell address that contains the original fee for sick notes (B17) changed relative to the destination (row 17).

12 Click a few other cells in column F to view the formula. Notice that in each cell, the address for cell F9 remains the same while the cell address for column B always changes relative to the destination row.

13 Copy the formula in cell G12 and paste it into cells G16:G19, G22, G27:G29, and G34 by completing steps similar to those in Steps 8–11.

14 Copy the formula in cell E38, paste it into cell G38, and then AutoFit the column width.

15 Make cell A40 the active cell, type **Increase in January Revenue:**, make cell G40 the active cell, type **=G38-E38**, and then press Enter.

> The increased revenue, *$1,324.00*, does not meet the $1,500.00 goal.

16 Make cell F9 the active cell and edit the value to read *6%*.

17 Look at the updated value in cell G40. Notice that the increased revenue of $1,588.80 now meets the goal set by Dr. Yarborough.

18 Use Format Painter to copy the formatting from cell E10 to the range of cells F10:G10 and then turn on the display of formulas.

19 Save, print, and then close **EMedS2-CVPRevYarborough.xlsx**.

In Addition

Understanding Absolute Addressing

The following table provides examples of different variations on absolute addressing. Pressing F4 repeatedly causes Excel to move through each of these variations for the selected cell address.

Example	Action
=$A$12*.01	Neither the column nor the row will change.
=$A12*.01	The column will remain fixed at column A, but the row will change.
=A$12*.01	The column will change, but the row remains fixed at row 12.
=A12*.01	Both the column and row will change.

Features Summary

Feature	Ribbon Tab, Group	Button	Quick Access Toolbar	Keyboard Shortcut
Accounting format	HOME, Number	$		
align left	HOME, Alignment			
align right	HOME, Alignment			
bold	HOME, Font	B		Ctrl + B
borders	HOME, Font			Ctrl + Shift + &
cell styles	HOME, Styles			
center	HOME, Alignment			
clear cell	HOME, Editing			
clip art	INSERT, Illustrations			
Comma format	HOME, Number	,		
copy	HOME, Clipboard			Ctrl + C
cut	HOME, Clipboard			Ctrl + X
decrease decimal	HOME, Number	.00 →.0		
decrease indent	HOME, Alignment			
delete cell, column, or row	HOME, Cells			
fill color	HOME, Font			
find	HOME, Editing			Ctrl + F
font	HOME, Font	Calibri		Ctrl + 1
font color	HOME, Font	A		Ctrl + 1
font size	HOME, Font	11		Ctrl + 1
Format Painter	HOME, Clipboard			
freeze panes	VIEW, Window			
increase decimal	HOME, Number	←.0 .00		
increase indent	HOME, Alignment			
insert cell, column, or row	HOME, Cells			

Feature	Ribbon Tab, Group	Button	Quick Access Toolbar	Keyboard Shortcut
italic	HOME, Font	*I*		Ctrl + I
merge and center	HOME, Alignment			
middle-align	HOME, Alignment			
paste	HOME, Clipboard			Ctrl + V
picture from file	INSERT, Illustrations			
repeat				Ctrl + Y
replace	HOME, Editing			Ctrl + H
Spelling	REVIEW, Proofing	ABC		F7
theme	PAGE LAYOUT, Themes	Aa		
theme colors	PAGE LAYOUT, Themes			
theme fonts	PAGE LAYOUT, Themes	A		
Thesaurus	REVIEW, Proofing			Shift + F7
undo an action			↶	Ctrl + Z
zoom	VIEW, Zoom			

Knowledge Check

Completion: In the space provided at the right, write in the correct term, command, or option.

1. Click this button to search for clip art at Office.com.
2. Click this button in the Illustrations group to insert an image stored in a file.
3. Use this feature to remove everything from a cell, including text and formatting.
4. To insert a new row between rows 11 and 12, make active any cell in this row.
5. To insert a new column between columns E and F, make active any cell in this column
6. This is the term for adjusting the width of a column to the length of the longest entry.
7. This is the name for the feature that shows how a formatting option from a drop-down gallery will look when applied to a cell or worksheet.
8. By default, cells are initially set to this numeric format.

9. Click this button in the Alignment group on the HOME tab to center the contents of a cell vertically between the top and bottom cell boundaries. _____

10. Click this button in the Clipboard group on the HOME tab to copy the formatting of the active cell. _____

11. This feature stores predefined cell formatting options that can be applied with one click. _____

12. This feature stores sets of colors, fonts, and effects that can be applied to the entire worksheet with one click. _____

13. To freeze rows 1 through 5, begin by making this cell active. _____

14. List two ways to adjust the zoom so that more cells are visible in the current window. _____

Skills Review

Review 1 Inserting an Image; Editing and Clearing Cells; Deleting Columns and Rows

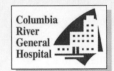

1. Open **CRGHLabReqRpt.xlsx**.
2. Save the workbook with the name **EMedS2-R-CRGHLabReqRpt**.
3. Make cell A1 the active cell and then insert **CRGHLogo.png**.
4. Resize and move the image so that it is positioned at the right side of cell A1.
5. Change the value in cell E30 from *17.87* to *16.55*.
6. Clear the contents and formatting of the range of cells A3:A4.
7. Clear the contents of the range of cells J40:P40.
8. Change the label in cell A26 from *Other* to *Immunology*.
9. Make cell B6 the active cell and then type **12 hr fast**.
10. Make cell B24 the active cell and then type **30 min rest**.
11. Delete row 3 and column C.
12. Save **EMedS2-R-CRGHLabReqRpt.xlsx**.

Review 2 Moving and Copying Cells; Inserting and Deleting Rows; Freezing Panes

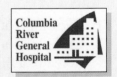

1. With **EMedS2-R-CRGHLabReqRpt.xlsx** open, move the contents of cell A2 to cell A3 and then merge and center the range of cells A3:F3.
2. Move the contents of cell E44 to cell A44.
3. Make cell G5 the active cell and then freeze panes.
4. Copy the formula in cell F44 and then paste it into cells I44, K44, M44, and N44.
5. Delete row 2.
6. Delete the row for which no requisitions were ordered in January (*Other Swabs*).
7. Insert a new row between *Other Tests* and *HDL & LDL* and then type **Antiphospholipid Antibodies** in column A of the new row.

8. Add the following data for Antiphospholipid Antibodies:

Lab Code:	**29011**	Fee:		**38.57**	
Reqs:	**2**	Insured Reqs:		**0**	
Third Party Bill Reqs:	**0**	Patient Direct Bill Reqs:	**2**		

9. Enter the formulas required to finish the total calculations for antiphospholipid antibodies requisitions.
10. Unfreeze the panes.
11. Save **EMedS2-R-CRGHLabReqRpt.xlsx**.

Review 3 Adjusting Column Width; Replacing Data; Formatting Numbers; Indenting Text

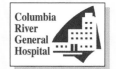

Columbia River General Hospital

1. With **EMedS2-R-CRGHLabReqRpt.xlsx** open, AutoFit columns A, B, and C.
2. Change the width of column G to *1.00 (16 pixels)*.
3. Select columns E, H, J, and L and then change the width to *6.00 (61 pixels)*.
4. Use the Replace feature to replace all occurrences of the value *15.45* with *16.25*.
5. Apply the Comma format to the values in columns I, K, M, and N.
6. Apply the Accounting format to the values in column F.
7. Format the values in column O to display with two decimal places.
8. Select the ranges of cells A4:A15, A18:A22, A25:A29, A32:A36, and A39:A41 and then click the Increase Indent button once.
9. Save **EMedS2-R-CRGHLabReqRpt.xlsx**.

Review 4 Changing Font, Font Attributes, and Alignment; Applying Cell Styles; Adding Borders and Shading; Using Format Painter

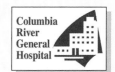

Columbia River General Hospital

1. With **EMedS2-R-CRGHLabReqRpt.xlsx** open, change the font in cell A1 to 36-point Bookman Old Style. *Note: If necessary, substitute another font, such as Times New Roman.*
2. Change the fill color in cell A1 to *Blue, Accent 5, Lighter 60%*.
3. Center the labels in the range of cells C3:O3 both horizontally and vertically.
4. Center horizontally the labels in the ranges of cells C17:D17, C24:D24, C31:D31, and C38:D38.
5. Select the range of cells A2:O2, apply bold formatting, and then change the fill color to *Blue, Accent 5, Lighter 80%*.
6. Select the range of cells C3:O3 and then apply the Accent1 cell style.
7. Make cell A3 the active cell and then apply the Accent3 cell style. Use Format Painter to copy the formatting from cell A3 to cells A17, A24, A31, and A38.
8. Add a top and bottom border to the range of cells A3:O3.
9. Add a top and double bottom border to cells F43, I43, K43, M43, and N43.
10. Make cell B3 the active cell and then type **Comments**. Use Format Painter to copy the formatting from cell C3 to cell B3.
11. Save **EMedS2-R-CRGHLabReqRpt.xlsx**.

Review 5 Inserting Comments; Changing the Zoom

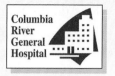

1. With **EMedS2-R-CRGHLabReqRpt.xlsx** open, make cell O6 the active cell and then insert the following comment:

    Check billings. Two extra reqs have been added to Insured, Third Party, or Patient Direct.

2. Make cell O14 the active cell and then add the same comment text as in Step 1.
3. Display the worksheet in the Print backstage area. Notice the worksheet will print on two pages.
4. Click the Back button to close the Print backstage area.
5. Change the zoom to *80%*.
6. Click the PAGE LAYOUT tab and then change the orientation to landscape.
7. In the Scale to Fit group, change the width to *1 page*.
8. In the Scale to Fit group, change the height to *1 page*.
9. Change the zoom to *100%*.
10. Print the worksheet. *Note: Check with your instructor if you submit your work in hard copy to see if you need to print two copies of this worksheet with one of the copies showing the cell formulas instead of the calculated results.*
11. Save and then close **EMedS2-R-CRGHLabReqRpt.xlsx**.

Skills Assessment

Assessment 1 Changing Zoom; Adjusting Column Width; Changing Font Color and Fill Color

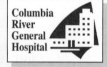

1. Tracy Fitzgerald, manager of support services at Columbia River General Hospital, has asked you to make changes to a worksheet containing recent Canadian healthcare statistical data. Tracy and Michelle Tan, CEO, will be presenting at a medical conference in Vancouver, British Columbia. Their presentation on the differences between patient costs and outcomes between the United States and Canada will rely heavily on the data in this worksheet. To begin, open **CRGHCdnHealthStats.xlsx**.
2. Save the workbook with the name **EMedS2-A1-CRGHCdnHealthStats.xlsx**.
3. Make the following changes:
    a. Change the zoom so you can view as much of the worksheet as possible to minimize horizontal scrolling. Make sure the cells are still readable. *Note: Depending on your monitor size and resolution settings, change the zoom to a value between 70% and 90%.*
    b. AutoFit all column widths to the length of the longest entry.
    c. Change the fill color behind the title *Total Healthcare Costs in Canada.* You determine the color.
    d. Change the font color and fill color for *Breakdown of Healthcare Costs by Procedures in Canada* and *Mortality Rates by Age/Sex in Canada by 100,000.* You determine the colors.
    e. Change the font color and fill color for *Leading Causes of Death in Canada 2014* and *Physical activity by age group and sex in Canada 2014.* You determine the colors.
4. Change the page orientation to landscape.
5. Save **EMedS2-A1-CRGHCdnHealthStats.xlsx**.

Assessment 2 Editing Cells; Inserting and Deleting Rows; Moving and Copying Cells; Formatting a Worksheet

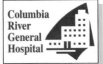

1. There is still work to be done on the Canadian healthcare statistical data worksheet before Tracy and Michelle can prepare the presentation for the conference in Vancouver. With **EMedS2-A1-CRGHCdnHealthStats.xlsx** open, edit the worksheet using the following information:
   a. In the *Total Healthcare Costs in Canada* section, for the year 2012, *Hospitals* should be *15326* instead of *14175.2*.
   b. In the *Total Healthcare Costs in Canada* section of the worksheet, insert a new column before *2011* and then enter the data as follows:

	2010
Hospitals:	**10299**
Other institutions:	**8204.7**
Physicians:	**21992**
Other professionals:	**21584.1**
Drugs:	**34669.8**
Other:	**15792.5**

   c. AutoFit column Q to the longest entry and then clear the formatting in cell Q1.
   d. The formula to sum total healthcare costs for each year is missing. Enter the correct formula for the first year, 2010 (Q10) and then copy the formula to cells R10, S10, T10, and U10. ***Hint: Be careful to sum to correct range***.
   e. Apply the Comma format with no decimal places to the numeric cells in the *Total Healthcare Costs in Canada* section of the worksheet.
   f. Type **in millions of dollars** in cell P2 and then apply bold and italic formatting.
   g. Merge and center cells A1, A25, I1, I29, and P1 over the columns in the respective sections.
   h. Change the alignment of any headings in the worksheet whose appearance could be improved.
   i. Move the contents of the range of cells P1:U10 (*Total Healthcare Costs in Canada* section) to cells I58:N67. Adjust the column widths as necessary after moving the cells.
   j. Apply font, border, and color formatting to enhance the appearance of the worksheet.
2. Save **EMedS2-A1-CRGHCdnHealthStats.xlsx**.

Assessment 3 Editing and Moving Cells; Entering Formulas; Formatting Numeric Cells

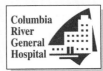

1. Tracy has reviewed the latest copy of the Canadian healthcare statistical data worksheet and noted the following changes to be made. With **EMedS2-A1-CRGHCdnHealthStats.xlsx** open, complete the worksheet using the following information:
   a. Type the following label in cell A60:
      Source: Statistics Canada, http://www.statcan.ca
   b. Cancer and cardiac disease are the two leading causes of death in Canada in 2014. In cell G3, create a formula to sum the male deaths from cancer and cardiac disease in the *Leading Causes of Death in Canada* section. In cell H3, create a formula to sum the female deaths from cancer and cardiac disease in the *Leading Causes of Death in Canada* section. In cell F3, calculate the total of cells G3 and H3 (male and female cardiac and cancer cases) as a percentage of cell E18.

c. Apply the Percent format with 1 decimal place to cell F3.

d. Enter a formula in cell B20 that will calculate the total deaths by psychoses and suicide as a percentage of cell E18. Format the result using the Percent format with 1 decimal place.

e. Enter a formula in cell B21 that will calculate the increase in total deaths by psychoses and suicide in the next year using the percent value in cell D21 as the increase percentage on the current total. Format the result using the Comma format.

2. Save **EMedS2-A1-CRGHCdnHealthStats.xlsx**.

Assessment 4 Performing Spell Check; Adjusting Column Width; Editing and Clearing Cells; Using Replace

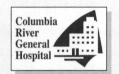

1. Further research at the Statistics Canada website has revealed that some input errors exist in the Canadian healthcare statistics worksheet. With **EMedS2-A1-CRGHCdnHealthStats.xlsx** open, make the following corrections:

a. Make cell A1 the active cell and then perform a spelling check and correct any errors.

b. AutoFit all column widths except the width of column F, which should be set to *8*.

c. Correct the following data entry errors in the *Physical activity by age group and sex in Canada 2014* section:

15–19 years, Females, Physically active:	430,212
20–24 years, Males, Physically inactive:	392,789
25–34 years, Males, Physically active:	472,345
35–44 years, Females, Physically inactive:	1,567,954

d. Clear the contents of the range of cells I4:N4.

e. Make cell N5 the active cell and then type the formula that will calculate the overall average from 2011 to 2014 for Major surgery healthcare costs: =SUM(J5:M5)/4. Copy this formula to the remaining rows in the section. If necessary, format the values to one decimal place.

f. Replace all occurrences of *Disease* with *Illness*. **Note: Do not use Replace All. Do not replace the text in cells in which other word forms of Disease (such as Diseases) exist.**

g. Make cell A62 active, type **Date:**, and then type today's date.

2. Click the PAGE LAYOUT tab and then change the *Width* option in the Scale to Fit group to *1 page*.

3. Print **EMedS2-A1-CRGHCdnHealthStats.xlsx**. *Note: Check with your instructor if you submit your work in hard copy to see if you need to print two copies of this worksheet with one of the copies showing the cell formulas instead of the calculated results.*

4. Save and then close **EMedS2-A1-CRGHCdnHealthStats.xlsx**.

Assessment 5 Finding Information on Dates

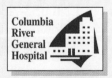

1. Use Excel's Help feature to find more information on how Excel stores dates and how they can be used in formulas.

2. Open **EMedS2-A1-CRGHCdnHealthStats.xlsx**.

3. Add the label *Presentation Date:* to cell A63.

4. Enter the date *April 13, 2016* in cell B63.

5. Add the label *Final Preparation Date:* to cell A64.

HELP

6. Create a formula in cell B64 that will subtract 5 days from the presentation date.
7. Use Save As to save the revised workbook with the name **EMedS2-A5-CRGHCdnHealthStats.xlsx**.
8. Print and then close **EMedS2-A5-CRGHCdnHealthStats.xlsx**. *Note: Check with your instructor if you submit your work in hard copy to see if you need to print two copies of this worksheet with one of the copies showing the cell formulas instead of the calculated results.*

Assessment 6 Locating Information on U.S. Healthcare Costs

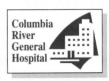

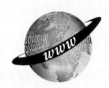

1. Tracy Fitzgerald has asked you to research healthcare costs in the United States for the presentation in Vancouver. Search the Internet for healthcare cost statistics for the United States. Consider narrowing your search to one area of focus, such as cancer or cardiac costs.
2. Create a workbook that summarizes the information you found.
3. Insert related clip art.
4. Create a formula that includes an absolute cell reference.
5. Include the sources for your data in the workbook.
6. Save the workbook with the name **EMedS2-A6-USHealthStats**.
7. Display formulas in the worksheet, print, and then close **EMedS2-A6-USHealthStats.xlsx**.

Marquee Challenge

Challenge 1 Preparing a Weekly Staffing Schedule for Neurology

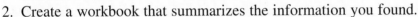

1. Create the worksheet shown in Figure E2.2 on page 302, including all formatting options. The worksheet shown has the Circuit theme applied. Use your best judgment to determine font, font size, font and fill colors, column widths, and/or row heights.
2. Insert **CRGHLogo.png** into the worksheet and then size and position it as desired.
3. Change the page orientation to landscape.
4. Save the workbook with the name **EMedS2-C1-NeurologyStaffing**.
5. Print and then close **EMedS2-C1-NeurologyStaffing.xlsx**.

Challenge 2 Preparing a Radiology Requisition Form

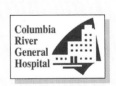

1. Open **CRGHRadiologyReq.xlsx**.
2. Edit and format the worksheet as shown in Figure E2.3 on page 302, including performing a spelling check. Use your best judgment to match as closely as possible the colors and fonts shown. The worksheet shown has the Circuit theme applied.
3. Save the workbook with the name **EMedS2-C2-CRGHRadiologyReq**.
4. Print and then close **EMedS2-C2-CRGHRadiologyReq.xlsx**.

FIGURE E2.2 Challenge 1

Columbia River General Hospital								Columbia River General Hospital

Neurology Staffing Worksheet

Beds:	6	Shift 1:	7am- 7pm			Rotation		
		Shift 2:	7pm- 7am			2 days followed by 2 nights; 4 on followed by 5 off		

Bed	Shift	Mon	Tue	Wed	Thu	Fri	Sat	Sun
1	1	McAllister	McAllister	Keller	Keller	Rashmi	Rashmi	Hillman
1	2	Yoshiko	Yoshiko	McAllister	McAllister	Huang	Huang	Baird
2	1	Hillman	Graham	Johan	Johan	McKenna	Petrovic	Zukic
2	2	Baird	Hillman	Hillman	Zukic	Zukic	Graham	Graham
3	1	Graham	Baird	Santos	Santos	Bernis	McKenna	Huang
3	2	Santos	Santos	Bernis	Bernis	Anatolius	Alvarez	Alvarez
4	1	Jorgensen	Jorgensen	Wei	Wei	Vezina	Zukic	Petrovic
4	2	McKenna	Wells	Wells	Jenkins	Johan	Johan	McKenna
5	1	Alvarez	Alvarez	Yoshiko	Yoshiko	Orlowski	Bernis	Jenkins
5	2	Petrovic	Petrovic	Jorgensen	Jorgensen	Jenkins	Anatolius	Lind
6	1	Huang	Biorje	Baird	Wells	Wells	Tomasz	Anatolius
6	2	Keller	Keller	Rashmi	Rashmi	Wei	Wei	Tomasz

FIGURE E2.3 Challenge 2

A	B	C	D	E
Columbia River General Hospital				
Radiology Requisition				
Patient Last Name		Date		
Patient First Name		Office use only		
Chart Number		Dept Charge Code		
Physician		Amount		
Technician			Left	Right
Esophagus		Ribs		
Upper G.I. Series		Sternoclavicular Joints		
Small Bowel		Clavicle		
Barium Enema		Shoulder		
		A.C. Joints		
Acute Abdomen		Scapula		
Chest		Humerus		
Sternum		Elbow		
Facial Bones		Forearm		
Mandible		Write		
Nasal Bones		Hand		
Skull		Finger or Thumb		
Sinuses		Hip		
T.M. Joints		Femur		
Cervical Spine		Knee		
Thoracic Spine		Tibia and Fibula		
Lumbosacral Spine		Ankle		
Pelvis		Heel		
Sacrum and Coccyx		Foot		
		Toe		
*Esophagus, Stomach, or Small Bowel		**Mammogram		
*Nothing to eat or drink after midnight prior to examination.				
**Wear separate blouse with skirt or slacks. No deodorant or talc.				

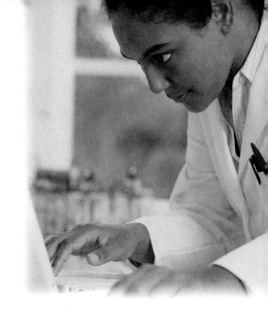

Excel SECTION 3

Using Functions, Adding Visual Elements, Printing, and Working with Tables

Student Resources

Before beginning the activities in Excel Section 3, copy to your storage medium the ExcelMedS3 folder from the Student Resources CD. This folder contains the data files you need to complete the projects in this Excel section.

Projects Overview

Calculate statistics and set print options for the standard exam room supplies report; compare discounts from two medical supply vendors and add graphics to the report; calculate dates in the dermatology patient tracking worksheet; and create charts summarizing dermatology diagnoses by age group of patient.

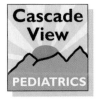

Revise the January fee summary report to calculate fee increases; calculate statistical functions, add dates, calculate expense variance, add a logo, sort, and set print options for a quarterly expense report; and create a chart, draw objects, and format a table in a rent and maintenance cost report.

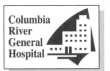

Finish a weekly adult cardiac bypass surgery report; calculate average standard costs for cardiac surgery patient stays; create charts, and change print options for a quarterly expense report; format, filter and sort the cardiac nurse casual call list; filter and sort the nursing professional development list; and create and format a patient cost report and a chart on U.S. cancer statistics.

303

Activity 3.1

Using Statistical Functions AVERAGE, COUNT, MAX, and MIN

So far, the only Excel function you have worked with is SUM. Excel includes numerous other built-in functions that are grouped into categories. The Statistical category contains several functions that can be used for data analysis purposes, such as calculating medians, variances, and frequencies, among others. The structure of a function formula begins with the equals sign (=), followed by the name of the function, and then the argument within parentheses. *Argument* is the term given to the values to be included in the calculation. The structure of the argument is dependent on the function being used and can include a single range of cells, multiple ranges, single cell references, or a combination thereof.

Project

Lee Elliott, office manager of North Shore Medical Clinic, would like you to compile statistics on the cost of supplies for eight exam rooms.

1. Open **NSMCSupplies.xlsx**.

2. Save the workbook in the ExcelMedS3 folder and name it **EMedS3-NSMCSupplies**.

3. Make cell F4 the active cell and then freeze the panes. Refer to Section 2, Activity 2.12, if you need assistance with this step.

4. Type the following labels in the cells indicated:

   A65:   **Average exam room standard cost:**
   A66:   **Maximum exam room standard cost:**
   A67:   **Minimum exam room standard cost:**
   A68:   **Count of exam room items:**

5. Make cell B65 the active cell.

   In the next steps, you will insert the AVERAGE function to determine the arithmetic mean of the totals in the cells in row 63. If an empty cell or a cell containing text is included in the argument, Excel ignores the cell when determining the result. If, however, the cell contains a zero value, it is included in the average calculation.

6. Click the HOME tab and then click the AutoSum button arrow in the Editing group.

7. Click *Average* at the drop-down list.

   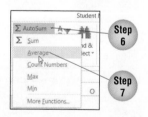

   Excel inserts the formula *=AVERAGE()* in the active cell with the insertion point positioned between the parentheses. Since no values exist immediately above or to the left of the active cell, Excel does not offer a suggested range. In the next step, you will drag to select the range in the formula.

8. Position the cell pointer over cell F63, hold down the left mouse button, drag right to cell M63, and then release the left mouse button. The range F63:M63 is inserted as the function argument.

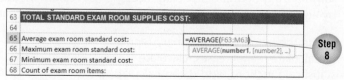

9 Press Enter or click the Enter button on the Formula bar.

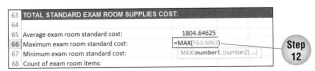

Step 9

> Excel returns the result *1804.64625* in cell B65.

10 If it is not already active, make cell B66 the active cell.

11 Click the AutoSum button arrow and then click *Max* at the drop-down list.

> The MAX function returns the largest value in the argument.

12 Type **F63:M63** and then press Enter.

> Excel returns the result *2191.58* in cell B66. Typing the range into the formula is sometimes faster if you are sure of the starting and ending cell references.

63	TOTAL STANDARD EXAM ROOM SUPPLIES COST:	
64		
65	Average exam room standard cost:	1804.64625
66	Maximum exam room standard cost:	=MAX(F63:M63)
67	Minimum exam room standard cost:	MAX(**number1**, [number2], ...)
68	Count of exam room items:	

Step 12

13 With cell B67 the active cell, type the function **=MIN(F63:M63)** and then press Enter.

> The MIN function returns the smallest value in the argument, *1381.27*. You can type the entire function directly into the cell if you know the name of the function you want to use and the structure of the argument.

64		
65	Average exam room standard cost:	1804.64625
66	Maximum exam room standard cost:	2191.58
67	Minimum exam room standard cost:	1381.27
68	Count of exam room items:	
69		

Step 13

14 With cell B68 the active cell, type the function **=COUNT(D4:D62)** and then press Enter.

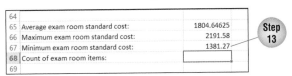

Step 14

> COUNT returns the number of cells that contain numbers or numbers that have been formatted as text and dates. Empty cells, text labels, or error values in the range are ignored.

15 Apply the Comma format to the range of cells B65:B67.

16 Click in any cell to deselect the range of cells B65:B67.

17 Save and then close **EMedS3-NSMCSupplies.xlsx**.

In Brief

Insert AVERAGE, MAX, MIN, or COUNT Functions
1. Make desired cell active.
2. Click AutoSum button arrow.
3. Click desired function.
4. Type or select argument.
5. Press Enter or click Enter button.

In Addition

Exploring Other Statistical Functions

Click *More Functions* at the AutoSum button drop-down list to open the Insert Function dialog box. This dialog box will allow you to access Excel's complete list of functions. A sampling of other statistical functions and their descriptions includes the following:

Function Name	Description
=COUNTA	counts the number of cells in a range (including those that contain labels); ignores empty cells
=COUNTBLANK	counts the number of empty cells in a range
=MEDIAN	returns the number in the middle of a range

Activity 3.2

Writing Formulas with Dates and Date Functions

Excel provides the TODAY and NOW date and time functions that insert the current date or date and time into a worksheet. The advantage to using the functions rather than just typing the date and/or time is that the functions automatically update the date and time when you open the worksheet. When you type a date in a cell, the date is stored as a serial number. Serial numbers in Excel begin with the number 1 (which represents January 1, 1900) and increase sequentially. Because dates are stored as numbers, they can be used in formulas. A date will appear in a cell based on how it is entered. Specify the appearance of dates in a worksheet with options at the Format Cells dialog box with the Number tab selected.

Project

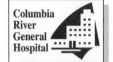

You will finish the weekly adult cardiac bypass surgery report for Columbia River General Hospital by entering dates and formulas to track patient movement from surgery to the follow-up visit at the surgeon's office 30 days later.

1. Open **CRGHCardiacSurgWk45.xlsx**.

2. Save the workbook in the ExcelMedS3 folder and name it **EMedS3-CRGHCardiacSurgWk45**.

3. Make cell I4 the active cell, type **=NOW()**, and then press Enter.

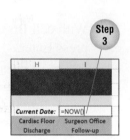

Step 3

   The current date and time are inserted in cell I4. In the next step, you will enter the TODAY function to see the difference between the two.

4. Make cell I4 the active cell, press Delete to clear the cell, type **=TODAY()**, and then press Enter.

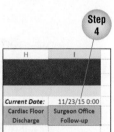

Step 4

   The current date is inserted in the cell with the time displayed as *0:00*. Normally, the time does not display when TODAY is used; however, since you entered the NOW function first, Excel retained the time format for the cell. In a later step, you will format the cell to display only the month, day, and year.

5. Make cell B4 the active cell, click the AutoSum button arrow in the Editing group, and then click *More Functions* at the drop-down list.

   The Insert Function dialog box opens. At this dialog box, you can search for a function by typing a phrase describing the type of formula you want in the *Search for a function* text box and then clicking the Go button or by selecting a category name and then browsing a list of functions.

6. Click the down-pointing arrow at the right of the *Or select a category* option box and then click *Date & Time* at the drop-down list.

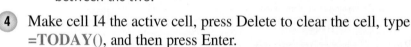

Step 6

Step 7

   The *Select a function* list box displays an alphabetical list of date and time functions. Clicking a function name causes the formula, its argument structure, and a description to appear below the list box.

7. With *DATE* selected in the *Select a function* list box, read the description of the formula and then click OK.

   The Function Arguments dialog box opens with a text box for each section of the function argument.

8 Type **2015** in the *Year* text box.

9 Press Tab to move the insertion point to the *Month* text box and then type **11**.

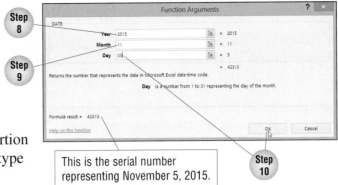

In Brief

Insert Date Functions
1. Make desired cell active.
2. Click AutoSum button arrow.
3. Click *More Functions*.
4. Change category to *Date & Time*.
5. Click desired function name.
6. Click OK.
7. Enter references in Function Arguments dialog box.
8. Click OK.

10 Press Tab to move the insertion point to the *Day* text box, type **05**, and then click OK.

This is the serial number representing November 5, 2015.

The Function Arguments dialog box displays the serial number for November 5, 2015, as *41218*. This is the value Excel stores in the cell. Notice that the formula in the Formula bar is *=DATE(2015,11,5)*.

11 Make cell D4 the active cell, type **=B4+6**, and then press Enter.

Excel displays the result *11/11/2015* in the cell (6 days from the week start date).

12 Make cell G6 the active cell, type **=F6+1**, and then press Enter.

During this report week, each patient moved through the system at normal speed, which is one day in the CSRU (Cardiac Surgery Recovery Unit).

13 Make cell H6 the active cell, type **=G6+4**, and then press Enter.

Bypass patients each spent four days on the cardiac floor after CSRU.

14 Make cell I6 the active cell, type **=E6+30**, and then press Enter.

Bypass patients attend a follow-up visit 30 days after their surgery date.

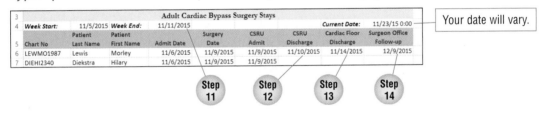

Your date will vary.

15 Select the range of cells G6:I6 and then use the fill handle to copy the formulas to the remaining rows (G7:I24).

16 Select the range of cells I6:I24.

In the next steps, you will format the date entries for the surgeon's follow-up visit to display the day of the week.

17 Click the Number Format button arrow in the Number group.

18 Click *Long Date* at the drop-down list.

19 AutoFit the width of column I.

You now need to change the dates of follow-up visits that fall on a Saturday or Sunday, since the surgeon's office is closed weekends.

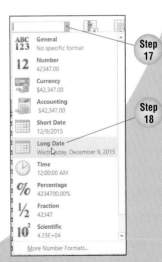

20 Make cell I15 the active cell, type **=DATE(2015,12,14)**, and then press Enter.

21 Copy cell I15 to each cell that resulted in a Saturday follow-up visit.

22 Make cell I21 the active cell, type **=DATE(2015,12,17)**, and then press Enter.

23 Copy the contents of cell I21 to each cell that resulted in a Sunday follow-up visit.

24 Save, print, and then close **EMedS3-CRGHCardiacSurgWk45.xlsx**.

Activity 3.3

Creating and Using Range Names

Assigning a name to a cell or a range of cells allows you to reference the cell(s) using a descriptive label rather than the cell or range address. This can save time and reduce confusion when creating formulas, printing, or navigating a large worksheet. Referencing by name also makes formulas easier to understand. For example, while a formula such as *=D3-D13* requires the reader to look at the labels next to the values in the cells in order to grasp its purpose, a formula such as *=Sales-Expenses* is easily and immediately understood. A range name can be a combination of letters, numbers, underscores, or periods up to 255 characters. The first character in a range name must be a letter, an underscore, or a backslash (\). Spaces are not valid in a range name. To create a range name, select the desired cells and then type the name in the Name box at the left of the Formula bar. When creating range names, consider the readability of the formula and use upper- and lowercase letters to facilitate comprehension.

Project

The November cardiac surgery cost report for Dr. Novak has been started. You have been asked to complete the *Standard Cost* column. You decide to begin by naming the cells to help you build the correct formula.

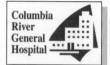

1. Open **CRGHNovakCardiacCosts.xlsx**.

2. Save the workbook in the ExcelMedS3 folder and name it **EMedS3-CRGHNovakCardiacCosts**.

   To begin, you want to name the cells in column D *Days*. The first step in naming a range is to select the range with which the name will be associated.

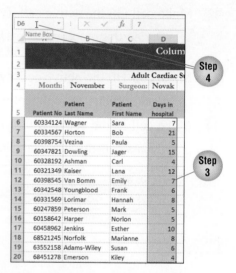

3. Select the range of cells D6:D20.

4. With the range of cells D6:D20 selected, point to the white box at the left side of the Formula bar (currently displays *D6*). Notice the ScreenTip that displays *Name Box*.

   The Name box displays the cell address of the active cell. If the active cell has been named, the name appears in the Name box instead. To assign a name to a cell or selected range, click in the Name box, type the desired name, and then press Enter.

5. Click in the Name box, type **Days**, and then press Enter.

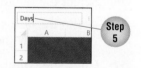

   The range name now appears in the Name box. In the next steps, you will assign a range name to individual cells that will be needed to calculate the standard cost.

6. Make cell G6 the active cell.

7. Click in the Name box, type **ShortCost**, and press then Enter.

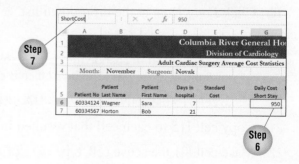

8. Make cell H6 the active cell, click in the Name box, type **LongCost**, and then press Enter.

9 Make cell I6 the active cell, click in the Name box, type **OvhShort**, and then press Enter.

10 Make cell J6 the active cell, click in the Name box, type **OvhLong**, and then press Enter.

11 Click the down-pointing arrow at the right of the Name box.

> A drop-down list of range names in the current workbook appears. To move the active cell to a named cell or range, click the name in the drop-down list.

12 Click *Days* at the drop-down list.

> The range D6:D20 is selected.

13 Make cell B24 the active cell, type **Average Days in Hospital:**, and then press Enter.

14 Make cell D24 the active cell, type **=AVERAGE(days)**, and then press Enter.

> Notice that range names are not case sensitive when used in a formula. When you type the range name *days* in the formula, notice that Excel color codes cells D6:D20 to show you the cells that are being referenced in the formula.

15 Format cell D24 to display zero decimal places.

16 Save **EMedS3-CRGHNovakCardiacCosts.xlsx**.

In Brief
Name Range
1. Select cell(s).
2. Click in Name box.
3. Type desired range name.
4. Press Enter.

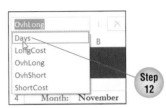

Step 12

Step 13 / Step 14

	A	B	C	D	E
5	Patient No	Patient Last Name	Patient First Name	Days in hospital	Standard Cost
6	60334124	Wagner	Sara	7	
7	60334567	Horton	Bob	21	
8	60398754	Vezina	Paula	5	
9	60347821	Dowling	Jager	15	
10	60328192	Ashman	Carl	4	
11	60321349	Kaiser	Lana	12	
12	60398545	Van Bomm	Emily	7	
13	60342548	Youngblood	Frank	6	
14	60331569	Lorimar	Hannah	8	
15	60247859	Peterson	Mark	5	
16	60158642	Harper	Norlon	5	
17	60458962	Jenkins	Esther	10	
18	68521245	Norfolk	Marianne	8	
19	63552158	Adams-Wiley	Susan	6	
20	68451278	Emerson	Kiley	4	
21					
22		Total Standard Cost:			
23					
24		Average Days in Hospital:		=AVERAGE(days)	
25					

In Addition

Managing Range Names

To edit or delete a range name, display the Name Manager dialog box, shown at the right. To do this, click the FORMULAS tab and then click the Name Manager button in the Defined Names group. The Name Manager dialog box displays the range names in the active workbook and provides buttons to edit or delete names.

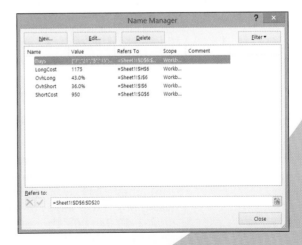

Activity 3.4

Using the Logical IF Function

The IF function returns one of two values in a cell based on a true-or-false answer to a question called a **logical test**. The format of an IF function is =*IF(logical_test,value_if_true,value_if_false)*. For example, assume a medical supplies salesperson earns a 3 percent commission if his or her sales are greater than or equal to $100,000 and a 2 percent commission if his or her sales are less than $100,000. Assume the sales value resides in cell B4. The statement B4>=100000 (*logical_test*) can only return a true or false answer. Depending on the answer, the salesperson's commission will be calculated at either B4*3% (*value_if_true*) or B4*2% (*value_if_false*). In this example, the IF function formula would be =*IF(B4>=100000,B4*3%,B4*2%)*.

Project

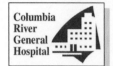

Columbia River General Hospital

Continuing your work on the November cardiac surgery cost report, you now need to calculate standard costs for patient stays. Standard costs are based on a daily cost rate and an overhead charge, both of which are dependent on the duration of the patient's stay.

1 With **EMedS3-CRGHNovakCardiacCosts.xlsx** open, make cell E6 the active cell.

2 Click the FORMULAS tab.

3 Click the Logical button ⬚ in the Function Library group and then click *IF* at the drop-down list.

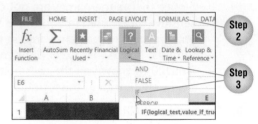

The Function Arguments dialog box for the IF statement opens. Notice the text boxes for the three arguments: *Logical_test, Value_if_true,* and *Value_if_false*. To begin, you want Excel to test whether the value in the Days range is less than or equal to 7. This test determines whether Excel calculates the standard cost at $950 per day and the overhead charge at 36% or $1175 per day with an overhead charge of 43%. You will use range names to make the IF statement easier to create and understand.

4 With the insertion point positioned in the *Logical_test* text box, type **days<=7** and then press Tab.

Watch the entries that appear at the right of each argument text box as you build the formula. Excel updates these entries to show you how the formula is working as you build each argument. Notice that next to the *Logical_test* text box you now see the TRUE and FALSE results Excel has calculated for each entry in the Days range.

5 With the insertion point positioned in the *Value_if_true* text box, type **(days*shortcost)+(days*shortcost*ovhshort)** and then press Tab.

If the Days value in cell D6 is less than or equal to 7, Excel calculates the standard cost as the days in hospital (D6) times 950 (G6) plus the days in hospital (D6) times 950 (G6) times a 36% overhead charge (I6). Another advantage to using range names is that by default, range names use absolute references. Since the formula will be copied to rows 7–20, absolute references are required for those cells that reference the daily cost and the percentages.

6 With the insertion point positioned in the *Value_if_false* text box, type **(days*longcost)+(days*longcost*ovhlong)**.

If the value in cell D6 is greater than 7, the formula calculates the standard cost as the days in hospital (D6) times 1175 (H6) plus the days in hospital (D6) times 1175 (H6) times a 43% overhead charge (J6). Notice that in the lower left corner of the dialog box, Excel shows the result that will be placed in the active cell (*Formula result = $9,044.00*). The value in cell D6 is 7, so the standard cost is calculated as (7*950)+(7*950*36%).

7 Click OK.

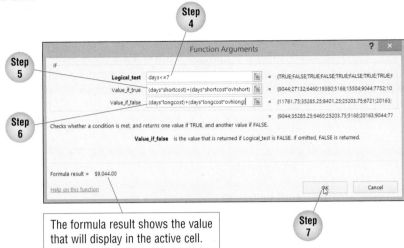

Step 4

Step 5

Step 6

The formula result shows the value that will display in the active cell.

Step 7

In Brief

Insert IF Function
1. Make desired cell active.
2. Click FORMULAS tab.
3. Click Logical button.
4. Click *IF*.
5. Type formula in *Logical_test* text box.
6. Type value or formula in *Value_if_true* text box.
7. Type value or formula in *Value_if_false* text box.
8. Click OK.

8 Drag the fill handle in cell E6 down to row 20 and then click in any cell to deselect the range.

9 Make cell E22 the active cell, click the AutoSum button in the Function Library group, and then press Enter to calculate the total standard cost for all of Dr. Novak's November surgeries.

10 Apply the Comma format to the range of cells E6:E20.

11 Click cell E6 and review the formula in the Formula bar: *=IF(Days<=7, (Days*ShortCost)+(Days*ShortCost*OvhShort),(Days*LongCost)+(Days*Long Cost*OvhLong))*.

The formula may be easier to comprehend if you include the range names when reading it to yourself.

Step 11

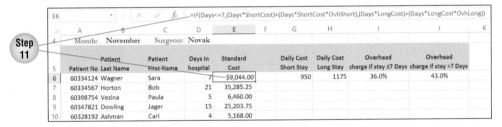

12 Save and then close **EMedS3-CRGHNovakCardiacCosts.xlsx**.

In Addition

Exploring the Benefits of the Function Arguments Dialog Box

One advantage to creating an IF function using the Function Arguments dialog box is that the formula automatically appears in the correct syntax. You do not have to worry about typing commas between arguments or the opening and closing brackets; these elements are automatically added to the formula. Another advantage is that the range names in the completed formula are also automatically displayed in the case used when the range name was created. For example, in this activity you typed *days*shortcost*, but the final formula displayed this entry as *Days*ShortCost*.

Activity 3.5

Creating a Column Chart

Numerical values are often more easily understood when presented visually in a chart. Excel includes several chart types, such as column, line, pie, bar, area, and scatter, with which you can graphically portray data. A chart can be placed in the same worksheet as the data or it can be inserted on its own sheet. To create a chart, select the cells containing the data you want to use and then choose the chart type. Excel charts the data in a separate object which can be moved, resized, and formatted.

Project

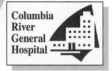

Hanna Moreland, manager of the Supplies Department at Columbia River General Hospital, has asked you to create a chart to compare operating expenses in each quarter.

1. Open **CRGHSuppliesDeptExp.xlsx**.

2. Save the workbook in the ExcelMedS3 folder and name it **EMedS3-CRGHSuppliesDeptExp**.

3. Select the range of cells A3:E9.

   The first step in creating a chart is to select the range of cells containing the data you want to chart. Notice that the range you just selected includes the row labels in column A. Labels are included to provide the frame of reference for each bar, column, or other chart marker. If you select multiple ranges, ensure that each range includes the same number of cells.

4. Click the INSERT tab.

5. Click the Insert Column Chart button in the Charts group.

6. Click the *3-D Clustered Column* option at the drop-down list (first column, first row in the *3-D Column* section).

   Excel graphs the data in a 3-D column chart and places the chart inside an object box in the center of the worksheet (see Figure E3.1).

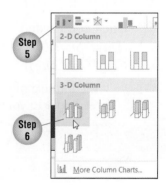

FIGURE E3.1 3-D Column Chart in an Object Box

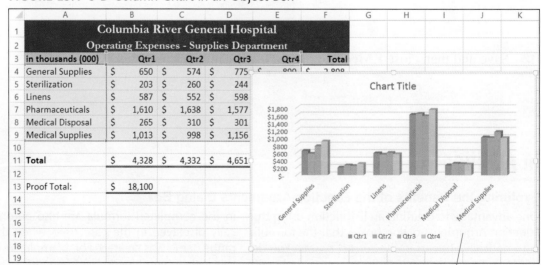

The 3-D column chart is placed in an object box that can be moved, resized, and formatted as needed.

7 Click the Move Chart button in the Location group on the CHART TOOLS DESIGN tab.

> **Need Help?**
> Can't see the CHART TOOLS DESIGN tab? You may have accidentally deselected the chart, causing the contextual tab to disappear. Click the chart to select the object. The CHART TOOLS DESIGN tab should reappear.

In Brief
Create Column Chart
1. Select cells.
2. Click INSERT tab.
3. Click Insert Column Chart button.
4. Click desired option.
5. Move and/or resize chart as desired.
6. Apply design options as desired.

8 At the Move Chart dialog box, click the *New sheet* option.

9 With *Chart1* selected in the *New sheet* text box, type **ColumnChart** and then click OK.

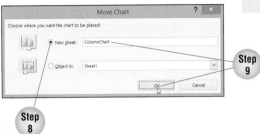

Step 8

Step 9

The chart object is moved to a new sheet in the workbook, titled *ColumnChart*. The chart is automatically scaled to fill the entire page in landscape orientation.

10 Click the Quick Layout button 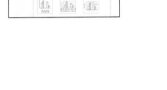 in the Chart Layouts group and then click the *Layout 3* option at the drop-down gallery.

Step 10

This layout adds a title to the top center of the chart and moves the legend to the bottom center.

11 Click *Chart Title* to select the title object, click at the beginning of the text to position the insertion point inside the chart title box, delete *Chart Title*, and then type **Operating Expenses by Quarter for Supplies Department**.

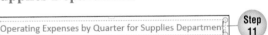 Step 11

12 Click inside the chart area to deselect the title text.

13 Click the More button in the Chart Styles group on the CHART TOOLS DESIGN tab.

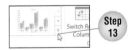 Step 13

14 Click the *Style 10* option in the drop-down gallery (second column, second row).

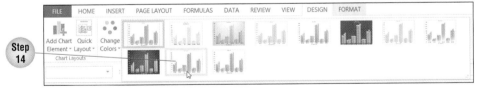

Step 14

15 Save **EMedS3-CRGHSuppliesDeptExp.xlsx**.

In Addition

Creating a Recommended Chart

If you are not sure what type of chart will best illustrate your data, consider letting Excel recommend a chart. To do this, select the data, click the INSERT tab, and then click the Recommended Charts button in the Charts group. This displays the data in a chart in the Insert Chart dialog box. Customize the recommended chart with options in the left panel of the dialog box and then click OK to insert the recommended chart in the worksheet. You can also insert a recommended chart in the worksheet with the keyboard shortcut Alt + F1.

Activity 3.6

Creating a Pie Chart

Pie charts illustrate each data point's size in proportion to the total of all items in the data source range. Each slice in a pie chart is a percentage of the whole pie. You can choose to display the percent values, the actual values used to generate the chart, or both values as data labels inside or outside the pie slices. Use a pie chart when you have only one data series to graph and there are no negative or zero values within the data range.

Project

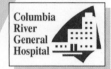

Hanna Moreland is pleased with the column chart you created for the quarterly operating expenses. Hanna would like you to create another chart that shows each expense as a proportion of the total expenses.

1. With **EMedS3-CRGHSuppliesDeptExp.xlsx** open, click the tab labeled *Sheet1* near the bottom left corner of the window and above the Status bar.

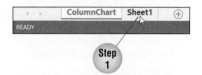

2. Click in any cell to deselect the range that was used to generate the column chart in the previous activity.

3. Select the range of cells A3:A9, hold down the Ctrl key, and then select the range of cells F3:F9.

4. Click the INSERT tab.

5. Click the Insert Pie or Doughnut Chart button in the Charts group.

6. Click the *3-D Pie* option in the *3-D Pie* section of the drop-down gallery.

7. Point to the border of the chart object until the pointer displays with the four-headed-arrow move icon attached, hold down the left mouse button, and then drag the chart below the data. Position the chart approximately centered below columns A–F with the top edge in row 16.

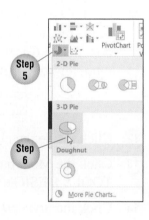

Need Help?

Before moving the chart, you may find it helpful to scroll down through the worksheet until you see several blank rows below row 16.

8. With the chart selected, click the Chart Elements button ✛ that displays at the right side of the chart.

9. Point to the *Data Labels* option that displays in the drop-down list and then click the expand triangle that displays at the right side of the option.

10. Click *More Options* at the side menu.

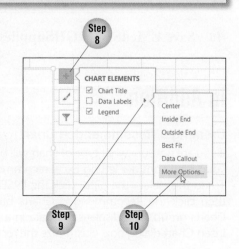

11 At the Format Data Labels task pane, click the *Percentage* check box below the *Label Contains* heading in the *LABEL OPTIONS* section to insert a check mark and then click the *Value* check box to remove the check mark.

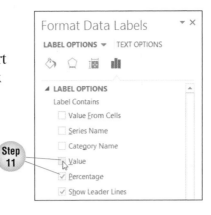

In Brief
Create Pie Chart
1. Select cells.
2. Click INSERT tab.
3. Click Insert Pie or Doughnut Chart button.
4. Click desired option.
5. Move and/or resize chart as desired.
6. Apply design options as desired.

12 Scroll down the Format Data Labels task pane (if necessary), click the expand arrow that displays at the left of *NUMBER*, click the down-pointing arrow at the right side of the *Category* option box, and then click *Percentage* at the drop-down list.

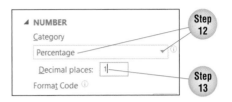

13 Select the number in the *Decimal places* text box and then type **1**.

14 Close the Format Data Labels task pane.

15 Click the Chart Styles button ✎ that displays at the right side of the chart.

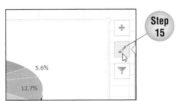

16 Click the *Style 3* option at the side menu.

17 Click the Chart Elements button, click the expand triangle that displays at the right side of the *Data Labels* option, and then click *Outside End* at the side menu.

Notice that the data labels move from inside the pie slices to the outer edges of the pie.

18 Change the chart title (currently displays as *Total*) to *Total Operating Expenses*.

Refer to Activity 3.5, Steps 11–12, if you need assistance with this step.

19 Click in the worksheet area outside the chart to deselect the chart.

20 Save **EMedS3-CRGHSuppliesDeptExp.xlsx**.

In Addition

Using Sparklines

Sparklines are miniature charts that you can insert within a cell to illustrate changes in a specific range of data within a row or column. For example, the sparkline chart shown below was created in cell G4 based on values in the range of cells B4:E4. To insert a sparkline chart, click the INSERT tab and then click the Line, Column, or Win/Loss buttons in the Sparklines group. At the Create Sparklines dialog box, select the data range that contains the values upon which you want to base the chart, select the cell in which to draw the chart, and then click OK.

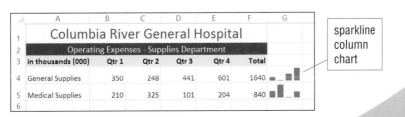

Activity 3.7

Modifying and Formatting Charts

To make changes to an existing chart, click inside a chart or chart element to display the translucent border around the perimeter of the chart object. Point to the border to move the chart or point to one of the eight sizing handles to resize the chart. When the chart is selected, the CHART TOOLS DESIGN and CHART TOOLS FORMAT tabs become available. Use these tabs to add new charts and/or delete or modify charts or chart elements as needed.

Project

Columbia River General Hospital

You will modify the charts created for the Operating Expenses worksheet by formatting the legend, applying bold formatting to the data labels, changing the font in the chart title, and changing the chart type for the column chart.

1. With **EMedS3-CRGHSuppliesDeptExp.xlsx** open, click anywhere inside the pie chart to select the chart object.

   When a chart is selected, the two contextual CHART TOOLS tabs become available: DESIGN and FORMAT.

2. Click inside the pie chart legend.

   Eight sizing handles appear around the legend, indicating that the object is selected. You can use these handles to resize the legend or you can drag the legend to a new location.

3. Click the CHART TOOLS FORMAT tab.

4. Click the Shape Outline button in the Shape Styles group and then click the *Light Blue* option in the drop-down gallery (seventh option from the left in the *Standard Colors* section).

   A thin light blue border appears around the legend.

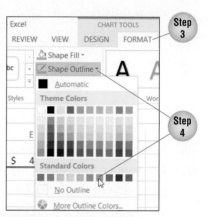

5. Click the chart title, select the text, and then use the Font and Font Size buttons on the Mini toolbar to change the title font to 16-point Verdana.

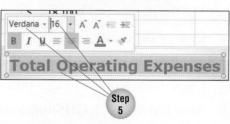

6. Click inside the chart area to deselect the chart title.

7. Click any one of the percent values around the edge of the pie.

   This selects all six data labels.

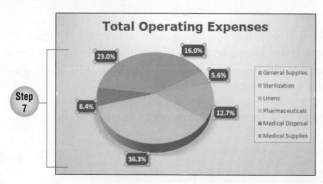

8 Click the HOME tab and then click the Bold button in the Font group to turn off bold formatting.

9 Click the ColumnChart tab near the bottom left corner of the window and then click inside the column chart to select the chart.

10 If necessary, click the CHART TOOLS DESIGN tab. Click the Change Chart Type button in the Type group.

11 At the Change Chart Type dialog box, click *Bar* in the left panel and then click the *3-D Clustered Bar* option (fourth option from the left at the top of the middle panel).

12 Click OK.

13 Click the More button in the Chart Styles group and then click the *Style 5* option at the drop-down gallery.

14 Print the bar chart.

15 Click the Sheet1 tab and then make cell A1 the active cell.

16 Display the Print backstage area.

17 Click the margins gallery in the *Settings* category (currently displays *Normal Margins*), click *Wide* at the drop-down list, and then click the Print button.

18 Save **EMedS3-CRGHSuppliesDeptExp.xlsx**.

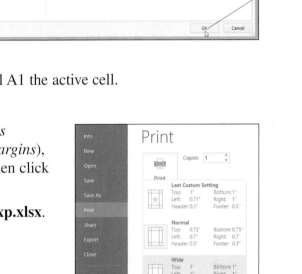

In Addition

Editing Chart Elements

Another way to make changes to a chart is to right-click the desired chart element to display a context-sensitive shortcut menu. For example, right-clicking an axis label in the bar chart displays the shortcut menu shown at the right. The bottom section of the shortcut menu changes depending on the element you click.

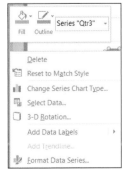

Inserting Shapes and Text Boxes

The Shapes button on the INSERT tab includes buttons with which you can draw lines, rectangles, basic shapes, block arrows, equation shapes, flowchart symbols, stars, banners, and callouts. Draw shapes or insert text boxes to add emphasis or create space for explanatory notes in a worksheet. Text can also be added to enclosed shapes.

Project An upcoming price increase from the hospital's medical waste disposal contractor is higher than expected. Hanna Moreland wants you to use a shape and a text box to add an explanatory note to the operating expenses worksheet.

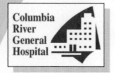

① With **EMedS3-CRGHSuppliesDeptExp.xlsx** open and the Sheet1 tab active, click the INSERT tab.

② Click the Shapes button in the Illustrations group and then click the *Arrow* option in the *Lines* section.

> When a shape has been selected from the Shapes button drop-down list, the pointer changes to crosshairs ➕.

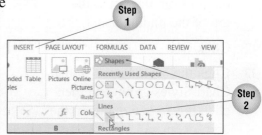

③ Position the crosshairs near the bottom left boundary of cell D12, click and drag up toward the value *310* in cell C8, and then release the mouse button. If you are not happy with the arrow, press Delete and then try again.

④ Click the Text Box button in the Insert Shapes group on the DRAWING TOOLS FORMAT tab.

> When the Text Box tool has been selected, the pointer changes to a downward-pointing arrow ↓.

⑤ Position the pointer at the top left boundary of cell D13 and then drag the pointer down and to the right to draw a text box of the approximate size shown in the image below.

> The insertion point is positioned inside the box when you release the left mouse button, indicating that you can begin typing text.

⑥ Type **Qtr2 next year will be 8% higher!** inside the text box.

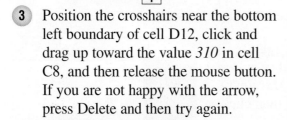

⑦ Click outside the text box to deselect the object. If necessary, resize the text box so that all of the text fits on one line.

8 Click the arrow shape to select it, hold down the Ctrl key, and then click the text box. Both drawn objects are now selected.

9 If necessary, click the DRAWING TOOLS FORMAT tab.

10 Click the Shape Outline button arrow in the Shape Styles group and then click the *Light Blue* option in the drop-down gallery (seventh option from the left in the *Standard Colors* section).

11 Click the Shape Outline button arrow a second time, point to *Weight*, and then click *1½ pt* at the side menu.

In Brief

Draw Shape
1. Click INSERT tab.
2. Click Shapes button.
3. Click desired shape.
4. Drag to create shape.
5. Move, resize, or format shape as desired.

Draw Text Box
1. Click INSERT tab.
2. Click Text Box button.
3. Drag to create text box.
4. Type text.
5. Click outside text box object.
6. Move, resize, or format text box as desired.

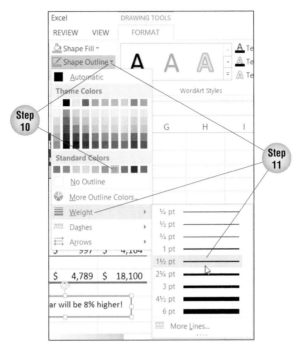

12 Click in any cell to deselect the drawn shapes.

Figure E3.2 shows the text box and arrow after formatting options have been applied.

13 Save **EMedS3-CRGHSuppliesDeptExp.xlsx**.

FIGURE E3.2 Formatted Text Box and Arrow

Columbia River General Hospital										
Operating Expenses - Supplies Department										
in thousands (000)		Qtr1		Qtr2		Qtr3		Qtr4		Total
General Supplies	$	650	$	574	$	775	$	899	$	2,898
Sterilization	$	203	$	260	$	244	$	298	$	1,005
Linens	$	587	$	552	$	598	$	564	$	2,301
Pharmaceuticals	$	1,610	$	1,638	$	1,577	$	1,743	$	6,568
Medical Disposal	$	265	$	310	$	301	$	288	$	1,164
Medical Supplies	$	1,013	$	998	$	1,156	$	997	$	4,164
Total	$	4,328	$	4,332	$	4,651	$	4,789	$	18,100
Proof Total:	$	18,100			Qtr2 next year will be 8% higher!					

Activity
3.9

Changing Page Layout Options

The PAGE LAYOUT tab contains buttons to modify the page setup and scaling options for printing purposes. You can also change printing options when previewing the worksheet at the Print backstage area. The margins of a worksheet are the blank areas between the top, bottom, left, and right edges of the page and the beginning of the printed text. The default margins in Excel are 0.75 inch at the top and bottom and 0.7 inch on the left and right sides. Smaller worksheets can be centered horizontally and/or vertically on the page to improve their appearance when printed. For larger worksheets, you can scale the size of printed text to force the printout to fit within a maximum number of pages.

Project

You will modify page layout options at the Print backstage area before printing the two worksheets you have been working on in this section.

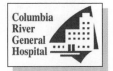
Columbia
River
General
Hospital

1 With **EMedS3-CRGHSuppliesDeptExp.xlsx** open, display the Print backstage area.

Notice the worksheet is not evenly balanced between the left and right margins. In the next steps you will change the margins to improve the page layout.

2 Click the margins gallery in the *Settings* category (currently displays *Wide Margins*).

3 Click *Custom Margins* at the drop-down list.

The Page Setup dialog box displays with the Margins tab active.

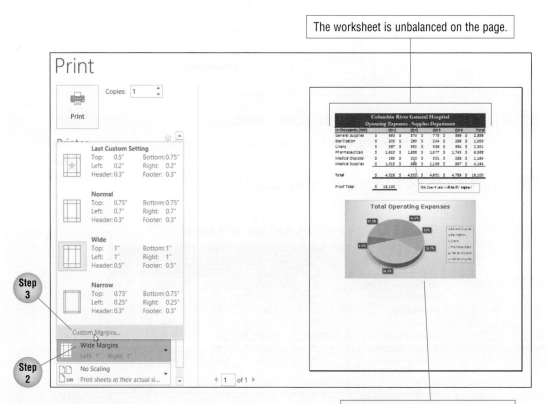

The worksheet is unbalanced on the page.

Your display may be in color if you are connected to a color printer.

4 Select the current entry in the *Top* measurement box, type **2.2**, select the current entry in the *Left* measurement box, type **1.25**, and then click OK.

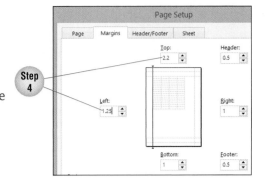

Step 4

> The preview pane in the Print backstage area shows the worksheet with the new margins applied. The page layout is improved for printing.

5 Click the Print button.

6 Save and then close **EMedS3-CRGHSuppliesDeptExp.xlsx**.

7 Open **EMedS3-CRGHNovakCardiacCosts.xlsx**.

8 Click the PAGE LAYOUT tab, click the Orientation button in the Page Setup group, and then click *Landscape* at the drop-down list.

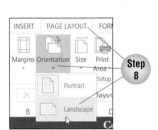

Step 8

9 Click the Margins button in the Page Setup group and then click *Custom Margins* at the drop-down list.

> The Page Setup dialog box displays with the Margins tab active. This is another way to display the same Page Setup dialog box you accessed via the margins gallery at the Print backstage area.

10 Click the *Horizontally* check box and the *Vertically* check box in the *Center on page* section and then click OK.

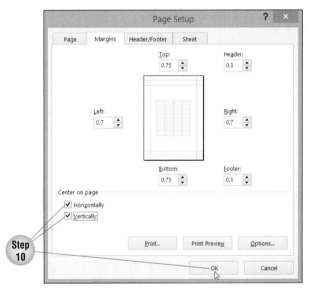

Step 10

> Centering the worksheet horizontally is another method that can be used to ensure the worksheet prints balanced between the left and right edges of the page. Clicking the *Vertically* check box means that the worksheet will also be centered between the top and bottom edges of the page.

11 Print the worksheet.

12 Save and then close **EMedS3-CRGHNovakCardiacCosts.xlsx**.

In Addition

Printing Column or Row Headings on Multiple Pages

Use the Print Titles button in the Page Setup group on the PAGE LAYOUT tab to specify column or row headings that you want printed at the top or left edge of every page. This will make the data in a multiple-page printout easier to understand and interpret.

Activity
3.10

Using Page Layout View; Inserting Headers and Footers

Page Layout view allows you to view the worksheet as it will look when printed, while still allowing you to make changes to the contents. When you are editing a worksheet in Page Layout view, horizontal and vertical rulers display to assist you with measurements.

A *header* is text that prints at the top of each page in a worksheet and a *footer* is text that prints at the bottom of each page in a worksheet. Excel includes predefined headers and footers, but you can also create your own custom header or footer.

Project

The operations manager at North Shore Medical Clinic would like a hard copy of the clinic supplies inventory worksheet. Since this is a long worksheet, you decide to add a header and footer to the report to include identifying information. You also decide to add page numbers and experiment with scaling options to fit the printout on two pages.

1. Open **EMedS3-NSMCSupplies.xlsx** and then click the Page Layout button located at the right side of the Status bar and to the left of the Zoom slider bar.

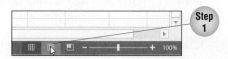

Step 1

2. At the Microsoft Office Excel message box indicating that freeze panes is not compatible with Page Layout view, click OK to unfreeze the panes and continue.

3. If necessary, use the horizontal and vertical scroll bars to adjust the view so that the top of the first page of the worksheet is visible in the window.

4. Click the text *Click to add header* near the top center of the page.

Headers and footers are divided into three sections. Click the left or right sections of the Header pane to type or insert header and footer elements in them. By default, text in the left section is left-aligned, text in the center section is centered, and text in the right section is right-aligned.

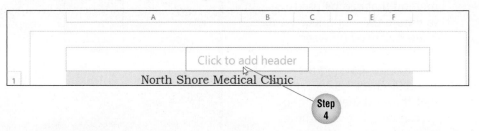

Step 4

5. Click in the left section of the header and then type your first and last names.

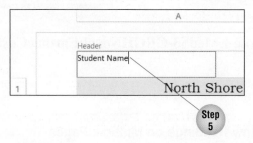

Step 5

6 Click in the right section of the header, type **Date Printed:**, and then press the spacebar once.

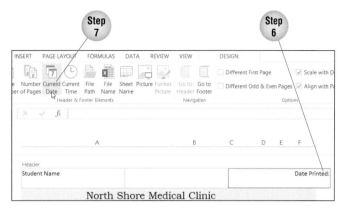

Step 7
Step 6

7 Click the Current Date button ⬚ in the Header & Footer Elements group on the HEADER & FOOTER TOOLS DESIGN tab.

> Excel inserts the code *&[Date]*, which is replaced with the current date when the worksheet is printed.

8 Click the Go to Footer button ⬚ in the Navigation group on the HEADER & FOOTER TOOLS DESIGN tab.

> The right section of the footer is selected for editing.

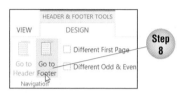

Step 8

9 Click in the center section of the footer to select it for editing.

10 Click the File Name button ⬚ in the Header & Footer Elements group.

> Excel inserts the code *&[File]*, which is replaced with the workbook file name when the worksheet is printed.

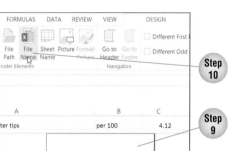

Step 10
Step 9

11 Click anywhere in the worksheet area outside the footer to close the footer section.

12 Scroll to the top of the worksheet to view the header. Notice that Excel now displays the current date in place of the *&[Date]* code.

13 Scroll down to the bottom of the worksheet and notice that Excel now displays the file name in place of the *&[File]* code.

14 Click the PAGE LAYOUT tab.

> By default, the header and footer margins are 0.3 inch. In the next step, you will adjust the header and footer margins to provide more white space at the top and bottom of the page.

15 Click the Margins button in the Page Setup group and then click *Custom Margins* at the drop-down list. At the Page Setup dialog box with the Margins tab active, change the margin settings as follows:

> *Top:* 1 *Header:* 0.5
> *Bottom:* 1 *Footer:* 0.5
> *Left:* 1

16 Click OK to close the Page Setup dialog box.

17 Review the new margin settings in Page Layout view.

18 Print the worksheet.

19 Click the Normal button located at the right side of the Status bar and to the left of the Zoom slider bar.

20 Save and then close **EMedS3-NSMCSupplies.xlsx**.

In Brief

Insert Header or Footer
1. Switch to Page Layout view.
2. Click *Click to add header* or *Click to add footer*.
3. Insert desired header and footer text and elements in left, center, or right sections.
4. Click in worksheet.

Activity 3.11

Formatting Data as a Table; Applying Table Style Options

Create a table in Excel to manage data independently from other cells in the worksheet, or to filter and sort a list. A worksheet can contain more than one range formatted as a table. By default, filter arrows appear in the first row of the table, a border surrounds the table range, and a sizing arrow appears in the bottom right corner. Excel includes a variety of predefined table styles to choose from when creating a table. The contextual TABLE TOOLS DESIGN tab becomes available when a range of cells is defined as a table.

Project

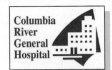

Luisa Gomez, Cardiac Nurse Manager, often uses a casual relief call list when a full-time nurse calls in sick. Luisa would like the list to be in a format that she can sort and filter based on shift preference and/or experience. You decide to use a table to accomplish this.

1. Open **CRGHCasualNurses.xlsx** and then save the workbook in the ExcelMedS3 folder and name it **EMedS3-CRGHCasualNurses**.

2. Select the range of cells A4:J35 and then click the Format as Table button 🖼️ in the Styles group on the HOME tab.

   The first step in defining a table is to specify the range of cells to be included. Do not include cells containing merged titles or other data that should not be included when you sort and filter the rows.

3. Click the *Table Style Medium 6* option (sixth column, first row in the *Medium* section) at the drop-down gallery.

   Excel includes 60 predefined table styles grouped into *Light*, *Medium*, and *Dark* sections. Use these styles to add color, borders, and shading to cells within a table. In addition, you can create your own custom table style and save it with the workbook.

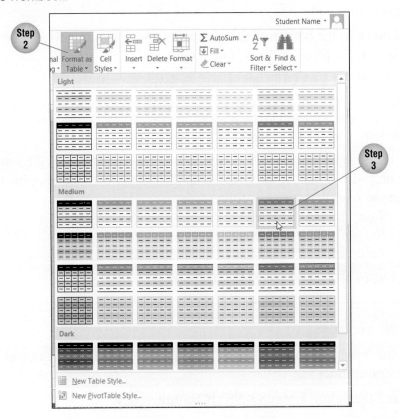

4 At the Format As Table dialog box, with =$A$4:$J$35 selected in the *Where is the data for your table?* text box, click OK.

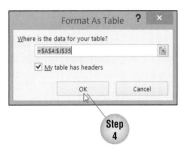

Step 4

Excel applies the table style formatting to the range, displays filter arrows in each cell in the first row of the table, adds a border to the table, and displays a sizing handle in the bottom right cell.

5 Click in any cell to deselect the range.

In the next step, you will add a new row to the table.

6 Right-click the row label for row 36, click *Insert* at the shortcut menu, and then type the new record in the columns indicated. Press Enter after typing the last cell.

Employee Number:	99823
Employee Last Name:	Awad
Employee First Name:	Rania
Hire Date:	=DATE(2015,1,31)
Telephone:	555-4652
Years Experience:	7
OR Experience:	Yes
Day Shift Only?:	No
Night Shift Only?:	No
Can Work Either Shift:	Yes

Since you typed data in the row immediately below the table, Excel automatically expands the table to include the new row. You can also insert a new row at the bottom of a table by selecting the last cell in the table and then pressing Tab.

7 If necessary, make cell J36 the active cell and then press Tab.

A new row is inserted at the bottom of the table.

8 Type the following text in the columns indicated in row 37. Press Enter after typing the last cell. (Do not press Tab, as this action will cause another new row to be added to the table.)

Employee Number:	99828
Employee Last Name:	Fernandez
Employee First Name:	Natalio
Hire Date:	=DATE(2015,1,31)
Telephone:	555-7643
Years Experience:	3
OR Experience:	Yes
Day Shift Only?:	No
Night Shift Only?:	Yes
Can Work Either Shift:	Weekends only

99754	Valdez	Linda	1/30/2015	555-3498	16	Yes	No	No	Yes
99823	Awad	Rania	1/31/2015	555-4652	7	Yes	No	No	Yes
99828	Fernandez	Natalio	1/31/2015	555-7643	3	Yes	No	Yes	Weekends only
ed:		31-Jan-15							

Steps 6-8

continues

9 Make active any cell within the table.

> The contextual TABLE TOOLS DESIGN tab is not available unless the active cell is positioned within the table.

10 If necessary, click the TABLE TOOLS DESIGN tab. Click the *Banded Rows* check box in the Table Style Options group to remove the check mark.

> When a table has banded rows, it means that every other row is formatted differently (for example, odd rows might be shaded in blue while even rows remain white). Banding makes it easier to read text across multiple columns in a list. The style of formatting for every other row is dependent on the table style that has been applied. Notice that once you remove the check mark from the check box, all rows are formatted the same.

11 Click the *Banded Columns* check box in the Table Style Options group to insert a check mark.

> Notice that every other column is now shaded in blue.

12 Click the *First Column* check box in the Table Style Options group to insert a check mark.

> The contents of the cells in the first column now appear in bold. The type of formatting applied by clicking the *First Column* check box depends on the table style.

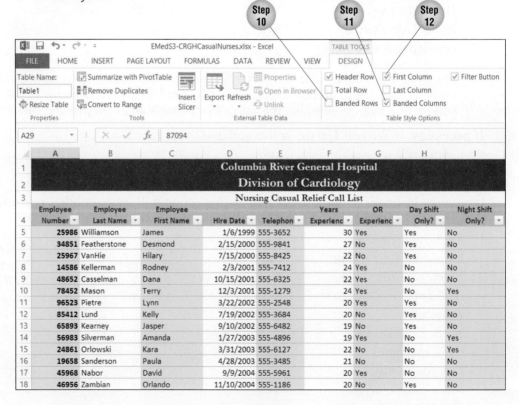

13 Select the range of cells E5:J37, click the HOME tab, and then click the Center button in the Alignment group.

14 Select the range of cells A4:J4 and then click the Middle Align button in the Alignment group.

Step 13

Step 14

Employee Number	Employee Last Name	Employee First Name	Hire Date	Telephone	Years Experience	OR Experience	Day Shift Only?	Night Shift Only?	Can Work Either Shift
25986	Williamson	James	1/6/1999	555-3652	30	Yes	Yes	No	Weekends only
34851	Featherstone	Desmond	2/15/2000	555-9841	27	No	Yes	No	Weekends only
25967	VanHie	Hilary	7/15/2000	555-8425	22	No	Yes	No	No
14586	Kellerman	Rodney	2/3/2001	555-7412	24	Yes	No	No	Yes
48652	Casselman	Dana	10/15/2001	555-6325	22	Yes	No	No	Yes
78452	Mason	Terry	12/3/2001	555-1279	24	Yes	No	Yes	No
96523	Pietre	Lynn	3/22/2002	555-2548	20	Yes	Yes	No	Weekends only
85412	Lund	Kelly	7/19/2002	555-3684	20	No	Yes	No	Weekends only
65893	Kearney	Jasper	9/10/2002	555-6482	19	No	Yes	No	No
56983	Silverman	Amanda	1/27/2003	555-4896	19	Yes	No	Yes	No
24861	Orlowski	Kara	3/31/2003	555-6127	22	No	No	Yes	No
19658	Sanderson	Paula	4/28/2003	555-3485	21	No	No	No	Yes
45968	Nabor	David	9/9/2004	555-5961	20	Yes	No	No	Yes
46956	Zambian	Orlando	11/10/2004	555-1186	20	No	Yes	No	No
38642	Ravi	Virginia	6/22/2005	555-6969	24	Yes	Yes	No	Weekends only
27846	Fairchild	Tina	8/10/2005	555-7822	11	Yes	No	Yes	No
68429	Quenneville	Rene	10/15/2005	555-4663	10	Yes	Yes	No	Weekends only

Columbia River General Hospital — Division of Cardiology — Nursing Casual Relief Call List

15 Click in any cell to deselect the range and then save **EMedS3-CRGHCasualNurses.xlsx**.

In Addition

Converting a Table to a Normal Range

A range that has been formatted as a table can be converted back to a normal range using the Convert to Range button in the Tools group on the TABLE TOOLS DESIGN tab (shown below). Convert a table to a range if you no longer need to treat the data range independently from the rest of the worksheet. For example, you may want to format a range as a table simply to apply the color, shading, and border effects that are available through table styles. Converting a table to a normal range preserves this formatting; however, features unique to a table, such as applying banding, adding a total row, and checking for duplicates, will no longer be available to the range.

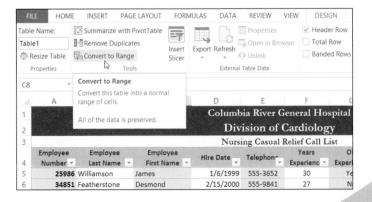

Activity 3.12

Sorting a Table by Single and Multiple Criteria

In Section 1 you learned to sort a payroll worksheet alphabetically by last name. Sorting rows in a table by single or multiple criteria involves many of the same steps. To sort by a single column, click in any cell in the column by which you wish to sort, click the Sort & Filter button, and then click either the *Sort A to Z* option or the *Sort Z to A* option at the drop-down list. To group the rows by one column and then sort them by another column, display the Sort dialog box. You can continue to group and sort by multiple criteria as needed.

Project

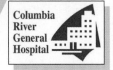

You decide to print the nursing casual relief call list with the data sorted alphabetically by last name. Next, you want to print the list grouped first in descending order by years of experience, second by OR experience, and third by whether the individual can work either shift.

1. With **EMedS3-CRGHCasualNurses.xlsx** open, in click any cell in column B of the table.

2. Click the Sort & Filter button in the Editing group on the HOME tab.

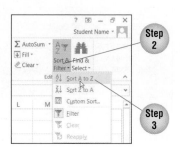

3. Click *Sort A to Z* at the drop-down list.

> The rows are arranged in ascending order by last name. An up-pointing black arrow displays in the filter arrow button to indicate that the table is sorted by the *Employee Last Name* column.

4. Print the worksheet.

5. Click the Sort & Filter button and then click *Custom Sort* at the drop-down list.

6. At the Sort dialog box, click the down-pointing arrow at the right of the *Sort by* option box in the *Column* section and then click *Years Experience* at the drop-down list.

7. Click the down-pointing arrow at the right of the *Order* option box (currently reads *Smallest to Largest*) and then click *Largest to Smallest* at the drop-down list.

8. Click the Add Level button.

9. Click the down-pointing arrow at the right of the *Then by* option box in the *Column* section and then click *OR Experience* at the drop-down list.

10. Click the down-pointing arrow at the right of the *Order* option box (currently reads *A to Z*) and then click *Z to A* at the drop-down list.

> If the employee has OR experience, you want them to come first within the group of employees with the same number of years of experience. Since cells in this column have only a Yes or No in the cell, sorting in descending order will ensure that those with OR experience are shown first.

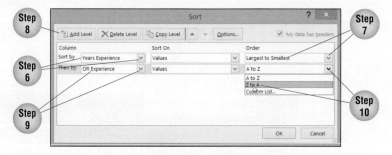

11 Click the Add Level button.

12 In the new row, click the down-pointing arrow at the right of the *Then by* option box in the *Column* section and then click *Can Work Either Shift* at the drop-down list.

13 Click the down-pointing arrow at the right of the *Order* option box (currently reads *A to Z*) and then click *Z to A* at the drop-down list.

> If the employee can work either shift, *Yes* will appear in the cell in the *Can Work Either Shift* column. Sorting in descending order will ensure that those who have no shift restrictions will be listed first within the groups of employees who have OR experience and the most years of experience.

14 Click OK to begin the sort.

In Brief

Sort Table by Single Column
1. Click in any row within column by which to sort.
2. Click Sort & Filter button.
3. Click *Sort A to Z* or *Sort Z to A*.

Sort Table by Multiple Columns
1. Click Sort & Filter button.
2. Click *Custom Sort*.
3. Select first column to sort by.
4. Select sort order.
5. Click Add Level.
6. Repeat Steps 3–5 for each sort column.
7. Click OK.

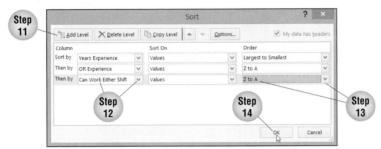

15 Examine the sorted worksheet and compare your results with Figure E3.3.

16 Print the worksheet.

17 Save **EMedS3-CRGHCasualNurses.xlsx**.

FIGURE E3.3 Sorted Partial Worksheet

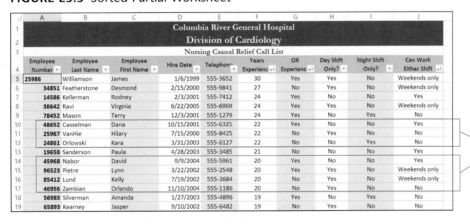

> Notice that if employees have the same years of experience and OR experience, those with *Yes* in the *Can Work Either Shift* column are listed before those who have a restriction on the shift they can work.

In Addition

Learning More about Sorting

By default, when you apply a sort in Excel, the values are sorted alphanumerically. Alphanumeric sorting arranges rows with entries that begin with symbols first, followed by numbers and then letters. The *Sort On* option box in the Sort dialog box also provides three additional methods by which you can group rows: *Cell Color*, *Font Color*, or *Cell Icon*.

Activity 3.13

Filtering a Table

A *filter* is used to display only those records within a table that meet certain criteria. When a filter is applied, the records that do not meet the criteria are temporarily hidden from view. Using a filter, you can view and/or print a subset of rows within a table. For example, you might want to print a list of employees who have OR experience. Once you have printed the list, you can remove the filter to redisplay all of the rows. To apply a filter, use the filter arrow buttons that display in the first row of the table.

Project

Luisa Gomez has asked you for two lists: one with employees who can only work the night shift and another with employees with OR experience who can work either shift.

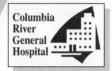

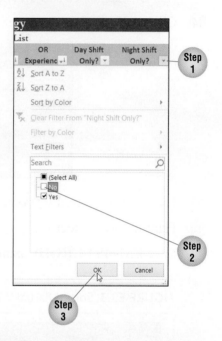

1 With **EMedS3-CRGHCasualNurses.xlsx** open, click the filter arrow button ▼ next to the column label *Night Shift Only?*

> A filter arrow button displays for each column in the table. Excel includes in the drop-down list that displays when you click this button each unique field value that exists within the column. In addition, the options *Sort A to Z*, *Sort Z to A*, and *Sort by Color* appear at the top of the list.

2 Click the *No* check box to remove the check mark.

> This causes rows with a *No* value to be hidden from view. Since the only other possible entry is *Yes*, the criterion for the filter is to display rows within the table that have the text entry *Yes* in column I.

3 Click OK.

> Excel hides any records that have a value other than *Yes* in column I, as shown in Figure E3.4. The row numbers of the matching items that were found are displayed in blue and a filter icon appears in the filter arrow button in cell I4 to indicate the column by which the table is filtered. The Status bar also indicates that 9 of 33 records were found. A filtered worksheet can be edited, formatted, charted, or printed.

The filter icon indicates that this column was used to filter the table.

Excel hides rows that do not meet the criterion. Matching row numbers are displayed in blue.

FIGURE E3.4 Filtered Worksheet

	A	B	C	D	E	F	G	H	I	J
1				Columbia River General Hospital						
2				Division of Cardiology						
3				Nursing Casual Relief Call List						
4	Employee Number	Employee Last Name	Employee First Name	Hire Date	Telephone	Years Experience	OR Experience	Day Shift Only?	Night Shift Only?	Can W Either
9	78452	Mason	Terry	12/3/2001	555-1279	24	Yes	No	Yes	N
12	24861	Orlowski	Kara	3/31/2003	555-6127	22	No	No	Yes	N
18	56983	Silverman	Amanda	1/27/2003	555-4896	19	Yes	No	Yes	N
23	27846	Fairchild	Tina	8/10/2005	555-7822	11	Yes	No	Yes	N
25	99576	Diaz	Anna	1/13/2014	555-9378	10	Yes	No	Yes	Ye
27	69417	LaPierre	Denis	4/23/2006	555-8643	10	Yes	No	Yes	N
30	34668	Fontana	Mario	7/31/2006	555-7433	10	No	No	Yes	N
31	99027	Kumar	Hashil	6/10/2013	555-2398	8	No	No	Yes	N
37	99828	Fernandez	Natalio	1/31/2015	555-7643	3	Yes	No	Yes	Weeken
38	**Updated:**	31-Jan-15								
39										

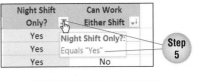

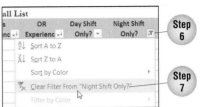

(4) Print the filtered worksheet.

(5) Point to the filter icon in the filter arrow button in cell I4. Notice that the filter criterion displays in the ScreenTip.

Step 5

(6) Click the filter arrow button in cell I4.

Step 6

(7) Click *Clear Filter From "Night Shift Only?"* at the drop-down list.

Step 7

All rows in the table are restored to view.

(8) Click the filter arrow button in cell G4.

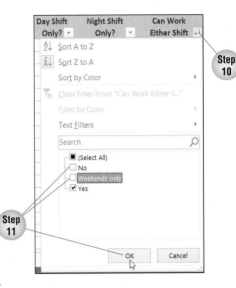

(9) Click the *No* check box to remove the check mark and then click OK.

Only the employees with OR experience are displayed.

Step 10

(10) Click the filter arrow button in cell J4.

(11) Click the *No* and *Weekends only* check boxes to remove the check marks and then click OK.

Only those employees with OR experience who can work either shift are now displayed (see Figure E3.5). Notice that you can continue to filter a table until only those records that meet your criteria are displayed.

Step 11

(12) Print the filtered worksheet.

(13) Redisplay all records for both filtered columns.

(14) Save and then close **EMedS3-CRGHCasualNurses.xlsx**.

FIGURE E3.5 Filtered Worksheet Using Two Criteria

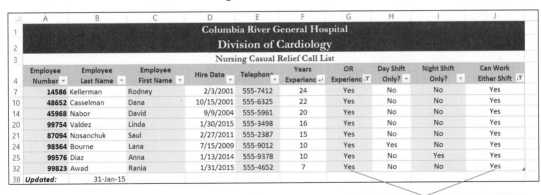

	A	B	C	D	E	F	G	H	I	J
1				Columbia River General Hospital						
2				Division of Cardiology						
3				Nursing Casual Relief Call List						
4	Employee Number	Employee Last Name	Employee First Name	Hire Date	Telephone	Years Experience	OR Experience	Day Shift Only?	Night Shift Only?	Can Work Either Shift
7	14586	Kellerman	Rodney	2/3/2001	555-7412	24	Yes	No	No	Yes
10	48652	Casselman	Dana	10/15/2001	555-6325	22	Yes	No	No	Yes
14	45968	Nabor	David	9/9/2004	555-5961	20	Yes	No	No	Yes
20	99754	Valdez	Linda	1/30/2015	555-3498	16	Yes	No	No	Yes
21	87094	Nosanchuk	Saul	2/27/2011	555-2387	15	Yes	No	No	Yes
24	98364	Bourne	Lana	7/15/2009	555-9012	10	Yes	Yes	No	Yes
25	99576	Diaz	Anna	1/13/2014	555-9378	10	Yes	No	Yes	Yes
32	99823	Awad	Rania	1/31/2015	555-4652	7	Yes	No	No	Yes
38	Updated:		31-Jan-15							

Only those employees with OR experience who can work either shift are shown.

In Addition

Filtering Data Not Formatted as a Table

Data in a worksheet that has not been formatted as a table can also be filtered using techniques similar to those you learned in this activity. Select the range of cells that you wish to filter, click the Sort & Filter button in the Editing group on the HOME tab, and then click *Filter* at the drop-down list. Excel displays filter arrow buttons in each column of the first row of the selected range.

Features Summary

Feature	Ribbon Tab, Group	Button
change chart type	CHART TOOLS DESIGN, Type	
change margins	PAGE LAYOUT, Page Setup OR FILE, *Print*	
create a column chart	INSERT, Charts	
create a pie chart	INSERT, Charts	
Date & Time functions	FORMULAS, Function Library	
draw a shape	INSERT, Illustrations	
draw a text box	INSERT, Text	
filter table	HOME, Editing	
format table	HOME, Styles	
header or footer	INSERT, Text OR Page Layout View	
Logical functions	FORMULAS, Function Library	
move chart	CHARTS TOOLS DESIGN, Location	
Normal view	VIEW, Workbook Views	OR
Page Layout view	VIEW, Workbook Views	OR
scale page width and/or height	PAGE LAYOUT, Scale to Fit OR FILE, *Print*	
sort table	HOME, Editing	
Statistical functions	FORMULAS, Function Library	

Knowledge Check

Completion: In the space provided at the right, write in the correct term, command, or option.

1. AVERAGE and COUNT are two of the functions in this category. _____
2. This Date and Time function inserts the current date (without the time) in the active cell. _____
3. To display the Insert Function dialog box, click this button on the HOME tab and then click *More Functions* at the drop-down list. _____
4. Enter a range name in this box at the left side of the Formula bar. _____
5. The IF function returns one of two values based on this criterion. _____
6. This type of chart illustrates each value as a proportion of the total. _____

7. When a chart is selected, these two contextual CHART TOOLS tabs appear. _____

8. The mouse pointer changes to this when you draw a shape. _____

9. To center a worksheet horizontally and vertically, click this tab in the Page Setup dialog box. _____

10. A header is text that prints here. _____

11. Footers are divided into this number of sections. _____

12. Click this button in the Styles group on the HOME tab to define an area of a worksheet as an independent range that can be formatted and managed separately from the rest of the worksheet. _____

13. Select this option from the Sort & Filter button drop-down list to display a dialog box where you can define more than one sort column. _____

14. This term refers to temporarily hiding rows that do not meet a specified criterion. _____

Skills Review

Review 1 **Inserting Statistical Functions**

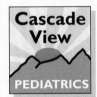

1. Open **CVPOpExp.xlsx**.
2. Save the workbook with the name **EMedS3-R-CVPOpExp**.
3. Make cell A15 the active cell.
4. Type **Average Expense** and then press Enter.
5. Type **Maximum Expense** and then press Enter.
6. Type **Minimum Expense** and then press Enter.
7. Make cell B15 the active cell and then create the formula that will calculate the average of the expense values in the range of cells B4:B9.
8. Make cell B16 the active cell and then create the formula that will return the maximum expense value within the range of cells B4:B9.
9. Make cell B17 the active cell and then create the formula that will return the minimum expense value within the range of cells B4:B9.
10. Copy the formulas in the range of cells B15:B17 to the range of cells C15:F17.
11. Apply the Comma format with zero decimal places to the range of cells B15:F17.
12. Save **EMedS3-R-CVPOpExp.xlsx**.

Review 2 **Inserting Date Functions**

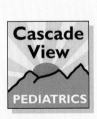

1. With **EMedS3-R-CVPOpExp.xlsx** open, make cell A19 the active cell.
2. Type **Date Created:** and then press the Right Arrow key.
3. With cell B19 the active cell, use the DATE function to insert the current date. *Note: You do not want to use the TODAY function, because you do not want the date to update each time you open the file.*
4. Format cell B19 to display the date in the format *14-Mar-12* (dd-mm-yy).
5. Make cell A20 the active cell.
6. Type **Next Revision Date:** and then press the Right Arrow key.
7. With cell B20 the active cell, type the formula **=B19+360** and then press Enter.
8. Save **EMedS3-R-CVPOpExp.xlsx**.

Review 3 Naming Ranges; Using the IF Function

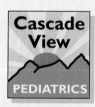

1. With **EMedS3-R-CVPOpExp.xlsx** open, insert three rows above row 19.
2. Make cell A19 the active cell, type **Current Target**, and then press Enter.
3. With cell A20 the active cell, type **Expense Over Target** and then press Enter.
4. Sydney Larsen has set a quarterly target of $960,000 for total expenses. Make cell B19 the active cell and then type **960**. Apply the Comma format with no decimal places to cell B19 and then name the cell *Target*.
5. Sydney wants you to insert a formula that, when applicable, will show the amount by which a quarter's total expenses have been exceeded. Make cell B20 the active cell and then enter the following IF function using the Function Arguments dialog box or by typing the formula directly into the cell: **=IF(B11>target,B11-target,0)**
6. Drag the fill handle from cell B20 to the range of cells C20:E20.
7. In the space provided below, write the values displayed in the cells indicated.

   B20: _____

   C20: _____

   D20: _____

   E20: _____

8. In the space provided, write in your own words a brief explanation of the IF function you entered in cell B20.

   _____

   _____

   _____

9. Change the value in cell B19 from *960* to *955*.
10. Save **EMedS3-R-CVPOpExp.xlsx**.

Review 4 Inserting a Picture; Sorting a List; Setting Print Options

1. With **EMedS3-R-CVPOpExp.xlsx** open, change the height of row 1 to *44.40 (74 pixels)*.
2. Select the range of cells A1:F1 and then change the fill color to *White, Background 1*.
3. Make cell A1 the active cell and then insert **CVPLogo.png** from your ExcelMedS3 folder.
4. Adjust the size and position of the logo until it is centered over columns A through F in row 1.
5. Select the range of cells A3:F9 and then sort the range in ascending order. Click in any cell to deselect the range.
6. Change the top margin to 2 inches.
7. Create a header that will print your first and last names in the left section and the current date and time (separated by one space) in the right section.
8. Create a footer that will print the word *Page* followed by the page number (separated by one space) in the center section.
9. Save, print, and then close **EMedS3-R-CVPOpExp.xlsx**. *Note: If you submit your work in hard copy, check with your instructor to see if you need to print two copies of this worksheet with one of the copies showing the cell formulas instead of the calculated results.*

Review 5 Creating and Modifying a Chart; Drawing an Arrow and Text Box; Formatting a Table

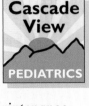

Cascade View

PEDIATRICS

1. Open **CVPRent&Maint.xlsx**.
2. Save the workbook with the name **EMedS3-R-CVPRent&Maint**.
3. Select the range of cells A3:E10 and then create a 3-D Clustered Column chart. Apply the Layout 3 quick layout, change the chart title to *Rent and Maintenance Costs*, and then move the chart to a new sheet titled *ColumnChart*.
4. With ColumnChart the active sheet, draw an arrow pointing to the column in the chart representing clinic cleaning for the fourth quarter. Draw a text box anchored to the end of the arrow and then type the following text inside the box: **Includes price increase from new contractor Universal Cleaning Corporation.**
5. Change the font of the text in the text box to 10-point Candara and then apply a dark red shape outline to the text box.
6. Apply a dark red shape outline to the arrow.
7. Display Sheet1 and then select the range of cells A3:F10. Format the range as a table using Table Style Light 20 (sixth column, third row in the *Light* section). Band the columns instead of the rows. Click the HOME tab, click the Sort & Filter button in the Editing group, and then click *Filter* at the drop-down list to remove the filter arrows from the labels in row 3.
8. Save **EMedS3-R-CVPRent&Maint.xlsx**.
9. Print the entire workbook and then close **EMedS3-R-CVPRent&Maint.xlsx**.

Skills Assessment

Note: If you submit your work in hard copy, check with your instructor before completing these assessments to find out if you need to print two copies of each worksheet with one of the copies showing the cell formulas instead of the calculated results.

Assessment 1 Using Statistical and IF Functions

1. Lee Elliott, Office Manager, has started a worksheet that includes the clinic's 15 most frequent medical supply purchases. Lee wants to calculate purchase quantity discounts from the clinic's two preferred medical supply vendors. Both vendors charge the same unit price, but each offers a discount plan with different percentages and quantity levels. Lee has asked for your help in writing the correct formulas to calculate the savings from each vendor. Specifically, Lee wants to know which supplier provides the better offer. To begin, open **NSMC15Supplies.xlsx**.
2. Save the workbook with the name **EMedS3-A1-NSMC15Supplies**.
3. In cell E4, create a formula to calculate the discount from AllCare Medical Supplies using the following criteria:
   - AllCare offers a 1.75% discount on the product's unit price for zero to four units ordered.
   - The discount rises to 2.5% when five or more units are ordered.
   - Create appropriate range names to reference the percentage values in cells B21 and B22 within your IF statement.

4. In cell F4, create a formula to calculate the discount from BestCare Health Supply using the following criteria:
   - BestCare offers a 1.8% discount on the product's unit price for zero to five units ordered.
   - The discount rises to 2.25% when six or more units are ordered.
   - Create appropriate range names to reference the percentage values in cells B23 and B24 within your IF statement.
5. Copy the formulas to the remaining rows in columns E and F.
6. Calculate the total discount value for all 15 supplies in cells E19 and F19.
7. Apply formatting options as needed.
8. Enter an appropriate label and create a formula to calculate the average discount below the total row for each vendor.
9. Print the worksheet in landscape orientation, centered horizontally.
10. Save and then close **EMedS3-A1-NSMC15Supplies.xlsx**.

Assessment 2 Changing Print Options; Using Date and IF Functions

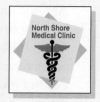

1. Darrin Lancaster, CMA, has asked you to finish the worksheet he started in order to track Dr. Hydall's dermatology patient records. To begin, open **NSMCDermPatients.xlsx**.
2. Save the workbook with the name **EMedS3-A2-NSMCDermPatients**.
3. Medical records are completed on the system 12 days after Dr. Hydall's report has been mailed to the referring physician. Create a formula in cell H4 that calculates the date the system report should be filed.
4. Copy the formula to the remaining rows in column H.
5. Create a formula for a recall date in column I using the following information:
   - If *Repeat Assessment* contains *Y* for Yes, then calculate the recall date 45 days from the date of the consultation visit.
   - If *Repeat Assessment* does not contain *Y*, instruct Excel to place the words *Not required* in the cell. ***Hint: Use quotation marks before and after a text entry in an IF statement. For example, =IF(G4="Y",...).***
   - Format the column to display the date in the same format as other dates within the worksheet.
   - Expand the column width as necessary.
6. Set the following print options:
   a. Change the orientation to landscape.
   b. Change the top margin to 1.75 inches and center the worksheet horizontally.
   c. Create a header that will print your name in the left header box and the current date in the right header box.
   d. Scale the worksheet to fit on one page.
7. Apply any other formatting changes to improve the worksheet's appearance.
8. Save, print, and then close **EMedS3-A2-NSMCDermPatients.xlsx**.

Assessment 3 Creating and Formatting Charts; Drawing an Arrow and a Text Box

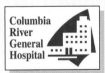

1. Dr. Hydall has asked you to create charts from the dermatology patient analysis report for a presentation to the local members of the American Academy of Dermatology. Dr. Hydall has specifically requested a column chart depicting the patient numbers for all diagnoses by age group and a pie chart summarizing all of the diagnoses by total patients. To begin, open **NSMCDermStats.xlsx**.
2. Save the workbook with the name **EMedS3-A3-NSMCDermStats**.
3. On a new sheet labeled *ColumnChart*, create a column chart that will display the values for patients aged 0–12 through 51+ for each diagnosis. Include an appropriate chart title. Include any other chart elements that will make the chart data easier to interpret.
4. Create a 3-D pie chart that will display the number of patients in each age group as a percentage of 100. ***Hint: Select the ranges of cells B3:G3 and B9:G9 before selecting the 3-D pie option.*** Include an appropriate chart title and display percentages as the data labels. Place the pie chart at the bottom of the worksheet starting in row 12 and resize the chart so that its width extends from the left edge of column A to the right edge of column H.
5. Draw an arrow pointing to the 13–20 age group slice in the pie chart. Create a text box at the end of the arrow containing the text *This age group growing 10% per year!*
6. If necessary, move and/or resize the arrow and text box. Change the font color of the text inside the text box to red and the outline color of the text box to blue.
7. Change the line color of the arrow to the same blue you used for the text box.
8. Center the worksheet horizontally.
9. Print the entire workbook.
10. Save and then close **EMedS3-A3-NSMCDermStats.xlsx**.

Assessment 4 Working with Tables

1. Laura Latterell, Education Director, has started a worksheet in which she tracks professional development completion for full-time nursing staff. Laura assists nurses with selection of professional development activities and plans workshops throughout the year to provide in-service training. Laura would like the worksheet to be used to provide printouts she needs for planning upcoming workshops. To begin, open **CRGHNursePD.xlsx**.
2. Save the workbook with the name **EMedS3-A4-CRGHNursePD**.
3. Format the range of cells A4:H32 as a table. You determine the table style.
4. Filter the table to obtain a list of nurses who are RNs and work in the ICU unit.
5. Sort the list in ascending order by last name.
6. Print the filtered list, changing print options as necessary to fit the printout on 1 page.
7. Redisplay all records.
8. Filter the list to obtain a list of nurses working in the PreOp unit who are not current with professional development (PD) activities.
9. Sort the list in ascending order by last name.
10. Print the filtered list.
11. Redisplay all records.
12. Sort the entire list first by *PD Current?*, then by *Years Experience*, and then by *Employee Last Name*, all in ascending order.
13. Print the sorted list.
14. Save and then close **EMedS3-A4-CRGHNursePD.xlsx**.

Assessment 5 Finding Information on Inserting, Renaming, and Deleting Worksheets

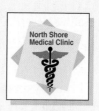

1. Use the Help feature to find out how to insert, rename, and delete worksheets.
2. Open **EMedS3-A3-NSMCDermStats.xlsx**.
3. Save the workbook with the name **EMedS3-A5-NSMCDermStats**.
4. Change the name of the *ColumnChart* sheet to *AgeStatsChart*.
5. Change the name of the *Sheet1* sheet to *DiagnosisByAgeGroup*.
6. Create a footer on each sheet that prints the file name followed by the sheet name separated by a comma and one space in the center section. ***Hint: Use the Page Setup dialog box to create a footer in a chart sheet.***
7. Print the entire workbook.
8. Save and then close **ExcelMedS3-A5-NSMCDermStats.xlsx**.

HELP

Assessment 6 Researching and Calculating Conference Costs

1. Visit the website for the American Association of Medical Assistants (AAMA) and find the dates and location for the upcoming annual convention.
2. The local chapter of the AAMA is willing to sponsor a student to attend the conference. As part of the application for sponsorship, you need to submit a detailed expense estimate.
3. Use the Internet to research airfare, hotel accommodations, conference registration fees, and any other expenses related to attending the conference.
4. Create an Excel worksheet that summarizes the cost of the conference.
5. Apply formatting enhancements to produce a professional quality worksheet.
6. Preview the worksheet and then adjust print options as necessary to improve the printed appearance and minimize paper usage.
7. Save the workbook and name it **EMedS3-A6-AAMAConference**.
8. Print and then close **EMedS3-A6-AAMAConference.xlsx**.

Marquee Challenge

Challenge 1 Preparing a Patient Cost Record

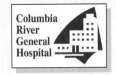

1. Create the worksheet shown in Figure E3.6 on page 340, including all formatting options. Use your best judgment to determine font, font size, font color, fill color, column widths, and/or row heights. Also note the following specifications:
   a. For all date entries, use a DATE function.
   b. Use a formula to calculate Length of Stay.
   c. Use a formula to calculate Direct Overhead at 15% of Total Direct Charges.
   d. Use a formula to calculate Indirect Overhead at 10% of Total Direct Charges.
   e. Use a formula to calculate TOTAL COST as the sum of Total Direct Charges, Direct Overhead, and Indirect Overhead.
2. Center the worksheet horizontally.
3. Create a header to print your name in the left section and the current date in the right section.
4. Create a footer to print the workbook name in the center section.
5. Make any other required changes to page layout options to ensure the cost report will print on one page.
6. Save the workbook and name it **EMedS3-C1-CRGHCost70176345**.
7. Print and then close **EMedS3-C1-CRGHCost70176345.xlsx**.

Challenge 2 Charting 10-Year New Cancer Rate Statistics

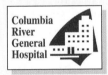

1. Open **USCancerStats.xlsx**.
2. Save the workbook with the name **EMedS3-C2-USCancerStats**.
3. Using the data in the worksheet, create the chart shown in Figure E3.7 on page 341 in its own sheet including all formatting options and drawn objects. Use your best judgment to determine colors and chart style.
4. Create a header to print your name in the left section and the current date in the right section.
5. Create a footer to print the workbook name in the center section.
6. Save **EMedS3-C2-USCancerStats.xlsx**.
7. Print the entire workbook and then close **EMedS3-C2-USCancerStats.xlsx**.

FIGURE E3.6 Challenge 1

Columbia River General Hospital
Patient Cost Record

Date of Cost Report	25-Feb-15		TOTAL COST		$	27,143.53
Patient Chart #	70176345		Attending Physician			Dr. Ruby Priyanka
PIN #	2365		Diagnosis/ Principal Procedure			Hip Replacement
Patient Last Name	**Nguyen**		Admit Date	9-Feb-15		
Date of Birth	Mary		Discharge Date	13-Feb-15		
	22-Oct-76		Length of Stay	4.0		

Department	Dept Code	Service Code	Description		Charges	
Patient Registration	521	13	IP Registration		$	65.15
Health Records	534	17	Clerical			187.50
Food Services	341	67	Patient Meals			375.15
Nursing	122	27	Orthopaedics			4,576.12
Operating Room	431	26	OR			6,548.55
Operating Room	431	31	Respiratory Therapy			235.00
Recovery Room	658	87	Recovery Level 4			678.23
Laboratory Services	377	18	Lab Requisitions			349.00
General Radiology	876	35	HIP LT AP			134.66
General Radiology	876	44	Pelvis & HIP LT			175.33
General Radiology	876	64	Ultrasound			133.28
Pharmacy	912	38	Inpatient Drugs			873.44
Physiotherapy	765	29	Physiotherapy			673.44
Occupational Therapy	844	28	Occupational Therapy			534.22
Physician Service	115	34	OR Surgeon			3,587.75
Inpatient Ward	239	12	General Ward			2,588.00
			Total Direct Charges		$	21,714.82
			Direct Overhead		$	3,257.22
			Indirect Overhead		$	2,171.48

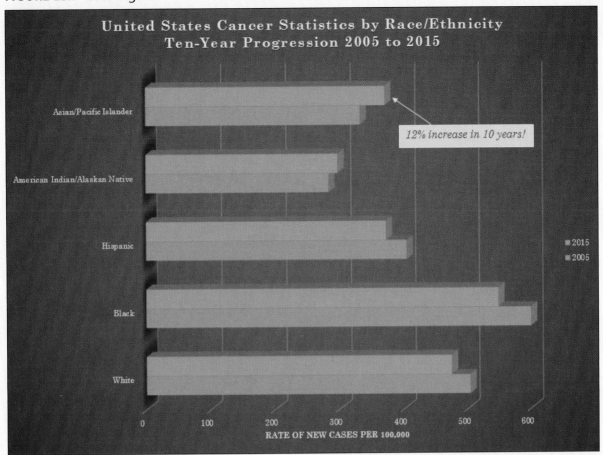

Integrating Programs
Word and Excel

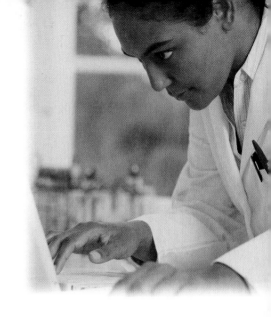

Skills

- Copy and paste Word data into an Excel worksheet
- Link an Excel worksheet with a Word document
- Update linked data
- View linked data as an icon
- Link an Excel chart with a Word document
- Embed an Excel worksheet into a Word document
- Edit an embedded worksheet

Student Resources

Before beginning the activities in this section, copy to your storage medium the IntegratingMed1 folder from the Student Resources CD. This folder contains the data files you need to complete the projects in this section.

Projects Overview

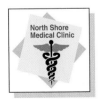

Copy and paste quarterly statistics on new patients; calculate depreciation values, edit data, and link an equipment worksheet to a Word document; link and update a chart depicting actual and projected expenditures to an Operations Report in Word; and embed a flu shot clinic form from Excel into a Word document.

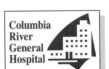

Copy and paste volunteer information from a worksheet to a Word document; link and update tuition fee billing data and a chart from a worksheet to a Word document; and embed a fact sheet into a hospital foundation document.

Copying and Pasting Word Data into an Excel Worksheet

Microsoft Office is a suite that allows for *integration*, which is the combining of data from two or more programs into one document. One way that integration can occur is by copying and pasting data between programs. The program containing the data to be copied is called the *source* program and the program where the data is pasted is called the *destination* program. For example, you can copy data from a Word document into an Excel worksheet. Copy and paste data between programs in the same manner as you would copy and paste data within a program.

Project

You will copy data on new patients at North Shore Medical Clinic from a Word document into an Excel worksheet and then use Excel to total the number of patients per month and per specialty.

1. Open Word and then open **NSMCNewPatientRpt.docx**.

2. Open Excel and then open **NSMCNewPatients-Qtr1.xlsx**.

3. Save the workbook with the name **Int1Med-NSMCNewPatients-Qtr1**.

4. Click the Word button on the Taskbar.

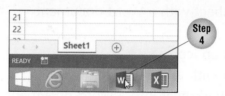

5. Select the last six rows of the table, as shown below.

6. Click the Copy button in the Clipboard group on the HOME tab.

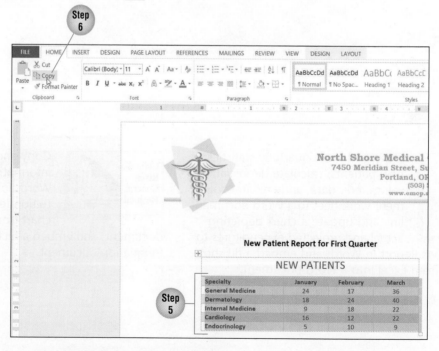

Specialty	January	February	March
General Medicine	24	17	36
Dermatology	18	24	40
Internal Medicine	9	18	22
Cardiology	16	12	22
Endocrinology	5	10	9

7. Click the Excel button on the Taskbar.

8 Make sure cell A5 is the active cell and then click the Paste button 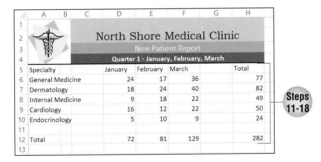 in the Clipboard group.

9 Click the Paste Options button and then click the Match Destination Formatting button.

10 Click in any cell to deselect the range.

11 Select the range of cells B5:D10 and then move the range to cells D5:F10.

12 Make cell H5 the active cell and then type **Total**.

13 Make cell H6 the active cell, click the AutoSum button ∑ in the Editing group on the HOME tab, and then press Enter to calculate the total of the range of cells D6:G6.

14 Use the fill handle to copy the formula in cell H6 down to the range of cells H7:H10.

15 Make cell A12 the active cell and then type **Total**.

16 Make cell D12 the active cell and then use the AutoSum button in the Editing group to calculate the total of the range of cells D6:D11.

17 Use the fill handle to copy the formula in cell D12 to the range of cells E12:H12.

18 Clear the contents of cell G12 to remove the zero.

Step 8

Step 9

Steps 11-18

In Brief

Copy Data from One Program to Another
1. Open desired programs and documents.
2. Select data in source program.
3. Click Copy button.
4. Click button on Taskbar representing destination program.
5. Click Paste button.

Specialty	January	February	March		Total
General Medicine	24	17	36		77
Dermatology	18	24	40		82
Internal Medicine	9	18	22		49
Cardiology	16	12	22		50
Endocrinology	5	10	9		24
Total	72	81	129		282

19 Apply formatting changes as desired to improve the appearance of the worksheet.

20 Save, print, and then close **Int1Med-NSMCNewPatients-Qtr1.xlsx**.

21 Click the Word button on the Taskbar.

22 Close **NSMCNewPatientRpt.docx**. If prompted to save changes to the document, click Don't Save.

In Addition

Cycling between Open Programs

Switch among open programs by clicking the button on the Taskbar representing the desired program. You can also cycle through open programs by pressing Alt + Tab. Pressing Alt + Tab causes a window to display. As you hold down the Alt key, continue pressing the Tab key until the desired program icon is selected in the window and then release the Tab key and the Alt key.

Activity 1.2

In the previous activity, you copied data from a Word document and pasted it into an Excel worksheet. If you updated the data in the Word document, you would need to copy and paste the updated data into the Excel worksheet to keep the worksheet current. If you often update data that is shared among different files, consider copying and linking the data. When data is linked, the data exists in the source program and is represented by a code in the destination program. This code identifies the name and location of the source program and document and the location of the data in the document. Since the data is located only in the source program, changes made to the data in the source program are automatically reflected in the destination program. Links are automatically updated whenever you open the destination program or edit the linked data in the destination program.

Project

You will open a worksheet with equipment purchase information, use a function to calculate straight-line depreciation, and then copy and link the data to a Word document.

1 With Word the active program, open **NSMCEquipGERm3-SLD.docx**.

2 Save the document with the name **Int1Med-NSMCEquipGERm3-SLD**.

3 Make Excel the active program and then open **NSMCEquipGERm3.xlsx**.

4 Save the workbook with the name **Int1Med-NSMCEquipGERm3**.

In the next steps, you will use Excel's SLN function to calculate the annual depreciation value to be recorded for each equipment item. Straight-line depreciation requires three values: the equipment's original cost, the estimated value of the equipment when taken out of service (salvage), and the expected number of years the clinic will use the item (life).

5 Make cell H6 the active cell and then click the Insert Function button f_x on the Formula bar.

6 Type **straight-line depreciation** in the *Search for a function* text box and then press Enter or click Go.

7 If necessary, click to select *SLN* in the *Select a function* list box and then click OK.

8 With the insertion point positioned in the *Cost* text box, type **E6** and then press Tab.

9 Type **F6** in the *Salvage* text box and then press Tab.

10 Type **G6** in the *Life* text box and then press Enter.

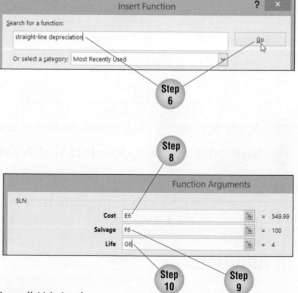

Excel returns the value *$112.50* in cell H6. In the Formula bar, the function is *=SLN(E6,F6,G6)*.

11 Copy the formula in cell H6 to the range of cells H7:H10.

12 Make cell H11 the active cell and then use the AutoSum button to calculate the total of the range of cells H6:H10.

13 Select the range of cells A5:H11 and then click the Copy button in the Clipboard group on the HOME tab.

14 Click the Word button on the Taskbar.

15 Press Ctrl + End to move the insertion point to the end of the document.

16 Click the Paste button arrow and then click *Paste Special* at the drop-down list.

17 Click *Microsoft Excel Worksheet Object* in the *As* list box, click the *Paste link* option, and then click OK.

G	H
al Clinic	
lule	
Room 3	
r 31, 2016	
Estimated Life (Yrs)	Straight-Line Depreciation
4	$112.50
3	$1,100.00
2	$89.98
2	$112.50
3	$146.67
	$1,561.64

Step 11

Step 12

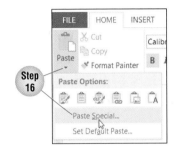

Step 16

Step 17

Paste Special

Source: Microsoft Excel Worksheet
Sheet1!R5C1:R11C9

As:
- Microsoft Excel Worksheet Object
- Formatted Text (RTF)
- Unformatted Text
- Picture (Windows Metafile)
- Bitmap
- Word Hyperlink
- HTML Format
- Unformatted Unicode Text

○ Paste:
● Paste link:

☐ Display as icon

Result
Inserts the contents of the Clipboard as a picture.
Paste Link creates a shortcut to the source file. Changes to the source file will be reflected in your document.

OK   Cancel

In Brief
Link Data between Programs
1. Open desired programs and documents.
2. Select data in source program.
3. Click Copy button.
4. Click button on Taskbar representing destination program.
5. Click Paste button arrow.
6. Click *Paste Special*.
7. Click object in *As* list box.
8. Click *Paste link*.
9. Click OK.

18 Save, print, and then close **Int1Med-NSMCEquipGERm3-SLD.docx**.

19 Click the Excel button on the Taskbar.

20 Press the Esc key to remove the marquee around the range of cells A5:H11 and then click any cell to deselect the range.

21 Save, print, and then close **Int1Med-NSMCEquipGERm3.xlsx**.

In Addition

Linking Data within a Program

Linking does not have to occur between different programs—you can also link data between files in the same program. For example, you can create an object in a Word document, such as a table or chart, and then link the object with another Word document (or several Word documents). If you make a change to the object in the original document, the linked object in the other document (or documents) will automatically be updated.

Activity 1.3

Updating Linked Data; Viewing a Link

The advantage of linking data over copying it is that editing the data in the source program will automatically update the data in the destination program. To edit linked data, open the document in the source program, make the desired edits, and then save the document. The next time you open the document in the destination program, the data will be updated. The display of the linked data in the destination program can be changed to an icon. The icon represents the document and program to which the object is linked.

Project

Lee Elliott, office manager for North Shore Medical Clinic, has given you revised estimates for salvage value and estimated life for two equipment items in the linked worksheet. You will open the worksheet, update the values, and then view the updated information in Word.

1. With Excel the active program, open **Int1Med-NSMCEquipGERm3.xlsx**.

   The salvage value and estimated life numbers for the AudioScope have been revised to *$75.00* and *3*, respectively.

2. Make cell F6 the active cell and then change the contents to *$75.00*.

3. Make cell G6 the active cell and then change the contents to *3*.

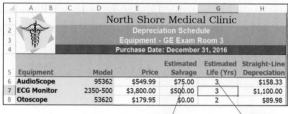

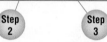

4. Save and close **Int1Med-SMCEquipGERm3.xlsx** and then close Excel.

5. With Word the active program, open **Int1Med-NSMCEquipGERm3-SLD.docx**.

6. Click Yes at the message asking if you want to update the document with the data from the linked files.

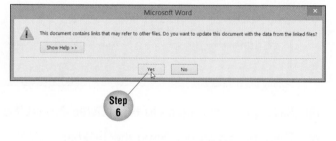

   The document opens and is automatically updated to reflect the changes you made in **Int1Med-NSMCEquipGERm3.xlsx**.

7. Review the Word document. Notice that the estimated salvage and estimated life values for the AudioScope have been updated.

   Another way to edit linked data is to double-click the linked object in the destination program.

8. Position the mouse pointer over the linked object and then double-click the left mouse button.

   Excel opens and displays **Int1Med-NSMCEquipGERm3.xlsx** in the Excel window. The linked range is highlighted. You need to change the salvage value and estimated life for the Wall Transformer to *$50.00* and *2*, respectively.

9. Make cell F10 the active cell and then change the contents to *$50.00*.

10. Make cell G10 the active cell and then change the contents to *2*.

11. Click the Save button on the Quick Access toolbar and then close Excel.

12 Notice that the values in the linked object in Word have been updated.

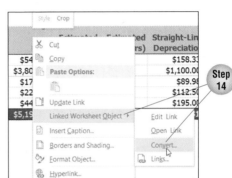

Equipment Purchase – GE Exam Room 3					
Purchase Date: December 31, 2016					
Straight-Line Depreciation Schedule					
Equipment	Model	Price	Estimated Salvage	Estimated Life (Yrs)	Straight-Line Depreciation
AudioScope	95362	$549.99	$75.00	3	$158.33
ECG Monitor	2350-500	$3,800.00	$500.00	3	$1,100.00
Otoscope	53620	$179.95	$0.00	2	$89.98
ThermoScan	40560	$225.00	$0.00	2	$112.50
Wall Transformer	652-A	$440.00	$50.00	2	$195.00
Total		$5,194.94			$1,655.81

Step 12

13 Save and then print **Int1Med-NSMCEquipGERm3-SLD.docx.**

14 Display the linked table as an icon. Begin by right-clicking the table, pointing to *Linked Worksheet Object*, and then clicking *Convert* at the side menu.

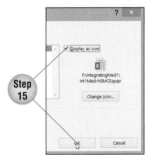

Step 14

15 At the Convert dialog box, click the *Display as icon* check box to insert a check mark and then click OK.

> Notice how the table changes to an icon representing the linked document.

16 Print **Int1Med-NSMCEquipGERm3-SLD.docx.**

17 Make sure the linked object icon is selected and then redisplay the table. To begin, right-click the icon, point to *Linked Worksheet Object*, and then click *Convert* at the side menu.

Step 15

18 At the Convert dialog box, click the *Display as icon* check box to remove the check mark and then click OK.

19 Save and then close **Int1Med-NSMCEquipGERm3-SLD.docx.**

In Brief

Update Linked Data
1. Open document in source program.
2. Make desired edits.
3. Save and close document.
4. Open document in destination program.
5. Click Yes to update links.
6. Save and close document.

Display Linked Object as an Icon
1. Select object.
2. Right-click in object.
3. Point to *Linked Worksheet Object* and then click *Convert*.
4. At Convert dialog box, click *Display as icon* check box.
5. Click OK.

In Addition

Breaking a Link

The link between an object in the destination and source programs can be broken if necessary. To break a link, right-click the linked object in the destination program, point to *Linked Worksheet Object*, and then click *Links*. At the Links dialog box, click the Break Link button. At the question asking if you are sure you want to break the link, click Yes.

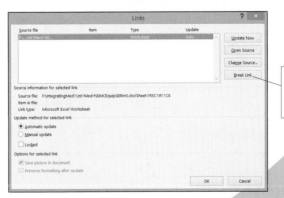

Click here to break the link for a selected object.

Activity 1.4

Linking an Excel Chart with a Word Document

While a worksheet does an adequate job of representing data, certain types of data are more effectively represented in a chart. A *chart* is a visual representation of numeric data. Charts, like worksheets, can be linked to a document in another program. Link a chart in the same manner as you would link a worksheet.

Project You will link an Excel chart depicting North Shore Medical Clinic's projected and actual expenditures with the Operations Report document saved in Word. After linking the chart, you will update the data used to generate the chart.

① With Word the active program, open **NSMCOpRpt.docx**.

② Save the document with the name **Int1Med-NSMCOpRpt**.

③ Make Excel the active program and then open **NSMCQtrlyExp.xlsx**.

④ Save the workbook with the name **Int1Med-NSMCQtrlyExp**.

⑤ Click the chart to select it. (A border displays around the chart.)

> Make sure you do not select an individual chart element when you select the chart. If you see a thin border with sizing handles around a chart element, click outside the chart and select the chart again. Click a white area around the inside perimeter to select the chart without selecting an individual chart element.

⑥ Click the Copy button in the Clipboard group on the HOME tab.

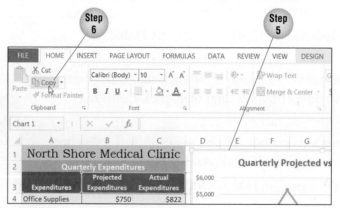

⑦ Click the Word button on the Taskbar.

⑧ Press Ctrl + End to move the insertion point to the end of the document.

⑨ Click the Center button ≡ in the Paragraph group on the HOME tab.

⑩ Click the Paste button arrow in the Clipboard group and then click *Paste Special*.

⑪ Click *Microsoft Excel Chart Object* in the *As* list box, click *Paste link*, and then click OK.

⑫ Save **Int1Med-NSMCOpRpt.docx**.

13 Make Excel the active program and then press the Esc key to remove the border from the chart.

> The actual expenditure value for Diagnostics is incorrect. You will enter the correct value and then examine the change in the chart in both Excel and Word.

14 Make cell C8 the active cell and then change the contents to *$3,400*.

15 Examine the revised chart in Excel.

16 Save and then close **Int1Med-NSMCQtrlyExp.xlsx**.

17 Make Word the active program.

18 Update the chart by clicking the FILE tab, scrolling down the Info backstage area, and then clicking *Edit Links to Files* at the bottom right side of the backstage area.

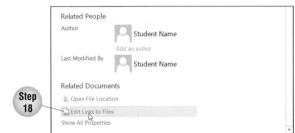

19 At the Links dialog box with the linked object selected in the list box, click the Update Now button.

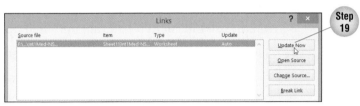

20 Click OK to close the Links dialog box.

21 Click the Back button to return to the document.

22 Change the percent value in the second-to-last sentence in the paragraph above the chart to *16.7%*. The sentence should now read *Overall, the clinic spent 16.7% more on operations than projected.*

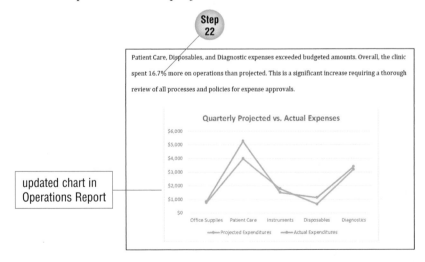

updated chart in Operations Report

23 Save, print, and then close **Int1Med-NSMCOpRpt.docx**.

Activity 1.5

Embedding an Excel Worksheet into a Word Document

In addition to copying and linking, another way to integrate data among different files in the same or different programs is by embedding it. While a linked object resides in the source program and is represented by a code in the destination program, an embedded object resides in the source program and in the destination program. When you make a change to an embedded object in the source program, the change is not made to the object in the destination program. Since an embedded object is not automatically updated, unlike a linked object, the only advantage to embedding rather than simply copying and pasting is that you can edit an embedded object in the destination program using the tools of the source program.

Project

You will copy and embed a flu shot clinic form created by Heather Mitsui, RMA at North Shore Medical Clinic, from an Excel worksheet into a Word document.

1. With Word the active program, open **NSMCShotClinics.docx**.

2. Save the document with the name **Int1Med-NSMCShotClinics**.

3. Make Excel the active program and then open **NSMCShotForm.xlsx**.

4. Save the workbook with the name **Int1Med-NSMCShotForm**.

   Heather Mitsui used Excel to create a flu shot dispensing record form for the upcoming flu shot clinics. You decide to embed Heather's form into a Word document, since the Word document has the clinic's letterhead at the top of the page.

5. Select the range of cells A9:K29 and then click the Copy button in the Clipboard group on the HOME tab.

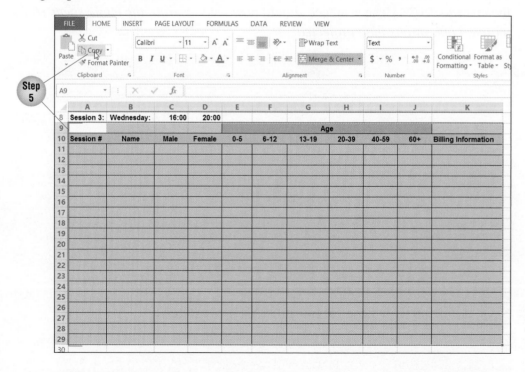

6 Make Word the active program and then press Ctrl + End to move the insertion point to the end of **Int1Med-NSMCShotClinics.docx**.

7 Click the Paste button arrow in the Clipboard group and then click *Paste Special*.

8 Click *Microsoft Excel Worksheet Object* in the *As* list box.

> Make sure you do not click the Paste link option.

9 Click OK.

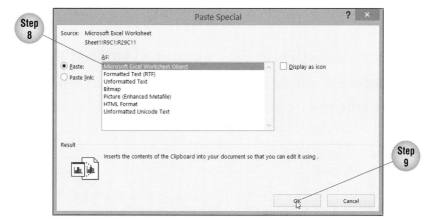

10 Display the Print backstage area to see how the form will look when printed.

11 Click the Back button to return to the form.

12 Save, print, and then close **Int1Med-NSMCShotClinics.docx**.

13 Make Excel the active program and then press the Esc key to remove the marquee from the selected range.

14 Click in any cell to deselect the range.

15 Close **Int1Med-NSMCShotForm.xlsx** and then close Excel.

In Brief

Embed Data
1. Open desired programs and documents.
2. Select data in source program.
3. Click Copy button.
4. Click button on Taskbar representing destination program.
5. Click Paste button arrow.
6. Click *Paste Special*.
7. Click object in *As* list box.
8. Click OK.

In Addition

Inserting an Embedded Object from an Existing File

In this activity, you embedded an Excel worksheet in a Word document using the Copy button and options at the Paste Special dialog box. Another method is available for embedding an object from an existing file. In the destination program file in Word, Excel, or PowerPoint, position the insertion point where you want the object embedded and then click the Object button in the Text group on the INSERT tab. At the Object dialog box, click the Create from File tab. At the Object dialog box with the Create from File tab selected, as shown at the right, type the desired file name in the *File name* text box or click the Browse button and then select the desired file from the appropriate folder. At the Object dialog box, make sure the *Link to file* check box does not contain a check mark and then click OK.

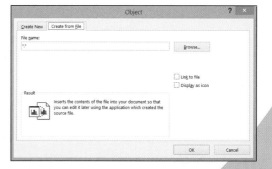

Activity 1.6

Editing an Embedded Worksheet

An embedded object can be edited in the destination program using the tools of the source program. Double-click the embedded object in the file in the destination program and the ribbon from the source program becomes active. For example, if you double-click an Excel worksheet that is embedded in a Word document, the Excel ribbon displays at the top of the Word document window.

Project

After embedding the flu shot clinic form into Word, you decide to make some changes to the form's layout.

North Shore Medical Clinic

1. With Word the active program, open **Int1Med-NSMCShotClinics.docx**.

2. Save the document with the name **Int1Med-NSMCShotClinics-Edit**.

3. Change the start time for the Session 3 clinic from *04:00 pm* to *06:30 pm.*

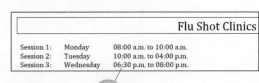

Flu Shot Clinics

Session 1:	Monday	08:00 a.m. to 10:00 a.m.
Session 2:	Tuesday	10:00 a.m. to 04:00 p.m.
Session 3:	Wednesday	06:30 p.m. to 08:00 p.m.

Step 3

4. Double-click anywhere in the embedded worksheet.

   In a few seconds, the worksheet displays surrounded by column and row designations and the Excel ribbon displays at the top of the Word window.

5. Click in any cell within the embedded worksheet to deselect the range.

6. Select columns E through J and then change the column widths to *6.00 (61 pixels)*.

Step 6

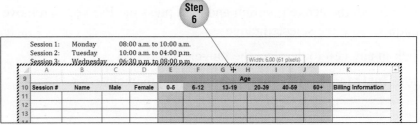

7. Click in any cell to deselect the columns.

8. Select the range of cells A9:D9 and cell K9 and then apply Lavender, Accent 4, Darker 25% fill color (eighth column, fifth row in the *Theme Colors* section).

Step 8

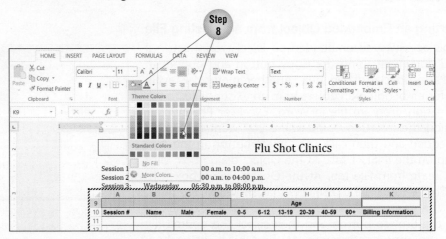

9 Insert a new column between columns D and E and then change the width of the new column to *6.00 (61 pixels)*.

10 Type the label **0-1** in cell E10.

11 Change the label in cell F10 from *0-5* to *2-5*.

12 If necessary, drag the middle right sizing handle of the embedded worksheet to the right to make sure columns A through L are visible within the object's border.

13 Merge and center the label *Age* over columns E through K.

14 Select cell E9 (contains the label *Age*) and then apply an outside border.

15 Select the range of cells A9:L9 and then apply an outside border.

16 Make sure the only cells visible within the embedded object border are in the range of cells A9:L29. If any other cells from the source worksheet are visible, use the horizontal and vertical scroll arrows to adjust the window.

> Figure I1.1 illustrates a portion of the embedded worksheet with the revised formatting applied in Steps 8 through 15. If this portion of your worksheet does not appear as shown in Figure I1.1, review Steps 8 through 15 to determine if you have missed a step. Also note that you may need to scroll within the worksheet to ensure that columns A through L and rows 1 through 29 are visible within the object's border.

17 Click outside the worksheet to deselect the embedded object.

18 Save, print, and then close **Int1Med-NSMCShotClinics-Edit.docx**.

In Brief
Edit Embedded Object
1. In source program, double-click embedded object.
2. Make desired edits.
3. Click outside object.

FIGURE I1.1 Excel Worksheet Embedded in a Word Document

Session 1:	Monday	08:00 a.m. to 10:00 a.m.									
Session 2:	Tuesday	10:00 a.m. to 04:00 p.m.									
Session 3:	Wednesday	04:00 p.m. to 08:00 p.m.									

	A	B	C	D	E	F	G	H	I	J	K	L
9								Age				
10	Session #	Name	Male	Female	0-1	2-5	6-12	13-19	20-39	40-59	60+	Billing Information
11												
12												
13												
14												
15												
16												
17												

In Addition

Troubleshooting Problems with Linking and Embedding

If you double-click a linked or embedded object and a message appears telling you that the source file or source program cannot be opened, consider the following troubleshooting options:

- Check to make sure that the source program is installed on your computer. If the source program is not installed, convert the object to the file format of a program that is installed.

- Try closing other programs to free up more memory and make sure you have enough memory to run the source program.

- Check to make sure the source program does not have any dialog boxes open.

- If you are trying to open a linked object, check to make sure no one else is working in the source file.

Skills Review

Review 1 Copying and Pasting Data

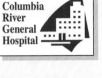

Columbia River General Hospital

1. Make Excel the active program and then open **CRGHVolunteers.xlsx**.
2. Make Word the active program and then open **CRGHVolPost.docx**.
3. Save the document with the name **Int1Med-R-CRGHVolPost**.
4. Make Excel the active program, select the range of cells C7:F28 and then click the Copy button in the Clipboard group on the HOME tab.
5. Make Word the active program and then press Ctrl + End to move the insertion point to the end of **Int1Med-R-CRGHVolPost**.
6. Paste the table into the Word document.
7. Select the table, display the Table Properties dialog box, center the table between the left and right margins, and then deselect the table.
8. View the document at the Print backstage area.
9. Click the Back button to return to the document.
10. Save, print, and then close **Int1Med-R-CRGHVolPost.docx**.
11. Make Excel the active program, remove the marquee, and then deselect the range.
12. Close **CRGHVolunteers.xlsx**.

Review 2 Linking an Object

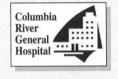

Columbia River General Hospital

1. Make Word the active program and then open **CRGH4thQtrFees.docx**.
2. Save the document with the name **Int1Med-R-CRGH4thQtrFees**.
3. Make Excel the active program and then open **CRGHQtrlyBilling.xlsx**.
4. Save the workbook with the name **Int1Med-R-CRGHQtrlyBilling**.
5. Select the range of cells A7:G16 and then link the cells to the end of the Word document **Int1Med-R-CRGH4thQtrFees.docx**.
6. Save, print, and then close **Int1Med-R-CRGH4thQtrFees.docx**.
7. Make Excel the active program, remove the marquee, and then deselect the range.
8. Close **Int1Med-R-CRGHQtrlyBilling.xlsx**.

Review 3 Creating and Linking a Chart

Columbia River General Hospital

1. With Excel the active program, open **Int1Med-R-CRGHQtrlyBilling.xlsx**.
2. Make Word the active program and then open **Int1Med-R-CRGH4thQtrFees.docx**. Click No when prompted to update links.
3. Make Excel the active program and then select the range of cells A7:A15 and G7:G15.
4. Create a 3-D pie chart with the following options:
   a. Insert *Fourth Quarter Tuition by Course* as the chart title.
   b. Apply the Style 3 chart style.
   c. Position the chart below the worksheet, starting in cell A18.
5. With the chart selected, copy and then link the chart to the Word document **Int1Med-R-CRGH4thQtrFees.docx**. Insert a triple space below the linked worksheet. If necessary, make changes to the chart or page layout options to fit the document on one page.

6. Save, print, and then close **Int1Med-R-CRGH4thQtrFees.docx**.
7. Make Excel the active program and then click any cell to deselect the chart.
8. Save, print, and then close **Int1Med-R-CRGHQtrlyBilling.xlsx**.

Review 4 **Editing Linked Objects**

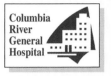

1. With Excel the active program, open **Int1Med-R-CRGHQtrlyBilling.xlsx**.
2. Make the following changes to the data in the specified cells:

B10:	575
D10:	1125
E10:	850
C14:	225
C15:	1175

3. Save, print, and then close **Int1Med-R-CRGHQtrlyBilling.xlsx**.
4. Make Word the active program and then open **Int1Med-R-CRGH4thQtrFees.docx**. Click Yes when prompted to update linked data.
5. Save, print, and then close **Int1Med-R-CRGH4thQtrFees.docx**.

Review 5 **Embedding and Editing an Object**

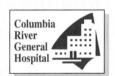

1. With Word the active program, open **CRGHFoundation.docx**.
2. Save the document with the name **Int1Med-R-CRGHFoundation**.
3. Make Excel the active program and then open **CRGHFactSheet.xlsx**.
4. Select the range of cells A6:H23 and then embed the cells at the end of the Word document **Int1Med-R-CRGHFoundation.docx**.
5. Make Excel the active program, remove the marquee, click any cell to deselect the range, and then close **CRGHFactSheet.xlsx**.
6. Close Excel.
7. Double-click the embedded object in **Int1Med-R-CRGHFoundation.docx**.
8. Select the range of cells A7:H23 and then apply Blue, Accent 1, Lighter 80% fill color (fifth column, second row in the *Theme Colors* section).
9. Change the value for *Volunteer & Auxiliary Members* to *812*.
10. Click outside the embedded object.
11. Save, print, and then close **Int1Med-R-CRGHFoundation.docx**.
12. Close Word.

Using POWERPOINT *in the* Medical Office

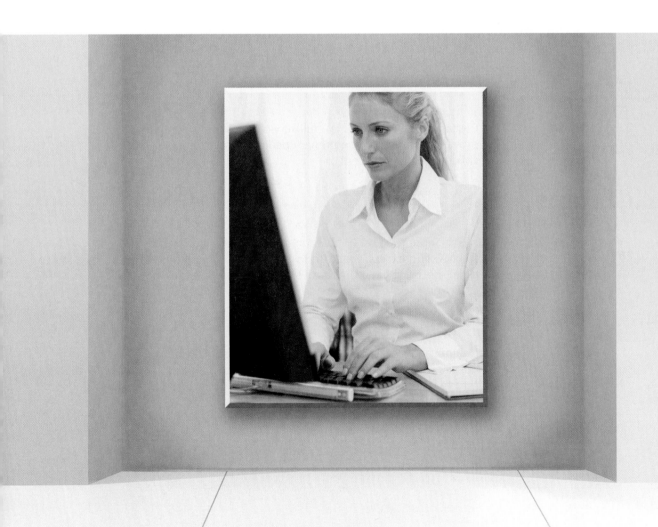

Introducing
POWERPOINT 2013

Create colorful and powerful presentations using PowerPoint, the full-featured presentation program included in the Microsoft Office suite. With PowerPoint, you can organize and display information and create visual aids. PowerPoint provides a wide variety of editing and formatting features as well as sophisticated visual elements such as photographs, clip art, WordArt, lines, shapes, and diagrams.

In Section 1, you will choose design templates for presentations; insert slides; choose slide layouts; select, move, and size placeholders; use the Help feature; check spelling in presentations; run presentations; and add transitions and sound to presentations. Section 2 focuses on editing slides and slide elements. In that section, you will rearrange, delete, and hide slides; cut, copy, and paste text within and between slides; apply font and font effects; apply formatting such as alignment, spacing, headers, and footers; change slide design themes; insert and format images, WordArt, and SmartArt graphics; and apply animation schemes.

In the two PowerPoint sections, you will prepare medical presentations for two clinics and a hospital as described below.

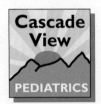

Cascade View Pediatrics is a full-service pediatric clinic that provides comprehensive primary pediatric care to infants, children, and adolescents.

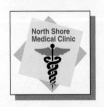

North Shore Medical Clinic is an internal medicine clinic dedicated to providing exceptional care to all patients. The physicians in the clinic specialize in a number of fields including internal medicine, family practice, cardiology, and dermatology.

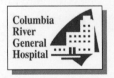

Columbia River General Hospital is an independent, not-for-profit hospital with the mission of providing high-quality, comprehensive care to patients and improving the health of members of the community.

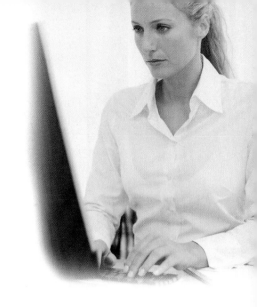

PowerPoint SECTION 1
Preparing a Presentation

Skills

- Complete the presentation cycle
- Choose a design theme
- Navigate in a presentation
- Insert a slide in a presentation
- Change the presentation view
- Change the slide layout
- Select, move, and size a placeholder
- Use the Help feature
- Check spelling in a presentation
- Use Thesaurus to display synonyms for words
- Run a presentation
- Use the pen and highlighter during a presentation
- Add transition and sound to a presentation
- Print and preview a presentation

Student Resources

Before beginning the activities in PowerPoint Section 1, copy to your storage medium the PowerPointMedS1 folder from the Student Resources CD. This folder contains the data files you need to complete the projects in this PowerPoint section.

Projects Overview

Prepare a presentation introducing PowerPoint 2013; prepare, edit, and format a presentation on diabetes; prepare a presentation on cystic fibrosis; and edit and format a presentation containing information on the clinic.

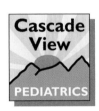

Prepare, edit, and format a presentation containing information on the clinic and prepare, edit, and format a presentation on chickenpox.

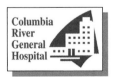

Prepare, edit, and format a presentation on fibromyalgia and prepare, edit, and format a presentation containing information on the hospital.

Activity 1.1

Completing the Presentation Cycle

PowerPoint is a presentation graphics program you can use to organize and present information. With PowerPoint, you can create a presentation and then print copies of the presentation for your audience to use as visual aids while you give the presentation.

Preparing a presentation in PowerPoint usually involves following a presentation cycle. The steps in the cycle vary but generally include opening PowerPoint; creating and editing slides; saving, printing, running, and closing the presentation; and then closing PowerPoint.

Project

You are an employee of North Shore Medical Clinic and Office 2013 has just been installed on your computer. You need to prepare a presentation in the near future, so you decide to open a presentation provided by PowerPoint and experiment with running the presentation.

North Shore Medical Clinic

1 At the Windows 8.1 Start screen, click the PowerPoint 2013 tile to open PowerPoint.

This step may vary. Check with your instructor for specific directions.

2 At the PowerPoint 2013 opening screen, click the *Welcome to PowerPoint* template.

If this template is not visible, you will need to search for it. To do this, click in the search text box, type **Welcome to PowerPoint**, and then press the Enter key.

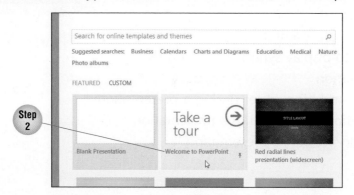

3 Click the Create button.

The Welcome to PowerPoint template opens in the PowerPoint window. Identify various elements of the PowerPoint 2013 window by comparing your screen with the image in Figure P1.1. Refer to Table P1.1 for a description of the window elements.

4 Run the presentation by clicking the Start From Beginning button on the Quick Access toolbar.

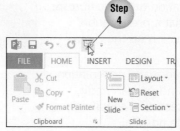

FIGURE P1.1 PowerPoint Window

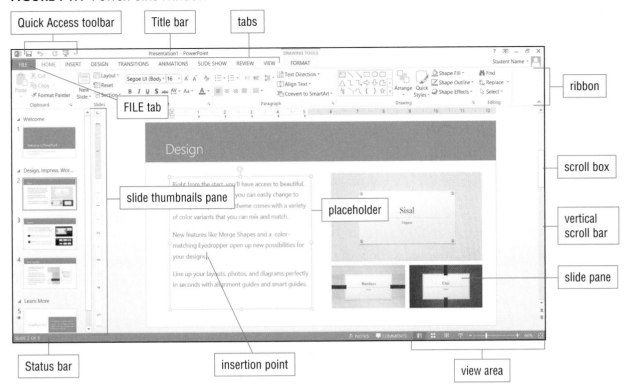

TABLE P1.1 PowerPoint Window Elements

Feature	Description
FILE tab	when clicked, displays backstage area with options for working with and managing files
I-beam pointer	used to move the insertion point or to select text
insertion point	indicates location of next character entered at the keyboard
placeholder	location on a slide with a dotted border that holds text or objects
Quick Access toolbar	contains buttons for commonly used commands
ribbon	area containing the tabs with commands and buttons divided into groups
slide pane	displays the slide and slide contents
slide thumbnails pane	left side of the screen that displays slide thumbnails
Status bar	displays slide number, view buttons, and Zoom slider bar
tabs	contain commands and features organized into groups
Title bar	displays file name followed by program name
vertical scroll bar	display specific slides using this scroll bar
view area	located toward right side of Status bar; contains buttons for changing the presentation view

continues

5 When the first slide fills the screen, read the information and then click the left mouse button. Continue reading the information in each slide and clicking the left mouse button to advance to the next slide. When a black screen displays, click the left mouse button to end the slide show.

6 Save the presentation by clicking the Save button 🖫 on the Quick Access toolbar.

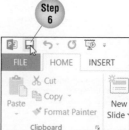

7 At the Save As backstage area, click the *OneDrive* option preceded by your name if you are saving to your OneDrive or click the *Computer* option if you are saving to the computer's hard drive or a USB flash drive.

8 Click the Browse button.

9 At the Save As dialog box, navigate to the PowerPointMedS1 folder on your storage medium, type **PMedS1-PowerPoint2013** in the *File name* text box, and then click the Save button or press Enter.

The Address bar in the Save As dialog box displays the active folder and the folder path.

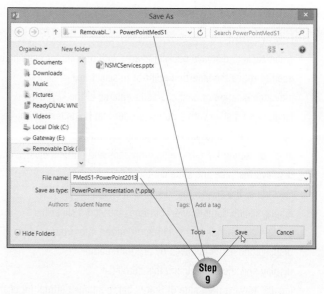

10 At the PowerPoint window, print the presentation information in outline view by clicking the FILE tab and then clicking the *Print* option.

> The FILE tab is located in the upper left corner of the screen at the left side of the HOME tab. When you click the FILE tab, the backstage area displays with options for working with and managing files. *Print* is one of these options.

11 At the Print backstage area, click the second gallery in the *Settings* category (contains the text *Full Page Slides*) and then click *Outline* in the *Print Layout* section of the drop-down list.

12 Click the Print button. *Note: Always check with your instructor before printing.*

13 Close the presentation by clicking the FILE tab and then clicking the *Close* option.

> If a message displays asking if you want to save the presentation, click Save.

14 Close PowerPoint by clicking the Close button that displays in the upper right corner of the screen.

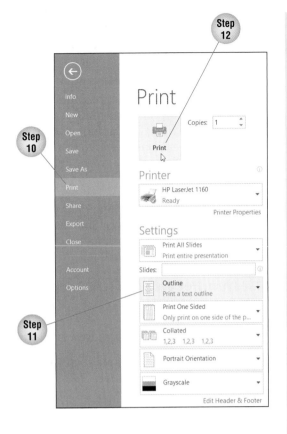

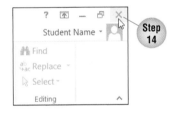

In Brief

Create Presentation from Template
1. Click FILE tab.
2. Click *New* option.
3. Click desired template.
4. Click Create button.

Save Presentation
1. Click Save button on Quick Access toolbar.
2. At Save As backstage area, click desired location.
3. Click Browse button.
4. At Save As dialog box, navigate to desired folder.
5. Type file name in *File name* text box.
6. Click Save or press Enter.

Run Presentation
Click Start From Beginning button on Quick Access toolbar.

Print Presentation
1. Click FILE tab.
2. Click *Print* option.
3. At Print backstage area, specify how you want presentation printed.
4. Click Print.

Close Presentation
1. Click FILE tab.
2. Click *Close* option.

In Addition

Using Tabs

Similar to the other applications in the Microsoft Office suite, the PowerPoint ribbon displays below the Quick Access toolbar. PowerPoint commands and features are organized into tabs that display in the ribbon area. The buttons and options in the ribbon area vary depending on the tab selected and the width of the window displayed on the screen. Commands and features are organized into groups within each tab. For example, the HOME tab, which is the default tab, contains the Clipboard, Slides, Font, Paragraph, Drawing, and Editing groups. When you hover the mouse over a button, a ScreenTip displays with the name of the button, a keyboard shortcut (if available), and a description of the purpose of the button.

Activity 1.2

Choosing a Design Theme and Creating Slides

Create a PowerPoint presentation using an installed template, as you did in the previous activity, or begin with a blank presentation and then apply a design theme or formatting of your own choosing. To display a blank PowerPoint presentation, click the FILE tab, click the *New* option, and then click the *Blank Presentation* template at the New backstage area. You can also display a blank presentation by pressing the keyboard shortcut Ctrl + N. The blank presentation displays in Normal view with the slide pane in the center and the slide thumbnails pane at the left side of the screen.

Project

Dr. St. Claire will be presenting information on diabetes at the Greater Portland Healthcare Workers Association meeting. She has asked you to prepare a PowerPoint presentation that she will use during the meeting. You decide to prepare the presentation using a design template provided by PowerPoint.

1. Open PowerPoint.

2. At the PowerPoint 2013 opening screen, click the *Blank Presentation* template.

3. At the PowerPoint window, click the DESIGN tab.

4. Click the More button ⟱ at the right side of the theme thumbnails in the Themes group.

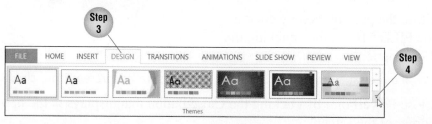

5. Click *Organic* in the *Office* section of the drop-down gallery. (Design thumbnails display in alphabetic order in the drop-down gallery.)

> The Themes drop-down gallery is equipped with the *live preview* feature, which means that when you hover your mouse pointer over one of the design themes, the slide in the slide pane displays with the design theme formatting applied. With the live preview feature, you can preview a design theme before actually applying it to the presentation.

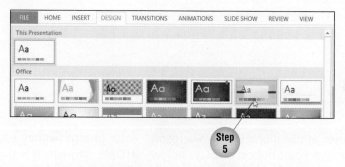

6. Click the fourth thumbnail from the left in the Variants group.

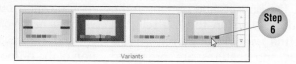

7 Click anywhere in the *Click to add title* placeholder that displays in the slide in the slide pane and then type **Understanding Diabetes**.

> A placeholder is a location on a slide marked with a border that holds text or an object.

8 Click anywhere in the *Click to add subtitle* placeholder that displays in the slide and then type **Greater Portland Healthcare Workers Association**.

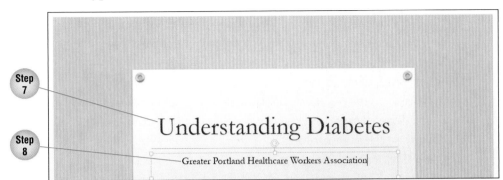

9 Click the HOME tab and then click the New Slide button [icon] in the Slides group.

> When you click the New Slide button, a new slide displays in the slide pane with the Title and Content layout. You will learn more about slide layouts in Activity 1.3.

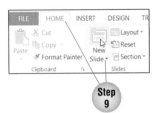

10 Click anywhere in the *Click to add title* placeholder that displays in the slide and then type **Statistics on Diabetes**.

11 Click anywhere in the *Click to add text* placeholder that displays in the slide and then type **Prevalence of diabetes in the United States**.

12 Press the Enter key and then type **Total number of people diagnosed with diabetes**.

13 Press the Enter key and then type **Diabetes by age group**.

> You can use keys on the keyboard to move the insertion point to various locations within a placeholder in a slide. Refer to Table P1.2 on page 368 for more information on how to do this.

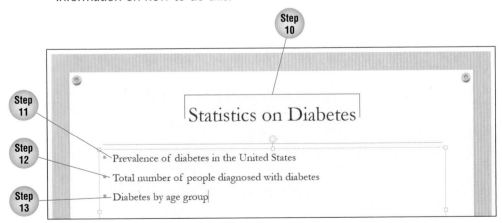

14 Click the New Slide button in the Slides group on the HOME tab.

continues

TABLE P1.2 Insertion Point Movement Commands

To move insertion point	Press
One character left	Left Arrow
One character right	Right Arrow
One line up	Up Arrow
One line down	Down Arrow
One word to the left	Ctrl + Left Arrow
One word to the right	Ctrl + Right Arrow
To end of a line of text	End
To beginning of a line of text	Home
To beginning of current paragraph in placeholder	Ctrl + Up Arrow
To beginning of previous paragraph in placeholder	Ctrl + Up Arrow twice
To beginning of next paragraph in placeholder	Ctrl + Down Arrow
To beginning of text in placeholder	Ctrl + Home
To end of text in placeholder	Ctrl + End

15 Click anywhere in the *Click to add title* placeholder that displays in the slide and then type **Types of Diabetes**.

16 Click anywhere in the *Click to add text* placeholder that displays in the slide and then type the bulleted text as shown in the image below. Press the Enter key after each item except the last item.

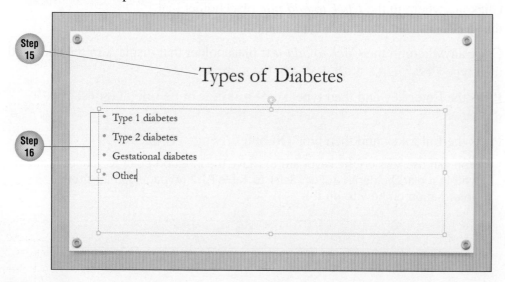

17 Click the New Slide button in the Slides group on the HOME tab.

18 Click anywhere in the *Click to add title* placeholder that displays in the slide and then type **Treatment of Diabetes**.

19 Click anywhere in the *Click to add text* placeholder that displays in the slide and then type the bulleted text as shown in the slide below. Press the Enter key after each item except the last item.

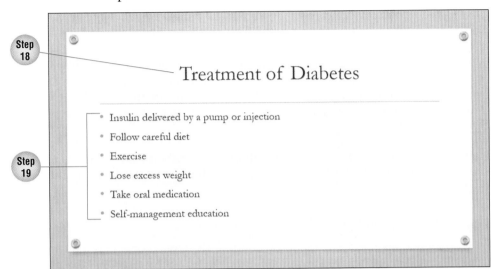

20 Click the Save button on the Quick Access toolbar.

21 At the Save As backstage area, click the desired location (for example, your OneDrive or the *Computer* option) and then click the Browse button.

22 At the Save As dialog box, navigate to the PowerPointMedS1 folder on your storage medium, type **PMedS1-Diabetes** in the *File name* text box, and then press Enter.

23 Close the presentation by clicking the FILE tab and then clicking the *Close* option.

In Addition

Planning a Presentation

Consider the following basic guidelines when preparing the content of a presentation:

- **Determine the main purpose of the presentation.** Do not try to cover too many topics. Identifying the main point of the presentation will help you stay focused and convey a clear message to the audience.
- **Determine the output.** To help decide the type of output needed, consider the availability of equipment, the size of the room where you will make the presentation, and the number of people who will be attending the presentation.
- **Show one idea per slide.** Each slide in a presentation should convey only one main idea. Too many ideas on a slide may confuse the audience and cause you to stray from the purpose of the slide.

- **Maintain a consistent design.** A consistent design and color scheme for slides in a presentation will create continuity and cohesiveness. Do not use too much color or too many pictures or other graphic elements.
- **Keep slides uncluttered and easy to read.** Keep slides simple and legible. Keep words and other items such as bullets to a minimum.
- **Determine printing needs.** Will you be providing audience members with handouts? If so, will these handouts consist of a printing of each slide? an outline of the presentation? a printing of each slide with space for taking notes?

Activity 1.3

Opening, Navigating, and Inserting Slides in a Presentation; Choosing a Slide Layout

Open a saved presentation by displaying the Open dialog box and then double-clicking the desired presentation. Display the Open dialog box by clicking the FILE tab and then clicking the *Open* option. At the Open backstage area, click the desired location (your OneDrive or the *Computer* option), and then click the Browse button. Navigate through slides in a presentation with buttons on the vertical scroll bar, by clicking desired slide thumbnails in Normal view, or by using keys on the keyboard. Insert a new slide with a specific layout by clicking the New Slide button arrow in the Slides group on the HOME tab and then clicking the desired layout at the drop-down list. Choose the layout that matches the type of text or object you want to insert in the slide.

Project

Dr. St. Claire has asked you to add more information to the diabetes presentation. You will insert a new slide between the third and fourth slides in the presentation and another at the end of the presentation.

1. Click the FILE tab and then click the *Open* option.

    You can also open a presentation by inserting the Open button on the Quick Access toolbar and then clicking the button. To insert the Open button, click the Customize Quick Access Toolbar button that displays at the right side of the toolbar and then click *Open* at the drop-down list.

2. At the Open backstage area, click the desired location and then click the Browse button.

3. At the Open dialog box, navigate to the PowerPointMedS1 folder on your storage medium and then double-click *PMedS1-Diabetes.pptx* in the Content pane.

4. With **PMedS1-Diabetes.pptx** open, click the Next Slide button ⏬ at the bottom of the vertical scroll bar.

    Clicking this button displays the next slide in the presentation, Slide 2. Notice that *SLIDE 2 of 4* displays at the left side of the Status bar.

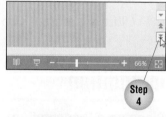

Step 4

5. Click the Previous Slide button ⏫ located toward the bottom of the vertical scroll bar to display Slide 1.

    When you click the Previous Slide button, *SLIDE 1 of 4* displays at the left side of the Status bar.

6. Display Slide 3 in the slide pane by clicking the third slide in the slide thumbnails pane (the slide titled *Types of Diabetes*).

7. Insert a new slide between Slides 3 and 4 by clicking the New Slide button in the Slides group on the HOME tab.

    When you select a slide in the slide thumbnails pane and then click the New Slide button, the new slide is inserted after the selected slide.

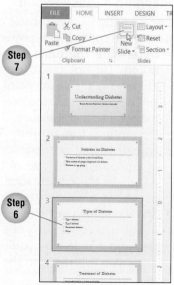

Step 7

Step 6

8 Click anywhere in the *Click to add title* placeholder in the slide in the slide pane and then type **Symptoms of Diabetes**.

9 Click anywhere in the *Click to add text* placeholder in the slide and then type the bulleted text as shown at the right. Press the Enter key after each item except the last item.

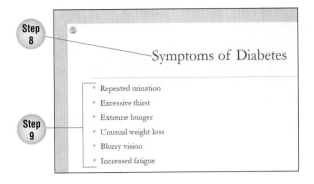

In Brief
Open Presentation
1. Click FILE tab.
2. Click *Open* option.
3. Click desired location.
4. Click Browse button.
5. At Open dialog box, double-click desired presentation.

10 Click below the Slide 1 thumbnail in the slide thumbnails pane.

When you click below the slide thumbnail, an orange horizontal line displays between Slides 1 and 2.

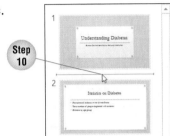

11 Click the HOME tab, click the New Slide button arrow, and then click the *Title Slide* option at the drop-down list.

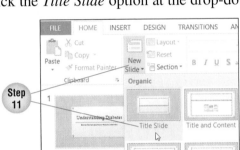

12 Click in the *Click to add title* placeholder and then type **What is Diabetes?**

13 Click in the *Click to add subtitle* placeholder and then type the text shown at the right.

14 Save **PMedS1-Diabetes.pptx**.

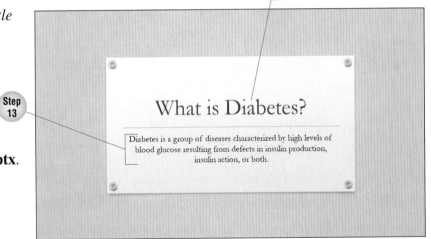

In Addition

Correcting Errors in PowerPoint

PowerPoint's AutoCorrect feature automatically corrects certain words as you type them. For example, type *teh* and press the spacebar and AutoCorrect changes it to *the*. PowerPoint also contains a spelling feature that inserts a wavy red line below words that are not found in the Spelling dictionary or not corrected by AutoCorrect. If a word with a red wavy line is correct, you can leave it as written since the red wavy line will not print. If the word is incorrect, change it.

Activity 1.4

PowerPoint provides different viewing options for a presentation. Change the view with buttons in the Presentation Views group on the VIEW tab or in the view area on the Status bar. The Normal view is the default view, and you can change the view to Outline view, Slide Sorter view, Notes Page view, or Reading view. Choose the view based on the type of activity you are performing in the presentation. For example, you can use Outline view to enter text in slides. When Outline view is active, the slide thumbnails pane changes to an outline pane for entering text. You can insert speaker's notes into a presentation using the notes pane, which can be displayed by clicking the NOTES button on the Status bar.

Project

After reviewing the diabetes presentation, Dr. St. Claire has asked you to edit a slide and add a new slide.

1 With **PMedS1-Diabetes.pptx** open, click the VIEW tab and then click the Outline View button in the Presentation Views group.

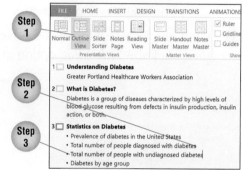

2 In the third slide, click immediately to the right of the text *Total number of people diagnosed with diabetes*.

3 Press the Enter key and then type **Total number of people with undiagnosed diabetes**.

4 Make Slide 4 the active slide, click anywhere in the text *Click to add notes* in the notes pane, and then type **Discuss other types of diabetes resulting from surgery, drugs, malnutrition, and infection.**

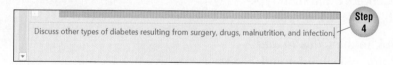

5 Display the slides in Notes Page view by clicking the Notes Page button in the Presentation Views group on the VIEW tab.

In Notes Page view, an individual slide displays on a page with any added notes displayed below the slide.

6 Click the Previous Slide button on the vertical scroll bar until Slide 1 displays.

7 Increase the zoom by clicking the Zoom button in the Zoom group on the VIEW tab, clicking the *100%* option at the Zoom dialog box, and then clicking OK.

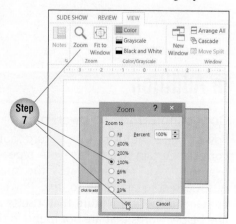

8 You can also change the zoom by using the Zoom slider bar. Position the mouse pointer on the Zoom slider bar button at the right side of the Status bar. Hold down the left mouse button, drag to the right until the zoom percentage at the left side of the Zoom slider bar displays as *136%*, and then release the mouse button.

In Brief
Display Presentation in Normal View
1. Click VIEW tab.
2. Click Normal button.

OR

Click Normal button in view area on Status bar.

Display Presentation in Outline View
1. Click VIEW tab.
2. Click Outline View button.

Display Presentation in Slide Sorter View
1. Click VIEW tab.
2. Click Slide Sorter button.

OR

Click Slide Sorter button in view area on Status bar.

Display Presentation in Notes Page View
1. Click VIEW tab.
2. Click Notes Page button.

9 Click the Zoom Out button at the left side of the Zoom slider bar until *70%* displays at the left side of the slider bar.

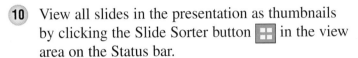

Step 9

> Click the Zoom Out button to decrease the zoom and click the Zoom In button to increase the zoom.

10 View all slides in the presentation as thumbnails by clicking the Slide Sorter button in the view area on the Status bar.

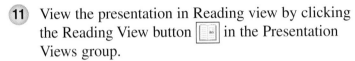

Step 10

11 View the presentation in Reading view by clicking the Reading View button in the Presentation Views group.

> Use Reading view to show a presentation to someone viewing the presentation on his or her own computer. You can also use Reading view to make it easier to navigate within a presentation. In Reading view, navigation buttons display in the lower right corner of the screen, immediately to the left of the view area on the Status bar.

12 View the presentation in Reading view by clicking the left mouse button on the slides until a black screen displays. At the black screen, click the mouse button again.

> This returns the presentation to the previous view—in this case, Slide Sorter view.

13 Return the presentation to Normal view by clicking the Normal button in the Presentation Views group.

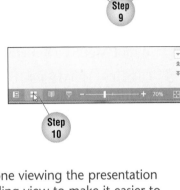

Step 13

14 If necessary, close the notes pane by clicking the NOTES button on the Status bar.

15 Save **PMedS1-Diabetes.pptx**.

In Addition

Navigating in a Presentation Using the Keyboard

You can also use the keyboard to navigate through slides in a presentation. In Normal view, press the Down Arrow key or the Page Down key to display the next slide or press the Up Arrow key or the Page Up key to display the previous slide in the presentation. Press the Home key to display the first slide in the presentation and press the End key to display the last slide in the presentation. Navigate in Outline view and Slide Sorter view by using the arrow keys on the keyboard. Navigate in Reading view by using the Right Arrow key to move to the next slide and the Left Arrow key to move to the previous slide.

Activity 1.5

Changing the Slide Layout; Selecting and Moving a Placeholder

So far, you have created slides based on a default slide layout. Change the slide layout by clicking the Layout button in the Slides group on the HOME tab and then clicking the desired layout at the drop-down list. Objects in a slide, such as text, charts, tables, or other graphic elements, are generally positioned in placeholders. Click the text or object to select the placeholder and a dashed border will surround the placeholder. You can move, size, and/or delete a selected placeholder.

Project

You have decided to make a few changes to the layout of the slides in the diabetes presentation.

1. With **PMedS1-Diabetes.pptx** open, make Slide 2 the active slide.

2. Click the HOME tab, click the Layout button 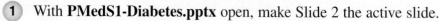 in the Slides group, and then click the *Title Only* option at the drop-down list.

    Position the mouse pointer on an option in the drop-down list and the name of the layout displays in a box. When you click the Title Only layout, the text is moved down in the slide and a bullet is inserted before the text describing diabetes.

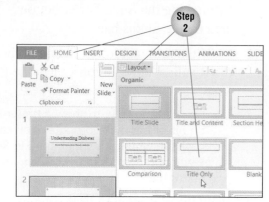

3. Click in the text describing diabetes to display the placeholder borders.

4. Move the placeholder by positioning the mouse pointer on the border of the placeholder until the mouse pointer displays with a four-headed arrow attached. Hold down the left mouse button, drag to the left until the text is positioned as shown in Figure P1.2, and then release the mouse button.

5. Click in the title *What is Diabetes?* and then move the title. To do this, position the mouse pointer on the border of the placeholder until the mouse pointer displays with a four-headed arrow attached, hold down the left mouse button, drag down until the title is positioned as shown in Figure P1.2, and then release the mouse button.

6. Click the Next Slide button on the vertical scroll bar until Slide 4 displays.

7. Click anywhere in the bulleted text to display the placeholder borders.

FIGURE P1.2 Slide 2

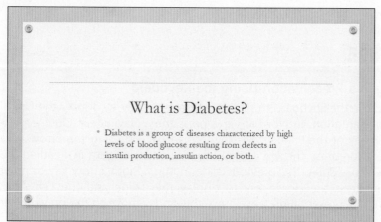

8 Decrease the size of the placeholder by positioning the mouse pointer on the bottom right sizing handle (displays as a white square) until the arrow pointer turns into a diagonal double-headed arrow.

9 Hold down the left mouse button, drag up and to the left until the placeholder displays as shown below, and then release the mouse button.

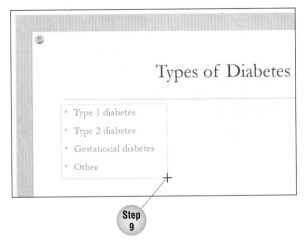

In Brief

Change Slide Layout
1. Make desired slide active.
2. Click HOME tab.
3. Click Layout button.
4. Click desired layout at drop-down list.

Move Placeholder
1. Click in placeholder.
2. Click placeholder border and drag with mouse to desired position.

Size Placeholder
1. Click inside placeholder.
2. Drag sizing handles to increase or decrease size as desired.

Step 9

10 Move the placeholder by positioning the mouse pointer on the border of the placeholder until the mouse pointer displays with a four-headed arrow attached. Hold down the left mouse button, drag to the right to the approximate location shown at the right, and then release the mouse button.

11 Click outside the placeholder to deselect it.

12 Save **PMedS1-Diabetes.pptx**.

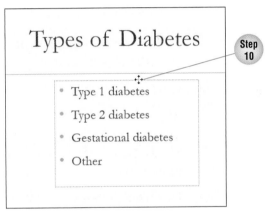

Step 10

In Addition

AutoFitting Text in Placeholders

If you decrease the size of a placeholder so much that the existing text no longer fits within the placeholder, PowerPoint will automatically decrease the size of the text to make it fit. If you click any character in the text whose size has been decreased, an AutoFit Options button displays at the left side of the placeholder. Click the AutoFit Options button and a list of choices for positioning objects in the placeholder displays, as shown at the right. The *AutoFit Text to Placeholder* option is selected by default and tells PowerPoint to fit text within the boundaries of the placeholder. Click the middle choice, *Stop Fitting Text to This Placeholder*, and PowerPoint will not automatically fit the text or object within the placeholder. Choose the last option, *Control AutoCorrect Options*, to display the AutoCorrect dialog box with the AutoFormat As You Type tab selected. Additional options may display depending upon the placeholder and the type of data it contains.

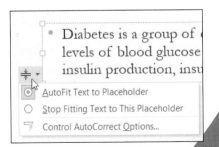

Activity 1.6

Using Help; Checking Spelling; Using the Thesaurus

Use the PowerPoint Help feature to display information about PowerPoint. To use the Help feature, click the Microsoft PowerPoint Help button (a question mark) located toward the upper right corner of the screen. At the PowerPoint Help window that displays, type the topic about which you want information and then press Enter or click the Search online help button. A list of topics related to the search text displays in the results window. Click the desired topic and information displays in the PowerPoint Help window.

Use PowerPoint's spelling checker to find and correct misspelled words and find duplicated words (such as *and and*). The spelling checker compares words in your slide with words in its dictionary. If a match is found, the word is passed over. If no match is found for the word, the spelling checker stops, selects the word, and offers replacements.

Use the Thesaurus to find synonyms, antonyms, and related words for a particular term. To use the Thesaurus, click the word for which you want to display synonyms and antonyms, click the REVIEW tab, and then click the Thesaurus button in the Proofing group. This displays the Thesaurus task pane with information about the word in which the insertion point is positioned.

Project

You have decided to create a new slide in the diabetes presentation. Because several changes have been made to the presentation, you know that checking the spelling of all the slide text is important, but you are not sure how to do it. You will use the Help feature to learn how to complete a spelling check and then use the Thesaurus to replace two words with synonyms.

1. With **PMedS1-Diabetes.pptx** open, display Slide 6 in the slide pane and then click the New Slide button in the Slides group on the HOME tab.

   This inserts a new slide at the end of the presentation.

2. Click in the *Click to add title* placeholder and then type **Complications of Diabetes**.

3. Click in the *Click to add text* placeholder and then type the text shown in Figure P1.3.

   Type the words exactly as shown. You will check the spelling in a later step.

FIGURE P1.3 Slide 7

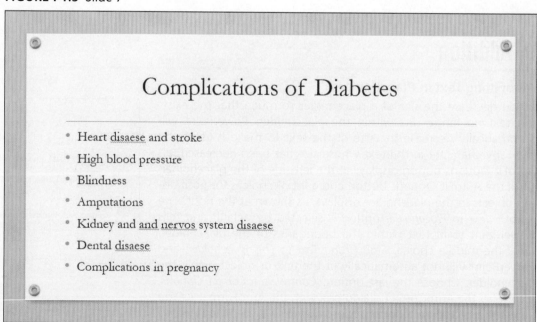

4 Learn how to complete a spelling check. Start by clicking the Microsoft PowerPoint Help button [?] located toward the upper right corner of the screen.

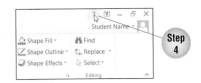

5 At the PowerPoint Help window, click in the search text box, type **check spelling**, and then press Enter.

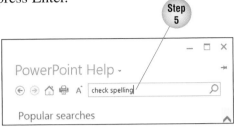

6 Click a hyperlink in the PowerPoint Help window that will display information on checking spelling.

7 Read the information about checking spelling and then click the Close button [×] in the upper right corner of the PowerPoint Help window.

8 Complete a spelling check by moving the insertion point to the beginning of the word *Heart*, clicking the REVIEW tab, and then clicking the Spelling button in the Proofing group.

9 When the spelling checker selects *disaese* in Slide 7 and displays *disease* in the list box in the Spelling task pane, click the Change All button.

Refer to Table P1.3 for a description of the buttons in the Spelling task pane.

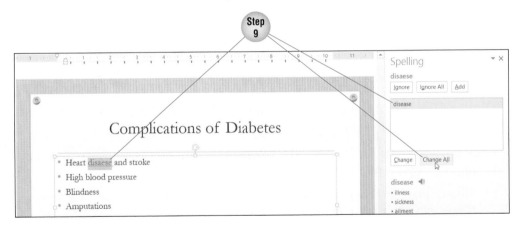

TABLE P1.3 Buttons in the Spelling Task Pane

Button	Function
Ignore	skips that occurrence of the word and leaves currently selected text as written
Ignore All	skips that occurrence and all other occurrences of the word in the presentation
Delete	deletes the currently selected word(s)
Change	replaces the selected word in the sentence with the selected word in the suggestions list box
Change All	replaces the selected word in the sentence and all other occurrences of the word in the presentation with the selected word in the suggestions list box
Add	adds the selected word to the main spelling check dictionary

continues

10 When the spelling checker selects *and* in Slide 7, click the Delete button.

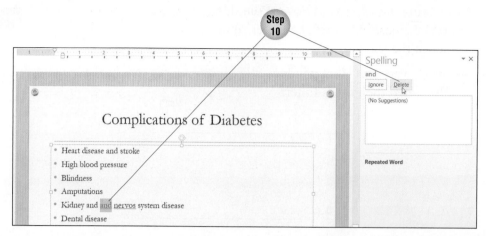

11 When the spelling checker selects *nervos* in Slide 7, click *nervous* in the list box in the Spelling task pane and then click the Change button.

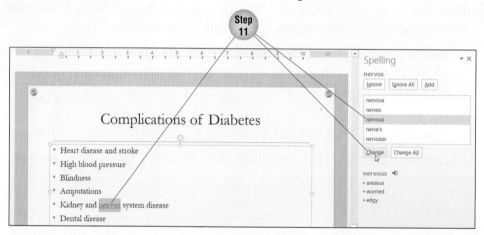

12 At the message telling you that the spelling check is complete, click OK.

13 Display Slide 5 in the slide pane and then click the word *Repeated* in the first bulleted item (*Repeated urination*).

14 Look up synonyms for *Repeated* by clicking the Thesaurus button 📖 in the Proofing group on the REVIEW tab.

> This displays the Thesaurus task pane, containing a list of synonyms for *Repeated*. Depending on the word you are looking up, the words in the Thesaurus task pane list box may display followed by *(n.)* for *noun*, *(adj.)* for *adjective*, or *(adv.)* for *adverb*. Antonyms may also display, generally at the end of the list of related synonyms, followed by the word *(Antonym)*.

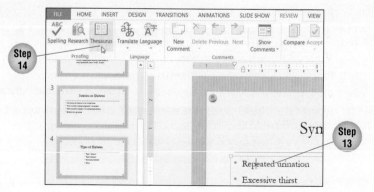

15 Position the mouse pointer on the word *Frequent* in the Thesaurus task pane, click the down-pointing arrow at the right of the word, and then click *Insert* at the drop-down list.

> This replaces *Repeated* with *Frequent*.

16 Close the Thesaurus task pane by clicking the Close button in the upper right corner of the task pane.

Step
16

In Brief

Use Help
1. Click Microsoft PowerPoint Help button.
2. Click in search text box.
3. Type desired text.
4. Press Enter.

Check Spelling
1. Click REVIEW tab.
2. Click Spelling button.
3. Change, ignore, or delete highlighted words.
4. When spelling check is complete, click OK.

Use Thesaurus
1. Click desired word.
2. Click REVIEW tab.
3. Click Thesaurus button.
4. Position mouse pointer on desired replacement word in Thesaurus task pane, click down-pointing arrow at right of word, and then click *Insert*.

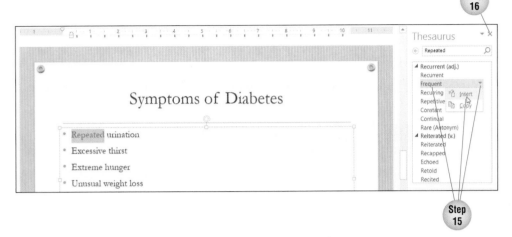

Step
15

17 Display Slide 7 in the slide pane, right-click the word *Complications* (located in the last bulleted item), point to *Synonyms* at the shortcut menu, and then click *Difficulties*.

> The shortcut menu offers another way to display synonyms of words.

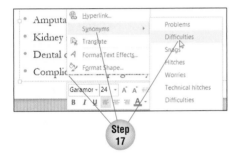

Step
17

18 Save **PMedS1-Diabetes.pptx**.

In Addition

Changing Spelling Options

Control spelling options at the PowerPoint Options dialog box with the *Proofing* option selected. Display this dialog box by clicking the FILE tab and then clicking *Options*. At the PowerPoint Options dialog box, click *Proofing* at the left side of the dialog box. With options in the dialog box, you can tell the spelling checker to ignore certain types of text, create custom dictionaries, and hide the red, wavy lines that indicate spelling errors in the presentation.

Editing While Checking Spelling

When checking the spelling in a presentation, you can temporarily leave the Spelling task pane by clicking in the slide. To resume the spelling check, click the Resume button in the Spelling task pane, as shown below.

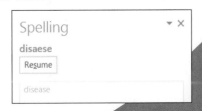

Activity
1.7

Running a Presentation

You can advance the slides in a PowerPoint presentation manually or automatically. You can also set up a slide show to run continuously for demonstration purposes. In addition to the Start From Beginning button on the Quick Access toolbar, you can run a slide show with the From Beginning button in the Start Slide Show group on the SLIDE SHOW tab or the Slide Show button in the view area on the Status bar. You can also run the presentation beginning with the currently active slide by clicking the From Current Slide button in the Start Slide Show group or by clicking the Slide Show button in the view area on the Status bar. Use the mouse or keyboard to advance through the slides. You can also use buttons on the Slide Show toolbar that displays when you move the mouse pointer while running a presentation.

Project

You are now ready to run the diabetes presentation. You will use the mouse to perform various actions while running the presentation.

1. With **PMedS1-Diabetes.pptx** open, click the SLIDE SHOW tab and then click the From Beginning button in the Start Slide Show group.

   Clicking this button starts the presentation. Slide 1 fills the entire screen.

2. After viewing Slide 1, click the left mouse button to advance to the next slide.

3. After viewing Slide 2, click the left mouse button to advance to the next slide.

4. At Slide 3, move the mouse pointer until the Slide Show toolbar displays dimmed in the lower left corner of the slide and then click the Previous button (displays as a left arrow) on the toolbar to display the previous slide (Slide 2).

   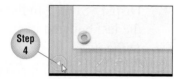

   With buttons on the Slide Show toolbar you can display the next slide, the previous slide, or another specific slide; use the pen, laser pointer, and highlighter to emphasize text on the slide; display slide thumbnails; and zoom in on elements of a slide. You can also display the Slide Show Help dialog box, shown in Figure P1.4, which describes all the navigation options available when running a presentation. Display this dialog box by clicking the More slide show options button on the Slide Show toolbar and then clicking *Help* at the pop-up list.

5. Click the right arrow button on the Slide Show toolbar to display the next slide (Slide 3).

6. Display the previous slide (Slide 2) by right-clicking anywhere in the slide and then clicking *Previous* at the shortcut menu.

   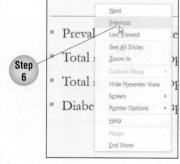

   Clicking the right mouse button causes a shortcut menu to display with a variety of options, including options to display the previous or next slide.

7. Display Slide 5 by typing the number *5* on the keyboard and then pressing Enter.

   Move to any slide in a presentation by typing the slide number and then pressing Enter.

8. Change to a black screen by typing the letter B on the keyboard.

   When you type the letter B, the slide is removed from the screen and the screen turns black. This feature can be useful in a situation where you want to discuss something with your audience that is unrelated to the slide.

FIGURE P1.4 Slide Show Help Dialog Box

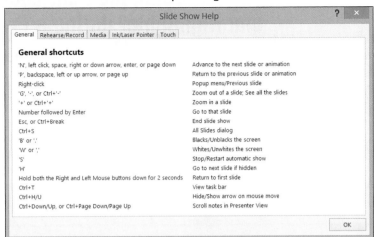

9 Return to Slide 5 by typing the letter B on the keyboard.

Typing the letter B switches between the slide and a black screen. Type the letter W if you want to switch between the slide and a white screen.

10 Zoom in on the bulleted items in Slide 5 by clicking the Zoom button (displays as a magnifying glass) on the Slide Show toolbar, hovering the magnification area over the bulleted items, and then clicking the left mouse button.

11 Press the Esc key to display Slide 5 without magnification.

12 Display thumbnails of all the slides in the presentation while viewing the slide show by clicking the See all slides button on the Slide Show toolbar.

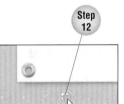

Step 12

13 Click the Slide 3 thumbnail on the screen.

This displays Slide 3 in the slide show.

14 Click the left mouse button to display Slide 4. Continue clicking the left mouse button until a black screen displays. At the black screen, click the left mouse button again.

This returns the presentation to Normal view.

15 Click Slide 2 in the slide thumbnails pane.

16 Click the From Current Slide button 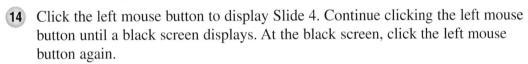 in the Start Slide Show group on the SLIDE SHOW tab.

Clicking this button starts the presentation from the currently active slide.

17 Click the left mouse button to advance to Slide 3 and then press the Esc key on the keyboard to end the presentation without viewing the remaining slides.

18 Save **PMedS1-Diabetes.pptx**.

In Addition

View a Presentation in Presenter View

If you are running a presentation using two monitors, you can display the presentation in Presenter view on one monitor. Use this view to control the slide show. For example, in Presenter view you can see your speaker notes, you have all the Slide Show toolbar options available, and you can advance slides and set slide timings. Press Alt + F5 to display the presentation in Presenter view.

Activity 1.8

Using the Pen, Laser Pointer, and Highlighter during a Presentation

Emphasize major points or draw the attention of the audience to specific items in a slide during a presentation by using the pen, laser pointer, or highlighter. To use the pen on a slide, run the presentation, and when the desired slide displays, move the mouse to display the Slide Show toolbar. Click the Pen button on the toolbar and then click *Pen* at the pop-up list. Use the mouse to draw in the slide to emphasize a specific element. If you want to erase the marks you made with the pen, click the Pen button and then click *Eraser* at the pop-up list. This causes the mouse pointer to display as an eraser. Drag through an ink mark to remove it. To remove all ink marks at the same time, click the *Erase All Ink on Slide* option at the Pen button pop-up list. When you are finished with the pen, press the Esc key to return the mouse pointer to an arrow. Options at the Pen button pop-up list also include a laser pointer and a highlighter.

Project

North Shore Medical Clinic

Dr. St. Claire would like to emphasize specific points within the presentation by highlighting and drawing. She wants you to learn how to use these features and then show her how to use them when she is giving a presentation.

1. With **PMedS1-Diabetes.pptx** open, click the From Beginning button in the Start Slide Show group on the SLIDE SHOW tab.

2. When the first slide fills the screen, click the left mouse button to advance to Slide 3. (This is the slide with the title *Statistics on Diabetes*.)

3. Move the mouse to display the Slide Show toolbar, click the Pen button, and then click *Laser Pointer* at the pop-up list.

    This turns the mouse pointer into a red, hollow, glowing circle.

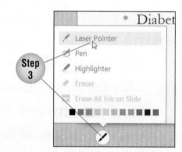

4. Practice moving the laser pointer around the screen.

5. Click the Pen button on the Slide Show toolbar and then click *Pen* at the pop-up list.

    This turns the mouse pointer into a small circle.

6. Using the mouse, draw a circle around the text *Total number of people with undiagnosed diabetes*.

7. Using the mouse, draw a line under *Diabetes by age group*.

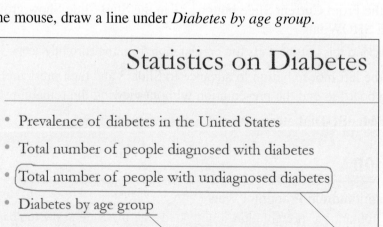

Statistics on Diabetes

- Prevalence of diabetes in the United States
- Total number of people diagnosed with diabetes
- Total number of people with undiagnosed diabetes
- Diabetes by age group

Step 7   Step 6

8 Erase the pen markings by clicking the Pen button on the Slide Show toolbar and then clicking *Erase All Ink on Slide* at the pop-up list. If the *Erase All Ink on Slide* option is dimmed so that you cannot access it, click in the slide to remove the pop-up list and then click the Pen button again.

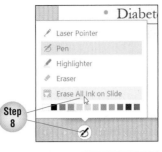

9 Change the color of the ink by clicking the Pen button and then clicking the *Blue* option at the pop-up list (third option from the right).

10 Draw a blue line under the words *United States*.

11 Return the mouse pointer back to an arrow by pressing the Esc key.

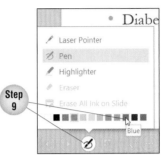

12 Click the left mouse button to advance to Slide 4.

13 Click the Pen button and then click *Highlighter* at the pop-up list.

This changes the mouse pointer to a light yellow rectangle.

14 Using the mouse, drag through the words *Type 1 diabetes* to highlight them.

15 Using the mouse, drag through the words *Type 2 diabetes* to highlight them.

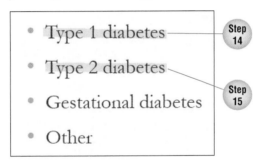

16 Return the mouse pointer back to an arrow by pressing the Esc key.

17 Press the Esc key on the keyboard to end the presentation without viewing the remaining slides. At the message asking if you want to keep your ink annotations, click the Discard button.

In Addition

Hiding and Displaying the Mouse Pointer

When running a presentation, the mouse pointer is set, by default, to be hidden automatically after three seconds of inactivity. The mouse pointer will appear again when you move the mouse. Change this default setting by clicking the More slide show options button on the Slide Show toolbar, clicking *Arrow Options,* and then clicking *Visible* if you want the mouse pointer to always be visible or *Hidden* if you do not want the mouse to display at all as you run the presentation. The *Automatic* option is the default setting.

Activity 1.9

Adding Transitions and Sound

You can enhance a presentation by applying transitions and sounds. A transition is how one slide is removed from the screen during a presentation and the next slide is displayed. Interesting transitions, such as fades, dissolves, pushes, covers, wipes, stripes, and bars can add excitement to your presentation. You can also insert sounds that you want to play at specific points during a presentation. Add transitions and sounds with options on the TRANSITIONS tab.

Project

Dr. St. Claire has asked you to enhance the presentation by adding transitions and sound to the slides.

1. With **PMedS1-Diabetes.pptx** open, click the TRANSITIONS tab.

2. Click the More button at the right side of the transition thumbnails that display in the Transition to This Slide group.

3. At the drop-down gallery, click the *Clock* option in the *Exciting* section of the drop-down gallery.

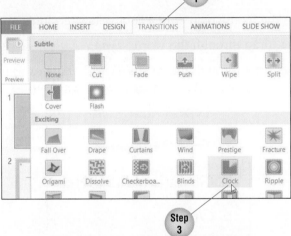

4. Click the Effect Options button in the Transition to This Slide group and then click *Wedge* at the drop-down list.

   The available effect options change depending on the transition selected.

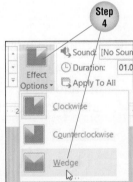

5. Click the down-pointing arrow at the right side of the Sound button option box in the Timing group.

6. At the drop-down gallery that displays, click *Click*.

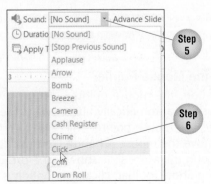

7. Set each slide transition to last for 3 seconds by clicking in the *Duration* measurement box, typing **3**, and then pressing Enter.

8. Click the Apply To All button 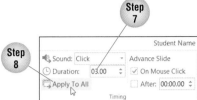 in the Timing group.

   Notice that a star icon displays below each slide number in the slide thumbnails pane.

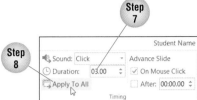

9. Click the Slide 1 thumbnail in the slide thumbnails pane.

10. Run the presentation by clicking the Slide Show button 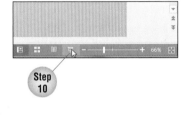 in the view area on the Status bar.

11. Click the left mouse button to move through the presentation.

12. At the black screen that displays after the last slide, click the left mouse button to return the presentation to Normal view.

13. Click the More button at the right side of the transition thumbnails that display in the Transition to This Slide group.

14. Click the *Wind* option in the *Exciting* section of the drop-down gallery.

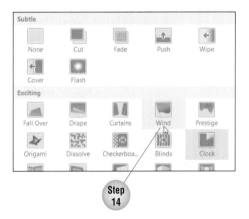

15. Click the down-pointing arrow at the right side of the Sound button option box and then click *Push* at the drop-down list.

16. Click the down-pointing arrow at the right of the *Duration* measurement box until *01.25* displays.

17. Click the Apply To All button in the Timing group.

18. With Slide 1 active, run the presentation.

19. Save **PMedS1-Diabetes.pptx**.

In Brief

Add Transition to All Slides in Presentation
1. Click TRANSITIONS tab.
2. Click More button at right side of transition thumbnails.
3. Click desired transition at drop-down gallery.
4. Click Apply To All button.

Add Transition Sound to All Slides in Presentation
1. Click TRANSITIONS tab.
2. Click arrow at right side of Sound button option box.
3. Click desired option at drop-down gallery.
4. Click Apply To All button.

In Addition

Running a Slide Show Automatically

Slides in a slide show can be advanced automatically after a specific number of seconds by inserting a check mark in the *After* check box in the Timing group and removing the check mark from the *On Mouse Click* check box. Change the time in the *After* measurement box by clicking the up- or down-pointing arrow at the right side of the measurement box or by selecting the text in the measurement box and then typing the desired time. If you want the transition time to affect all slides in the presentation, click the Apply To All button. In Slide Sorter view, the transition time displays below each affected slide. Click the Slide Show button to run the presentation. The first slide displays for the specified amount of time and then the next slide automatically displays.

Activity
1.10

Previewing and Printing a Presentation

You can print each slide in a presentation on a separate page; print each slide at the top of a separate page, leaving the bottom of the page for notes; print up to nine slides on a single piece of paper; or print the slide titles and topics in outline form.

Before printing a presentation, consider previewing it. Choose the desired print options and display a preview of the presentation in the Print backstage area. Display this view by clicking the FILE tab and then clicking the *Print* option. Click the Back button or press the Esc key to exit the backstage area.

Project Dr. St. Claire needs the slides in the diabetes presentation printed as handouts and as an outline. You will preview and then print the presentation in various formats.

North Shore
Medical Clinic

1 With **PMedS1-Diabetes.pptx** open, display Slide 1 in the slide pane.

2 Click the FILE tab and then click the *Print* option.

Slide 1 of your presentation displays at the right side of the screen as it will when printed. Use the Next Page button (right-pointing arrow) located below and to the left of the slide to view the next slide in the presentation, click the Previous Page button (left-pointing arrow) to display the previous slide in the presentation, use the Zoom slider bar to increase or decrease the size of the slide, and click the Zoom to Page button to fit the slide in the viewing area in the Print backstage area. The left side of the Print backstage area displays three categories—*Print*, *Printer*, and *Settings*. Galleries display below each category name. For example, the *Printer* category has one gallery that displays the name of the currently selected printer, and the *Settings* category has a number of galleries that describe how the slides will print.

3 Click the Next Page button located below and to the left of the preview slide to display the next slide in the presentation.

This displays Slide 2 in the backstage area.

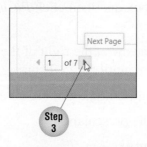

Step
3

4 Click twice on the Zoom In button that displays at the right side of the Zoom slider bar.

Clicking the Zoom In button increases the size of the slide, and clicking the Zoom Out button decreases the size of the slide.

5 Click the Zoom to Page button located at the right side of the Zoom slider bar.

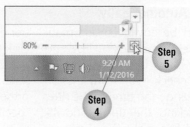

Step
5

Step
4

6 You decide to create handouts with all of the slides printed on one page, but first you want to preview how the slides will appear on the page. To do this, click the second gallery in the *Settings* category (contains the text *Full Page Slides*) and then click *4 Slides Horizontal* in the *Handouts* section.

> Notice how four slides display on the preview page.

7 Click the Print button in the *Print* category.

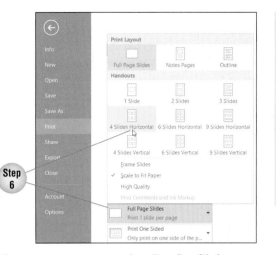

Step 6

In Brief

Print Presentation
1. Click FILE tab.
2. Click *Print* option.
3. At Print backstage area, specify desired printing options.
4. Click Print button.

Preview Presentation
1. Click FILE tab.
2. Click *Print* option.
3. View preview in right panel of Print backstage area.

8 You want to print all slide text as an outline on one page so that Dr. St. Claire can use the printout as a reference. To do this, click the FILE tab and then click the *Print* option.

9 At the Print backstage area, click the second gallery in the *Settings* category (contains the text *4 Slides Horizontal*) and then click *Outline* in the *Print Layout* section.

10 Click the Print button in the *Print* category.

> With the *Outline* option selected, the presentation prints on one page with slide numbers, slide icons, and slide text in outline form.

11 You need a printout of Slide 5. To do this, click the FILE tab and then click the *Print* option.

12 At the Print backstage area, click the second gallery in the *Settings* category (contains the text *Outline*) and then click *Full Page Slides* in the *Print Layout* section.

13 Click in the *Slides* text box located below the first gallery in the *Settings* category, type 5, and then click the Print button.

14 Save **PMedS1-Diabetes.pptx**.

15 Close the presentation by clicking the FILE tab and then clicking the *Close* option.

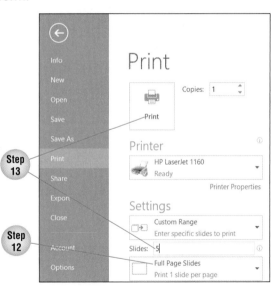

Step 13

Step 12

In Addition

Using Options at the Slide Size Dialog Box

You can adjust various slide characteristics with options at the Slide Size dialog box, shown at the right. Display this dialog box by clicking the DESIGN tab, clicking the Slide Size button in the Customize group, and then clicking *Customize Slide Size* at the drop-down list. With options at this dialog box, you can specify slide size; page width and height; slide orientation; and orientation for notes, handouts, and outlines.

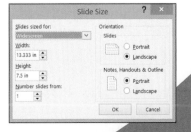

Features Summary

Feature	Ribbon Tab, Group	Button	FILE Tab Option	Keyboard Shortcut
apply transitions and sounds to all slides	TRANSITIONS, Timing			
close a presentation			*Close*	Ctrl + F4
close PowerPoint		✕		
Help		?		F1
layout	HOME, Slides			
new slide	HOME, Slides			Ctrl + M
Normal view	VIEW, Presentation Views			
Notes Page view	VIEW, Presentation Views			
Open backstage area			*Open*	Ctrl + O
open blank presentation				Ctrl + N
Outline view	VIEW, Presentation Views			
Print backstage area			*Print*	Ctrl + P
Reading view	VIEW, Presentation Views			
run presentation from current slide	SLIDE SHOW, Start Slide Show			Shift + F5
run presentation from Slide 1	SLIDE SHOW, Start Slide Show			F5
save			*Save*	Ctrl + S
Save As backstage area			*Save As*	F12
Slide Sorter view	VIEW, Presentation Views			
spelling checker	REVIEW, Proofing			F7
themes	DESIGN, Themes			
Thesaurus	REVIEW, Proofing			Shift + F7
transition duration	TRANSITIONS, Timing			
transitions	TRANSITIONS, Transition to This Slide			
transition sound	TRANSITIONS, Timing			
Zoom dialog box	VIEW, Zoom			

Knowledge Check

Completion: In the space provided at the right, write in the correct term, command, or option.

1. To run a presentation beginning with Slide 1, click this button on the Quick Access toolbar. _____
2. The Save button is located on this toolbar. _____
3. Normal view contains the slide thumbnails pane and this pane. _____
4. The New Slide button is located on this tab. _____
5. The Zoom slider bar is located at the right side of this bar. _____
6. Click the Microsoft PowerPoint Help button and this displays. _____
7. The Spelling button is located in the Proofing group on this tab. _____
8. Use this feature to find synonyms, antonyms, and related words for a particular term. _____
9. Move the mouse while running a presentation and this toolbar displays. _____
10. Press this key on the keyboard to change to a black screen while running a presentation. _____
11. Press this key on the keyboard to end a presentation without viewing all of the slides. _____
12. Add transitions and sounds to a presentation with options on this tab. _____
13. Specify the length of a transition using the *Duration* measurement box in this group on the TRANSITIONS tab. _____
14. You can print up to this number of slides on a single piece of paper. _____

Skills Review

Review 1 Applying a Design Theme and Creating Slides

Columbia River General Hospital

1. With a blank presentation open in PowerPoint, click the DESIGN tab, click the More button at the right of the theme thumbnails in the Themes group, and then click the *Basis* option.
2. Click the third variant in the Variants group (white with an orange border).
3. Type the title and subtitle for Slide 1 as shown in Figure P1.5.
4. Click the HOME tab and then click the New Slide button in the Slides group.
5. Apply the Title Slide layout. (You will arrange the text in the placeholder in the next review activity.)
6. Type the text in Slide 2 as shown in Figure P1.5.
7. Continue creating the slides for the presentation, using the text shown in Figure P1.5.
8. Save the presentation and name it **PMedS1-R-Fibromyalgia**.

FIGURE P1.5 Review 1

Slide 1	Title	Columbia River General Hospital
	Subtitle	Facts about Fibromyalgia
Slide 2	Title	What is Fibromyalgia?
	Subtitle	Fibromyalgia is an arthritis-related condition characterized by generalized muscular pain and fatigue.
Slide 3	Title	Who is Affected by Fibromyalgia?
	Bullets	• Approximately 1 in 50 Americans may be affected
		• Mostly women but men and children can also have the disorder
		• People with certain diseases such as rheumatoid arthritis, lupus, and spinal arthritis
		• People with a family member with fibromyalgia may be more likely to be diagnosed with the disorder
Slide 4	Title	Treatments for Fibromyalgia
	Bullets	• Medication to diminish pain and improve sleep
		• Exercise programs that stretch muscles
		• Relaxation techniques
		• Education programs to help understand the disorder

Review 2 Inserting a Slide; Changing the Slide Layout; Moving a Placeholder

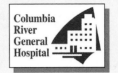

1. With **PMedS1-R-Fibromyalgia.pptx** open, insert a new Slide 3 between the current Slides 2 and 3 and type the text shown in Figure P1.6.
2. Display Slide 2 in the slide pane and then change the slide layout to *Title Only*.
3. Click in the text containing the description of fibromyalgia and then move the placeholder so it is centered horizontally and vertically on the slide.
4. Display Slide 3 in the slide pane, click in the bulleted text to select the placeholder, and then decrease the right side of the placeholder by dragging the middle right sizing handle to the left. (Do not decrease the width of the placeholder so much that the bulleted text has to wrap.)
5. Position the placeholder so that the bulleted text is centered on the slide.
6. Save **PMedS1-R-Fibromyalgia.pptx**.

FIGURE P1.6 Review 2

Slide 3	Title Bullets	Causes of Fibromyalgia • Infectious illness • Physical and/or emotional trauma • Muscle abnormalities • Hormonal changes • Repetitive injuries

Review 3 Adding Transitions and Sound; Running and Printing a Presentation

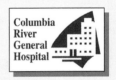

1. With **PMedS1-R-Fibromyalgia.pptx** open, click the TRANSITIONS tab.
2. Click the More button at the right side of the transition thumbnails that display in the Transition to This Slide group and then click a transition of your choosing.
3. Click the down-pointing arrow at the right of the Sound button option box and then click a transition sound of your choosing.
4. Apply the transition and sound to all slides in the presentation.
5. Make Slide 1 the active slide and then run the presentation.
6. Print the presentation as an outline.
7. Print the presentation with all five slides positioned horizontally on the page.
8. Save and then close **PMedS1-R-Fibromyalgia.pptx**.

Skills Assessment

Assessment 1 Preparing a Presentation for Columbia River General Hospital

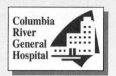

1. Prepare a presentation for Columbia River General Hospital with the information shown in Figure P1.7. (You determine the design template.)
2. Add a transition and sound of your choosing to all slides in the presentation.
3. Run the presentation.
4. Print the presentation with all five slides positioned horizontally on one page.
5. Save the presentation and name it **PMedS1-A1-CRGH**.
6. Close **PMedS1-A1-CRGH.pptx**.

FIGURE P1.7 Assessment 1

Slide 1	Title	Columbia River General Hospital
	Subtitle	Our mission is to provide comprehensive and high-quality care for all of our patients.
Slide 2	Title	Hospital Directives
	Bullets	• Highest-quality patient care
		• Exceptional customer services
		• Fully trained and qualified staff
		• Delivery of first-class health education
Slide 3	Title	Facilities
	Bullets	• 400 licensed beds
		• Level II adult trauma system
		• 14 operating rooms
		• 25-bed adult intensive care unit
		• Level III neonatal intensive care unit
		• 24-hour emergency services
Slide 4	Title	Physicians Clinics
	Bullets	• Division Street
		• Lake Oswego
		• Fremont Center
		• Oak Grove
Slide 5	Title	Health Foundation
	Subtitle	Columbia River General Hospital's Health Foundation is a nonprofit organization that promotes the well-being of adults and families served by the hospital.

Assessment 2 Preparing a Presentation for Cascade View Pediatrics

1. Prepare a presentation for Cascade View Pediatrics with the information shown in Figure P1.8. (You determine the design theme.)
2. Add a transition and sound of your choosing to all slides in the presentation.
3. Run the presentation.
4. Print the presentation with all five slides positioned horizontally on one page.
5. Save the presentation and name it **PMedS1-A2-CVP**.
6. Close **PMedS1-A2-CVP.pptx**.

FIGURE P1.8 Assessment 2

Slide 1	Title	Cascade View Pediatrics
	Subtitle	350 North Skagit
		Portland, OR 97505
		(503) 555-7700

Slide 2	Title	Doctor Consultations
	Bullets	• By appointment only
		• Monday through Friday, 9:00 a.m. to 5:30 p.m.
		• Monday and Wednesday, 6:30 to 8:00 p.m.
		• Saturday, 9:00 a.m. to noon

Slide 3	Title	Nurse Consultations
	Bullets	• By appointment only
		• Tuesday and Thursday, 2:00 to 4:30 p.m.
		• Monday and Wednesday, 6:30 to 8:00 p.m.

Slide 4	Title	Accepted Insurance Plans
	Bullets	• Premiere Group
		• Health Plus America
		• Madison Health
		• Healthwise Cooperative
		• Uniform Medical

Slide 5	Title	Education Programs
	Bullets	• Child development and therapy
		• Asthma education
		• Diabetes education
		• Positive parenting
		• Grandparents' workshop
		• First aid

Assessment 3 Finding Information on the Undo Button

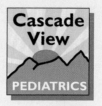

1. Open **PMedS1-A2-CVP.pptx** and then use the Help feature to learn how to undo an action.
2. After learning how to undo an action, make Slide 1 the active slide.
3. In the slide pane, click immediately right of the telephone number *(503) 555-7700* and then press Enter.
4. Type the email address CVP@emcp.cvpediatrics.com and then press Enter. (PowerPoint converts the email address to a hyperlink [changes the color and underlines the text].)

HELP

5. Undo the action that converted the text to a hyperlink.
6. Type Website: www.emcp.net/cvp.
7. Press the Enter key. (This converts the website to a hyperlink.)
8. Undo the action that converted the text to a hyperlink.
9. If necessary, increase the size of the placeholder to better accommodate the new text.
10. Print only Slide 1.
11. Save and then close **PMedS1-A2-CVP.pptx**.

Assessment 4 Finding Information on Setting Slide Show Timings

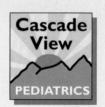

1. Open **PMedS1-A2-CVP.pptx**.
2. Use the Help feature or experiment with the options on the TRANSITIONS tab and learn how to set slide show timings manually.
3. Set up the presentation so that, when running the presentation, each slide advances after three seconds.
4. Run the presentation.
5. Save and then close **PMedS1-A2-CVP.pptx**.

HELP

Assessment 5 Locating Information and Preparing a Presentation on Chickenpox

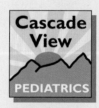

1. You need to prepare a presentation on chickenpox that includes information such as symptoms, treatment, incubation period, and infectious period. Use the information you prepared for **WMedS3-A7-Chickenpox.docx** and research additional information on the Internet.

2. Using PowerPoint, create a presentation about chickenpox that contains a title slide with Cascade View Pediatrics and the name you choose for your presentation. Include additional slides that cover a description of chickenpox and its symptoms, treatments, and incubation and infectious periods.
3. Run the presentation.
4. Print all of the slides horizontally on one page.
5. Save the presentation and name it **PMedS1-A5-Chickenpox**.
6. Close **PMedS1-A5-Chickenpox.pptx**.

Marquee Challenge

Challenge 1 Preparing a Presentation on Cystic Fibrosis

1. Prepare the presentation shown in Figure P1.9 using the Berlin design theme.
2. Save the completed presentation and name it **PMedS1-C1-CysticFib**.
3. Apply a transition and sound to all slides and then run the presentation.
4. Print the presentation as a handout with all six slides horizontally on one page.
5. Save and then close **PMedS1-C1-CysticFib.pptx**.

FIGURE P1.9 Challenge 1

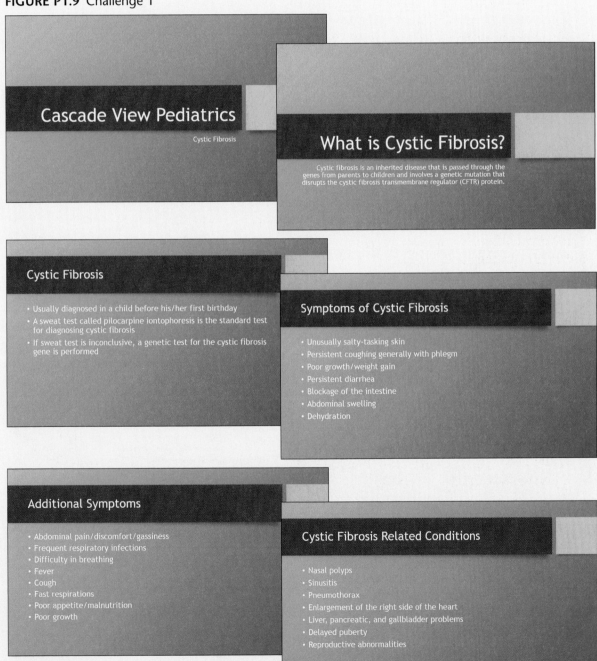

Challenge 2 Editing a Presentation on Clinic Services

1. Open **NSMCServices.pptx** and then save it with the name **PMedS1-C2-NSMCServices**.
2. Apply the Parallax design theme, change the slide layout for the second slide (allow the subtitle text to automatically wrap as you decrease the size of the placeholder), and then size and move the placeholders as shown in Figure P1.10.
3. Run the presentation.
4. Print the presentation as a handout with four slides horizontally per page.
5. Save and then close **PMedS1-C2-NSMCServices.pptx**.

FIGURE P1.10 Challenge 2

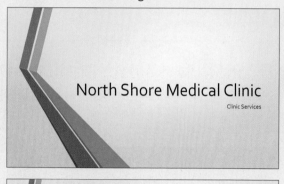

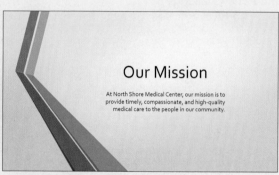

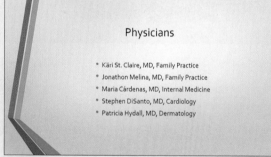

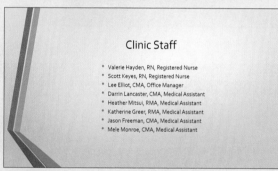

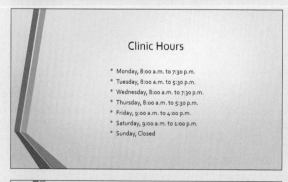

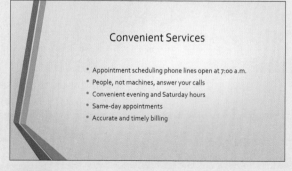

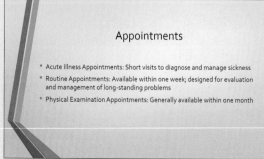

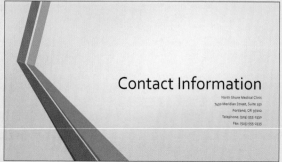

PowerPoint SECTION 2
Editing Slides and Slide Elements

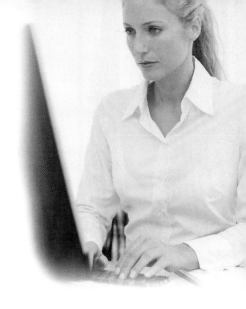

Skills

- Open a presentation and save it with a new name
- Rearrange, delete, and hide slides
- Increase and decrease the indent of text
- Select, cut, copy, and paste text
- Apply font and font effects
- Find and replace fonts
- Apply formatting with Format Painter
- Change alignment and line and paragraph spacing
- Draw text boxes and shapes
- Insert headers and footers
- Change the design theme, theme colors, and theme fonts
- Insert and format images
- Insert and format WordArt
- Insert and format a SmartArt graphic
- Apply an animation to an object in a slide

Student Resources

Before beginning the activities in PowerPoint Section 2, copy to your storage medium the PowerPointMedS2 folder from the Student Resources CD. This folder contains the data files you need to complete the projects in this PowerPoint section.

Projects Overview

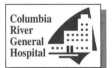

Open an existing presentation containing information on classes offered by the Education Department and then save, edit, and format the presentation; open an existing presentation containing information on the Community Commitment reorganization plan and then save, edit, and format the presentation.

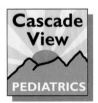

Open an existing presentation on opening a clinic in Vancouver, save the presentation with a new name, and then edit and format the presentation.

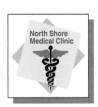

Open an existing presentation containing information on sickle cell anemia and then save, edit, and format the presentation; prepare a presentation on cholesterol.

Activity 2.1

Saving a Presentation with a New Name; Managing Slides

When you open an existing presentation and make changes to it, you can save it with the same name or a different name. Save an existing presentation with a new name at the Save As dialog box.

As you edit a presentation, you may need to rearrange, delete, or hide slides. PowerPoint provides various views for creating and managing a presentation. Manage slides in the slide thumbnails pane or in Slide Sorter view. Switch to Slide Sorter view by clicking the Slide Sorter button in the view area on the Status bar or by clicking the VIEW tab and then clicking the Slide Sorter button in the Presentation Views group.

Project

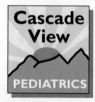

The doctors at Cascade View Pediatrics are considering expanding by opening a clinic in the Vancouver, Washington, area. Dr. Severin has prepared a presentation with facts about Vancouver and has asked you to edit the presentation.

1 With PowerPoint open, click the FILE tab and then click the *Open* option.

2 At the Open backstage area, click the *Computer* option or your OneDrive and then click the Browse button.

3 At the Open dialog box, navigate to the PowerPointMedS2 folder and then double-click *CVPVancouver.pptx*.

4 Click the FILE tab, click the *Save As* option, and then click the PowerPointMedS2 folder in the *Current Folder* section of the Save As backstage area.

5 At the Save As dialog box, press the Home key to move the insertion point to the beginning of the file name, type **PMedS2-** in the *File name* text box, and then press Enter. (The file name in the *File name* text box should display as *PMedS2-CVPVancouver.pptx*.)

Pressing the Home key saves you from having to type the entire file name.

6 Right-click Slide 3 in the slide thumbnails pane and then click *Delete Slide* at the shortcut menu.

You can also delete a selected slide by pressing the Delete key on the keyboard.

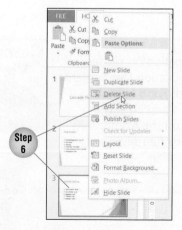

7 Click the Slide Sorter button ⊞ in the view area on the Status bar.

8 Click Slide 7 to make it active.

A selected slide displays with an orange border.

9 Position the mouse pointer on Slide 7, hold down the left mouse button, drag the slide to the right of Slide 2, and then release the mouse button.

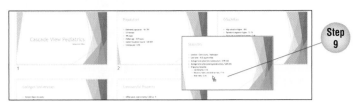

Step 9

10 Click the Normal button in the view area on the Status bar.

11 Position the mouse pointer on the Slide 6 thumbnail in the slide thumbnails pane, hold down the left mouse button, drag up until the slide displays immediately below the Slide 2 thumbnail, and then release the mouse button.

Step 11

12 Click Slide 4 in the slide thumbnails pane to make it active and then hide the slide by clicking the SLIDE SHOW tab and then clicking the Hide Slide button in the Set Up group.

When a slide is hidden, the slide thumbnail is dimmed and the slide number displays with a diagonal line through it.

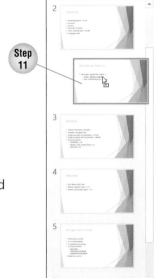

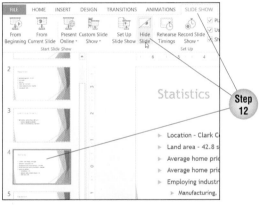

Statistics

Step 12

► Location - Clark C
► Land area - 42.8 s
► Average home pric
► Average home pric
► Employing industr
    ► Manufacturing,

13 Run the presentation by clicking the From Beginning button in the Start Slide Show group. Click the left mouse button until a black screen displays. At the black screen, click the left mouse button again.

14 Redisplay the hidden slide by making sure the Slide 4 thumbnail is selected in the slide thumbnails pane and then clicking the Hide Slide button in the Set Up group.

15 Save **PMedS2-CVPVancouver.pptx**.

In Addition

Copying Slides within a Presentation

Copying a slide within a presentation is similar to moving a slide. To copy a slide, position the arrow pointer on the desired slide in Slide Sorter view and then hold down the Ctrl key and the left mouse button. Drag to the location where you want the slide to appear, release the left mouse button, and then release the Ctrl key. When you drag with the mouse, the mouse pointer displays with a square and a plus symbol next to the pointer.

In Brief

Save Presentation with New Name
1. Click FILE tab.
2. Click *Save As* option.
3. Click desired folder.
4. Type presentation name.
5. Click Save or press Enter.

Delete Slide
1. Click Slide Sorter button in view area on Status bar.
2. Click desired slide.
3. Press Delete key.

OR

1. Right-click desired slide in slide thumbnails pane.
2. Click *Delete Slide*.

Move Slide
1. Click Slide Sorter button in view area on Status bar.
2. Click desired slide.
3. Drag slide to desired position.

Hide Slide
1. Click desired slide in slide thumbnails pane.
2. Click SLIDE SHOW tab.
3. Click Hide Slide button.

Activity 2.2

Increasing and Decreasing List Level

In Outline view, you can organize and develop the content of a presentation by rearranging text within a slide, moving slides, or increasing and decreasing the list level, or indent, of text. Click the Decrease List Level button in the Paragraph group on the HOME tab or press Shift + Tab to move text up to the previous level. Click the Increase List Level button in the Paragraph group or press the Tab key to move text down to the next level. You can also increase and/or decrease the indent of text in the slide in the slide pane.

Project

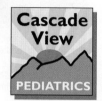

As you continue editing the Vancouver presentation, you will increase and decrease the indent of text in slides.

1. With **PMedS2-CVPVancouver.pptx** open, make sure the presentation displays in Normal view.

2. Display Slide 6 in the slide pane and then click the HOME tab.

3. Looking at the text in Slide 6, you realize that the school names below *University of Portland* should not be indented. To decrease the indent and move them up to the previous list level, start by positioning the insertion point immediately to the left of the *C* in *Clark* and then clicking the Decrease List Level button in the Paragraph group on the HOME tab.

   You can also decrease the indent by pressing Shift + Tab.

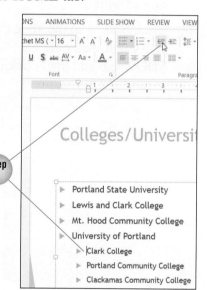

4. Position the insertion point immediately to the left of the *P* in *Portland Community College* and then move the text to the previous level by pressing Shift + Tab.

5. Use steps similar to those in either Step 3 or Step 4 to move *Clackamas Community College* to the previous level.

6. Make Slide 2 active. Move the two bulleted items below *Estimated population* down to the next level by clicking immediately left of the *5* in *51%* and then clicking the Increase List Level button in the Paragraph group on the HOME tab.

   You can also increase the indent by pressing the Tab key.

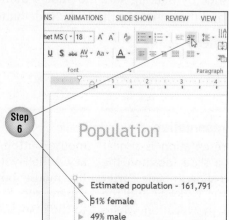

7 Position the insertion point immediately to the left of the *4* in *49%* and then press the Tab key.

8 Display Slide 4 in the slide pane.

9 Click the VIEW tab and then click the Outline View button in the Presentation Views group.

10 Looking at Slide 4, you notice that the slide contains too much text. You decide to move some of it to a new slide. To do this, click immediately to the left of the *E* in *Employing* in the outline pane (previously the slide thumbnails pane) and then press Shift + Tab.

> Pressing Shift + Tab moves the text to the previous level and creates a new slide with *Employing industries* as the title.

11 Change the title of the slide by typing **Employment** and then pressing Enter.

> As you type *Employment*, the text *Employing industries* moves to the right. When you press Enter, *Employing industries* moves to the next line and begins a new slide.

12 Move the text *Employing industries* by pressing the Tab key.

> The new slide now contains the title *Employment* with *Employing industries* as a bulleted item with three bulleted items below it.

13 Click the Normal button in the Presentation Views group on the VIEW tab.

14 If necessary, click the NOTES button on the Status bar to close the notes pane.

15 Save **PMedS2-CVPVancouver.pptx**.

In Brief

Decrease Text Indent
Click Decrease List Level button.
OR
Press Shift + Tab.

Increase Text Indent
Click Increase List Level button.
OR
Press Tab.

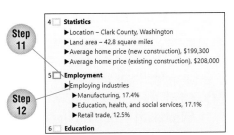

In Addition

Rearranging Text in Outline View

You can use the mouse to move text in the outline pane. To do this, position the mouse pointer on the slide icon or bullet at the left side of the text until the arrow pointer turns into a four-headed arrow. Hold down the left mouse button, drag the arrow pointer to the desired location (a thin horizontal line displays), and then release the mouse button. If you position the arrow pointer on the bullet and then hold down the left mouse button, all text following that bullet is selected. Dragging selected text with the mouse moves the text to a new location in the presentation. You can also copy selected text. To do this, click the slide icon or click the bullet to select the desired text. Position the arrow pointer in the selected text, hold down the Ctrl key, and then hold down the left mouse button. Drag the arrow pointer (displays with a light gray box and a plus sign attached) to the desired location, release the mouse button, and then release the Ctrl Key.

Activity 2.3

Selecting, Cutting, Copying, and Pasting Text

Text in a slide can be selected and then deleted from the slide, cut from one location and pasted into another, or copied from one location and pasted into another. Select text using the mouse or the keyboard. Use buttons in the Clipboard group on the HOME tab to cut, copy, and paste text.

Project As you review the Vancouver presentation again, you decide to delete, move, and copy specific text items.

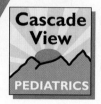

1. With **PMedS2-CVPVancouver.pptx** open, make sure the presentation displays in Normal view and then display Slide 7 in the slide pane.

2. Click anywhere in the bulleted text.

   Clicking in the bulleted text selects the placeholder containing the text.

3. Position the mouse pointer on the bullet that displays before *University of Portland* until the pointer turns into a four-headed arrow and then click the left mouse button.

   Refer to Table P2.1 for additional information on selecting text.

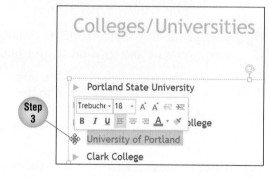

4. Click the Cut button in the Clipboard group on the HOME tab.

5. Position the insertion point immediately to the left of the *L* in *Lewis and Clark College* and then click the Paste button in the Clipboard group.

6. Position the mouse pointer on the bullet that displays before *George Fox University* until the pointer turns into a four-headed arrow and then click the left mouse button.

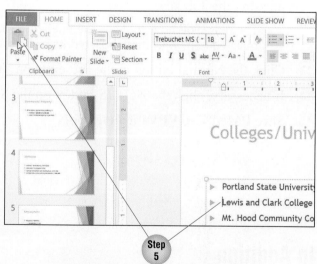

TABLE P2.1 Selecting Text

To select	Perform this action
entire word	Double-click word.
entire paragraph	Triple-click anywhere in paragraph.
entire sentence	Press Ctrl + click anywhere in sentence.
text mouse pointer passes through	Click and drag with mouse.
all text in selected object box	Press Ctrl + A or click Select button in Editing group and then click *Select All*.

7 Click the Cut button in the Clipboard group.

8 Position the insertion point immediately to the left of the *L* in *Lewis and Clark College* and then click the Paste button in the Clipboard group.

9 Make Slide 6 active, move the insertion point so it is positioned immediately to the right of *7.4%*, and then press the Enter key.

10 Type **Area Universities** and then press the Enter key.

11 Make Slide 7 active; select *Portland State University*, *University of Portland*, and *George Fox University*; and then click the Copy button 📋 in the Clipboard group.

> When selecting the text, do not include the space after *George Fox University*. If you include the space, which is actually an invisible paragraph symbol, you will get an extra blank line when you paste the text.

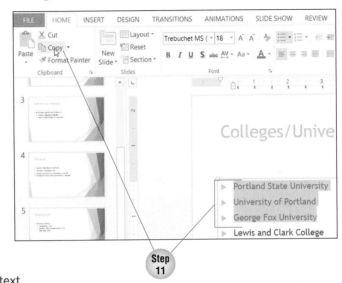

12 Make Slide 6 active and then click below the heading *Area Universities*.

> This selects the placeholder and positions the insertion point below the *Area Universities* heading.

13 Click the Paste button in the Clipboard group. If a blank line displays below *George Fox University*, press the Backspace key twice.

> If a blank line displays below *George Fox University*, it means that the invisible paragraph symbol after the text was selected when copying.

14 Increase the indent of the universities' names by selecting the three names (*Portland State University*, *University of Portland*, and *George Fox University*) and then clicking the Increase List Level button in the Paragraph group on the HOME tab.

15 Save **PMedS2-CVPVancouver.pptx**.

In Brief

Cut and Paste Text
1. Select text.
2. Click Cut button.
3. Position insertion point.
4. Click Paste button.

Copy and Paste Text
1. Select text.
2. Click Copy button.
3. Position insertion point.
4. Click Paste button.

In Addition

Copying a Slide between Presentations

You can copy slides within a presentation as well as between presentations. To copy a slide, click the slide you want to copy (either in Slide Sorter view or in the slide thumbnails pane in Normal view) and then click the Copy button in the Clipboard group on the HOME tab. Open the presentation into which the slide is to be copied (in either Slide Sorter view or Normal view). Click in the location where you want the slide to be positioned and then click the Paste button. The copied slide will take on the formatting of the presentation into which it is copied.

Activity 2.4

Applying Fonts and Font Effects

The Font group on the HOME tab consists of two rows of buttons. The top row contains buttons for changing the font and font size and a button for clearing formatting. The bottom row contains buttons for applying font effects such as bold, italic, underline, shadow, and strikethrough as well as buttons for changing the character spacing, case, and font color of selected text.

Project

As you continue working to improve the appearance of slides in the Vancouver presentation, you decide to apply font effects to specific text in the presentation.

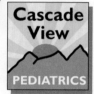

1. With **PMedS2-CVPVancouver.pptx** open, display Slide 1 in the slide pane.

2. Select the text *Cascade View Pediatrics*, click the Bold button **B** in the Font group on the HOME tab, and then click the Italic button **I**.

3. With the clinic name still selected, click the Decrease Font Size button **A˅** in the Font group.

4. Select the subtitle *Vancouver Clinic*, click the Bold button, and then click the Italic button.

5. With the subtitle still selected, click twice on the Increase Font Size button **A˄** in the Font group.

6. Make Slide 2 active, select *161,791*, and then click the Underline button **U** in the Font group.

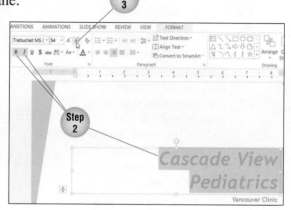

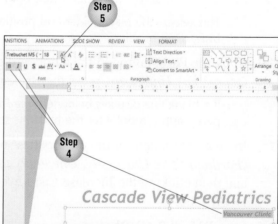

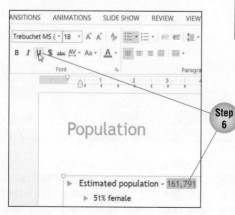

7 Make Slide 1 active and then select the text *Cascade View Pediatrics*.

8 Click the Font button arrow in the Font group, scroll down the drop-down gallery (fonts display in alphabetical order), and then click *Cambria*.

In Brief

Apply Font Effects
1. Select text.
2. Click desired button in Font group.

Change Font
1. Select text or placeholder.
2. Click Font button arrow.
3. Click desired font at drop-down gallery.

Change Font Size
1. Select text or placeholder.
2. Click Font Size button arrow.
3. Click desired size at drop-down gallery.

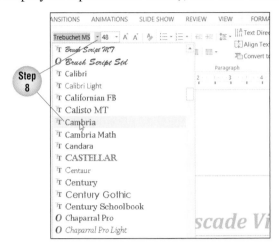

9 With the clinic name still selected, click the Font Size button arrow and then click *54* at the drop-down gallery.

10 Select the subtitle *Vancouver Clinic*, click the Font button arrow, and then click *Cambria* at the drop-down gallery.

> The drop-down gallery displays the most recently used fonts at the top.

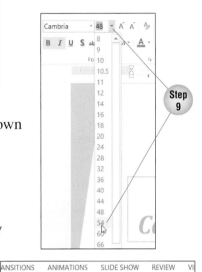

11 With the subtitle still selected, click the Font Color button arrow [A] and then click the *Blue, Accent 2, Darker 25%* option at the drop-down gallery (sixth column, fifth row in the *Theme Colors* section).

12 Print Slide 1.

13 Save **PMedS2-CVPVancouver.pptx**.

In Addition

Choosing Typefaces

A *typeface* is a set of characters with a common design and shape. PowerPoint refers to a typeface as a *font*. Fonts can be decorative or plain and are either monospaced or proportional. A monospaced font allots the same amount of horizontal space for each character, while a proportional font allots a varying amount of space for each character. Proportional fonts are divided into two main categories: serif and sans serif. A *serif* is a small line at the end of a character stroke. Consider using a serif font for text-intensive slides because the serifs help move the reader's eyes across the text. Use a sans serif font for titles, subtitles, headings, and short lines of text.

Activity 2.5

Changing the Font at the Font Dialog Box; Replacing Fonts

In addition to using the buttons in the Font group on the HOME tab, you can apply font formatting with options at the Font dialog box. With options at this dialog box, you can change the font; the font style, size, and color; and apply font effects such as underline, strikethrough, superscript, subscript, and all caps. If you decide to change a font that appears in all or many slides within a presentation, use the Replace Font dialog box to simplify this task.

Project

As you are still not satisfied with the font in the Vancouver presentation, you decide to change the font for the title and subtitle and replace the Trebuchet MS font on the remaining slides.

1. With **PMedS2-CVPVancouver.pptx** open, make sure Slide 1 is the active slide.

2. Select the text *Cascade View Pediatrics*.

3. Display the Font dialog box by clicking the Font group dialog box launcher 🗗 on the HOME tab.

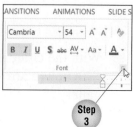

Step 3

4. At the Font dialog box, click the down-pointing arrow at the right side of the *Latin text font* option box and then click *Constantia* at the drop-down list. (You will need to scroll down the drop-down list to display *Constantia*.)

5. Click the down-pointing arrow at the right side of the *Font style* option box and then click *Bold* at the drop-down list.

6. Select the current measurement in the *Size* text box and then type **50**.

7. Click the Font color button in the *All text* section and then click the *Dark Blue* option (ninth option from the left in the *Standard Colors* section).

8. Click OK to close the Font dialog box.

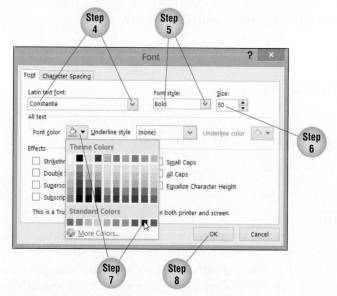

9. Select the subtitle *Vancouver Clinic*.

10. Click the Font group dialog box launcher.

11 At the Font dialog box, click the down-pointing arrow at the right side of the *Latin text font* option box and then click *Constantia* at the drop-down list. (You will need to scroll down the drop-down list to display *Constantia*.)

12 Click the down-pointing arrow at the right side of the *Font style* option box and then click *Bold* at the drop-down list.

13 Select the current measurement in the *Size* text box and then type 32.

14 Click OK to close the Font dialog box.

15 Make Slide 2 active.

16 You decide to replace all occurrences of the Trebuchet MS font with the Constantia font. To begin, click the Replace button arrow in the Editing group on the HOME tab and then click *Replace Fonts* at the drop-down list.

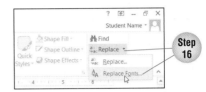

17 At the Replace Font dialog box, click the down-pointing arrow at the right of the *Replace* option box and then click *Trebuchet MS* at the drop-down list.

18 Click the down-pointing arrow at the right of the *With* option box and then click *Constantia* at the drop-down list. (You will need to scroll down the drop-down list to display *Constantia*.)

19 Click the Replace button and then click the Close button.

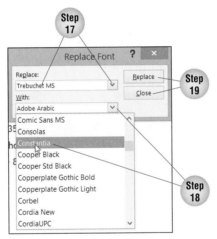

20 Save **PMedS2-CVPVancouver.pptx**.

In Brief

Change Font at Font Dialog Box
1. Select text.
2. Click Font group dialog box launcher.
3. Click desired options at Font dialog box.
4. Click OK.

Change All Occurrences of Font
1. Click Replace button arrow, then click *Replace Fonts*.
2. At Replace Font dialog box, click down-pointing arrow at right of *Replace* option and then click desired font.
3. Press Tab.
4. Click down-pointing arrow at right of *With* option and then click desired font.
5. Click Replace button.
6. Click Close button.

In Addition

Choosing Presentation Fonts

Choose a font for a presentation based on the tone and message you want the presentation to portray, as well as who your audience will be. For example, choose a more serious font, such as Constantia or Times New Roman, for a conservative audience, and choose a less formal font, such as Comic Sans MS, Lucida Handwriting, or Mistral, for a more informal or lighthearted audience. For text-intensive slides, choose a serif font, such as Cambria, Candara, Times New Roman, or Bookman Old Style. For titles, subtitles, headings, and short text items, consider a sans serif font such as Calibri, Arial, Tahoma, or Univers. Use no more than two or three different fonts in each presentation. To ensure legibility in a slide, choose a font color that contrasts with the slide background.

Activity 2.6

Formatting with Format Painter

Use the Format Painter feature to apply the same formatting in more than one location in a slide or slides. To use the Format Painter, apply the desired formatting to text, position the insertion point anywhere in the formatted text, and then double-click the Format Painter button in the Clipboard group on the HOME tab. Using the mouse, select the additional text to which you want to apply the formatting. After applying the formatting in the desired locations, click the Format Painter button to deactivate it. If you need to apply formatting to only one other location, click the Format Painter button once. The first time you select text, the formatting is applied and the Format Painter is deactivated.

Project

Improve the appearance of slides in the Vancouver presentation by applying a font and then using the Format Painter to apply the formatting to other text.

1. With **PMedS2-CVPVancouver.pptx** open, make sure Slide 2 is the active slide.

2. Select the title *Population*.

3. Click the Font group dialog box launcher.

4. At the Font dialog box, click the down-pointing arrow at the right side of the *Latin text font* option box and then click *Cambria* at the drop-down list.

5. Click the down-pointing arrow at the right side of the *Font style* option box and then click *Bold* at the drop-down list.

6. Click the Font color button in the *All text* section and then click the *Blue, Accent 2, Darker 25%* option (sixth column, fifth row in the *Theme Colors* section).

7. Click the *Small Caps* check box in the *Effects* section to insert a check mark.

8. Click OK to close the Font dialog box.

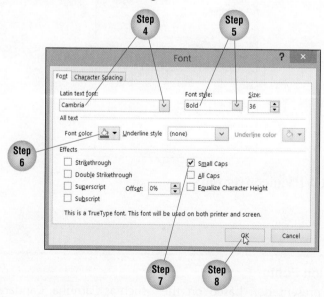

9. At the slide, click outside the selected text to deselect it.

10 Click anywhere in the title *POPULATION*.

11 Double-click the Format Painter button in the Clipboard group on the HOME tab.

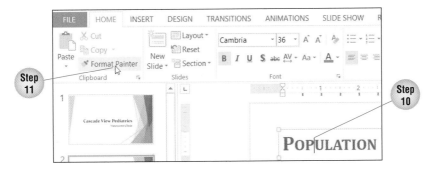

12 Click the Next Slide button to display Slide 3.

13 Using the mouse, select the words *Commercial Property*.

> The mouse pointer displays with a paintbrush attached. This indicates that the Format Painter feature is active. You can also apply the formatting to a single word by clicking any character in the word.

14 Click the Next Slide button to display Slide 4.

Need Help?

If the paintbrush is no longer attached to the mouse pointer, Format Painter has been turned off. Turn it back on by clicking in a slide title with the desired formatting and then double-clicking the Format Painter button.

15 Click any character in the title *Statistics*.

16 Click the Next Slide button to display Slide 5.

17 Click any character in the title *Employment*.

18 Apply formatting to the titles in the remaining three slides.

19 When formatting has been applied to all slide titles, click the Format Painter button in the Clipboard group on the HOME tab.

> Clicking the Format Painter button turns off the feature.

20 Save **PMedS2-CVPVancouver.pptx**.

In Addition

Choosing a Custom Color

Click the Font Color button at the Font dialog box and a palette of color choices displays. Click the *More Colors* option and the Colors dialog box displays with a honeycomb of color options. Click the Custom tab and the dialog box displays as shown at the right. With options at this tab, you can mix your own color. Click the desired color in the *Colors* palette or enter the values for the color in the *Red*, *Green*, and *Blue* measurement boxes. Adjust the luminosity of the current color by dragging the slider located at the right side of the color palette.

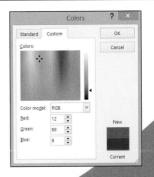

In Brief
Use Format Painter
1. Position insertion point on text containing desired formatting.
2. Double-click Format Painter button.
3. Select text to which you want to apply formatting.
4. Click Format Painter button.

Activity 2.7

Changing Alignment and Line and Paragraph Spacing; Drawing a Text Box and Shape

The slide design template generally determines the horizontal and vertical alignment of text in placeholders. Text may be left-aligned, center-aligned, or right-aligned in a placeholder, as well as aligned at the top, middle, or bottom of the placeholder. You can change the alignment of specific text with buttons in the Paragraph group on the HOME tab or with options at the Align Text button drop-down list. Use options at the Line Spacing button drop-down list or the *Line Spacing* option at the Paragraph dialog box to change line spacing. The

Paragraph dialog box also contains options for changing text alignment, indentation, and spacing before and after text.

If you want to add text to a slide but do not want to use the Title and Text layout, draw a text box in a slide and then type text inside the box. Use the Shapes button on the HOME tab or INSERT tab to draw shapes in a slide, such as squares, circles, block arrows, callouts, stars, and banners. Use options on the DRAWING TOOLS FORMAT tab to format and customize a text box or a shape.

Project

Change the alignment of specific text in slides and improve the appearance of text in slides by adjusting the vertical alignment and paragraph spacing. Dr. Severin has also asked you to insert a slide containing a description of Vancouver.

Cascade View PEDIATRICS

1. With **PMedS2-CVPVancouver.pptx** open, make Slide 1 active.

2. Click anywhere in the text *Cascade View Pediatrics* and then click the Center button ≡ in the Paragraph group on the HOME tab.

    You can also change text alignment with the keyboard shortcuts shown in Table P2.2.

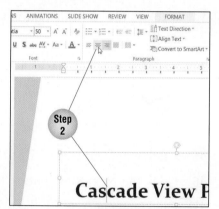

3. Select the subtitle *Vancouver Clinic* and then click the Center button in the Paragraph group.

4. Click the Align Text button in the Paragraph group and then click *Middle* at the drop-down list.

5. With Slide 1 active, click the New Slide button arrow and then click *Title Only* at the drop-down list.

6. Click in the *Click to add title* placeholder and then type **About Vancouver**.

7. Make Slide 3 active, click any character in the title *POPULATION*, and then click the Format Painter button in the Clipboard group.

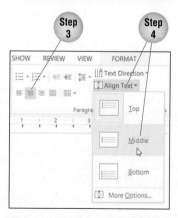

TABLE P2.2 Keyboard Shortcuts for Changing Alignment

Alignment	Keyboard Shortcut
left-align	Ctrl + L
center-align	Ctrl + E
right-align	Ctrl + R
justify-align	Ctrl + J

8 Make Slide 2 active and then select the title *About Vancouver*.

Format Painter applies the formatting and then deactivates automatically.

9 Draw a text box in the slide. Begin by clicking the INSERT tab and then clicking the Text Box button in the Text group.

10 Using the mouse, draw a box that is approximately the size shown at the right.

To draw a text box, hold down the mouse button as you drag in the slide.

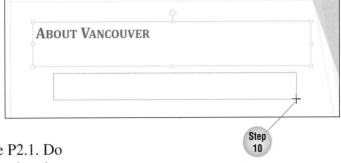

11 Type the text shown in Figure P2.1. Do not press the Enter key after typing the web address. If you do so accidentally, immediately click the Undo button.

12 Select all of the text in the text box and then change the font to 24-point Constantia.

13 Justify the text by clicking the Justify button in the Paragraph group.

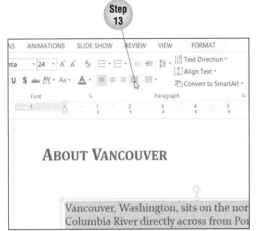

14 Make Slide 3 active, select the bulleted text, click the Line Spacing button in the Paragraph group, and then click *Line Spacing Options* at the drop-down list.

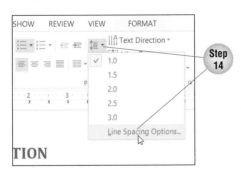

FIGURE P2.1 Step 11

Vancouver, Washington, sits on the north bank of the Columbia River directly across from Portland, Oregon. The Pacific Coast is less than 90 miles to the west. The Cascade Mountain Range rises on the east. Mount St. Helens National Volcanic Monument and Mt. Hood are less than two hours away. The spectacular Columbia River Gorge National Scenic Area lies 30 minutes to the east. (www.cityofvancouver.us)

continues

15 At the Paragraph dialog box, click the up-pointing arrow at the right side of the *After* measurement box in the *Spacing* section.

This displays *6 pt* in the *After* measurement box.

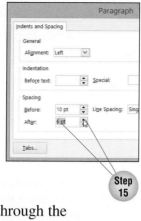

Step 15

16 Click OK to close the dialog box.

17 Make Slide 4 active (contains the title COMMERCIAL PROPERTY) and then select the bulleted text.

18 Click the Line Spacing button and then click *1.5* at the drop-down list.

19 Make Slide 5 active, select the text from the second bullet through the fourth bullet, click the Line Spacing button, and then click *Line Spacing Options* at the drop-down list.

20 At the Paragraph dialog box, click twice on the up-pointing arrow at the right of the *Before* measurement box in the *Spacing* section (this displays *18 pt* in the measurement box) and then click OK.

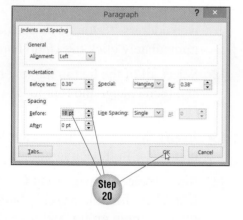

Step 20

21 Make Slide 6 active and then follow steps similar to those in Steps 19 and 20 to change the *Before* spacing to *18 pt*.

22 Make Slide 8 active and then select text from the second bullet through the eighth bullet. Display the Paragraph dialog box, change the *Before* spacing to *0 pt*, and then click OK to close the dialog box.

Step 24

23 Make Slide 9 active and then insert a new blank slide by clicking the New Slide button arrow and then clicking *Blank* at the drop-down list.

24 Draw a shape in the slide. Begin by clicking the INSERT tab, clicking the Shapes button in the Illustrations group, and then clicking *Bevel* at the drop-down list (first column, third row in the *Basic Shapes* section).

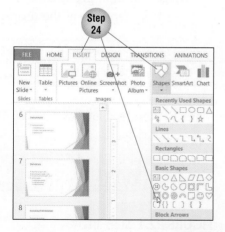

Shape options are also available in the Drawing group on the HOME tab.

25 Position the mouse pointer in the slide, hold down the left mouse button, drag to create the shape as shown at the right, and then release the mouse button.

If you are not satisfied with the size of the image, press the Delete key and then draw the image again.

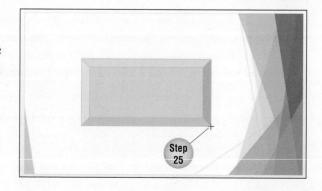

Step 25

26 With the shape selected, type the text **To schedule a tour of our clinic, please call (503) 555-7700.**

> When a shape is selected, text will automatically appear inside it when typed.

27 With the shape selected, click the More button at the right of the shape style thumbnails in the Shape Styles group on the DRAWING TOOLS FORMAT tab and then click the *Subtle Effect - Blue, Accent 2* option (third column, fourth row).

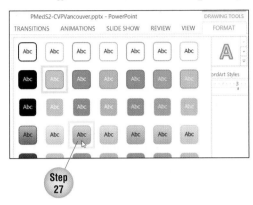

Step 27

In Brief

Change Horizontal Text Alignment
1. Select text or click in text paragraph.
2. Click desired alignment button in bottom row of Paragraph group.

Change Vertical Text Alignment
1. Select text or placeholder.
2. Click Align Text button.
3. Click desired alignment at drop-down list.

Change Line Spacing
1. Select text or placeholder.
2. Click Line Spacing button.
3. Click desired option at drop-down list.

OR

1. Select text or placeholder.
2. Click Line Spacing button.
3. Click *Line Spacing Options* at drop-down list.
4. At Paragraph dialog box, specify desired spacing.
5. Click OK.

Insert Text Box
1. Click INSERT tab.
2. Click Text Box button.
3. Click or drag in slide to create text box.

Draw Shape
1. Click INSERT tab.
2. Click Shapes button.
3. Click desired shape at drop-down list.
4. Drag in slide to draw shape.

28 Click the Shape Outline button arrow in the Shape Styles group and then click the *Dark Blue* option in the *Standard Colors* section.

29 Select the text in the shape, click the HOME tab, change the font to 40-point Candara, and then change the font color to *Blue, Accent 2, Darker 50%*.

Step 28

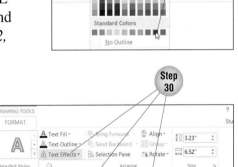

30 With the text still selected, click the DRAWING TOOLS FORMAT tab, click the Text Effects button in the WordArt Styles group, point to *Glow*, and then click the *Blue, 8 pt glow, Accent color 2* option (second column, second row in the *Glow Variations* section).

Step 30

31 Print Slide 2 and Slide 10.

32 Save **PMedS2-CVPVancouver.pptx**.

In Addition

Inserting a New Line

When creating bulleted text in a slide, pressing the Enter key causes the insertion point to move to the next line, inserting another bullet. Situations may occur where you want to create a blank line between bulleted items without creating another bullet. One way to do this is to use the New Line command, Shift + Enter. Pressing Shift + Enter inserts a new line that is considered part of the previous paragraph.

Activity 2.8

Inserting Headers and Footers

Insert information you want to appear at the top or bottom of individual slides or at the top or bottom of individual printed notes or handout pages using options at the Header and Footer dialog box. If you want the same types of information to appear on all slides, display the Header and Footer dialog box with the Slide tab selected. With options at this dialog box, you can insert the date and time, insert the slide number, and create a footer. To insert header or footer elements you want to print on all notes or handouts, choose options at the Header and Footer dialog box with the Notes and Handouts tab selected.

Project You decide to insert the current date and slide number in the Vancouver presentation and create a header for notes pages.

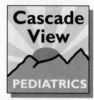

1. With **PMedS2-CVPVancouver.pptx** open, display Slide 1 in the slide pane.

2. Insert a footer that prints at the bottom of each slide. To begin, click the INSERT tab and then click the Header & Footer button in the Text group.

3. At the Header and Footer dialog box with the Slide tab selected, click the *Date and time* check box to insert a check mark. If it is not already selected, click the *Update automatically* option to select it.

4. Click the *Slide number* check box to insert a check mark.

5. Click the *Footer* check box and then type **Vancouver Clinic** in the *Footer* text box.

6. Click the Apply to All button.

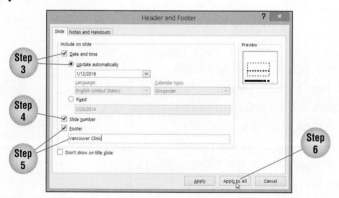

7. Make Slide 4 active.

8. Display the notes pane by clicking the NOTES buttons on the Status bar.

9. Click in the notes pane and then type **Contact two commercial real estate companies about available office space.**

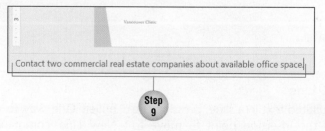

10. Insert a header that will print on notes and handouts pages by clicking the Header & Footer button in the Text group on the INSERT tab.

11   At the Header and Footer dialog box, click the Notes and Handouts tab.

12   Click the *Date and time* check box to insert a check mark and then, if necessary, click the *Update automatically* option to select it.

13   Click the *Header* check box and then type **Cascade View Pediatrics**.

14   Click the *Footer* check box and then type **Vancouver Clinic**.

15   Click the Apply to All button.

16   Print the presentation as handouts with six slides horizontally per page.

17   Print Slide 4 as a notes page. To do this, click the FILE tab, click the *Print* option, click the second gallery in the *Settings* category (contains the text *6 Slide Horizontal*), and then click *Notes Pages* in the *Print Layout* section.

18   Click in the *Slides* text box (located below the first gallery in the *Settings* category) and then type 4.

19   Click the Print button.

20   Remove the footer that displays on each slide. Begin by clicking the INSERT tab and then clicking the Header & Footer button in the Text group.

21   With the Slide tab selected, click the *Date and time* check box, the *Slide number* check box, and the *Footer* check box to remove the check marks.

22   Click the Apply to All button.

23   Click the NOTES button on the Status bar to close the notes pane.

24   Save **PMedS2-CVPVancouver.pptx**.

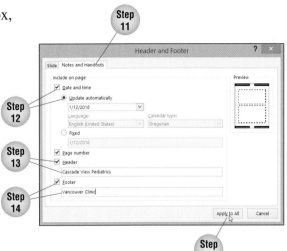

Step 11

Step 12

Step 13

Step 14

Step 15

Step 19

Step 18

Step 17

In Brief

Insert Header/Footer on Slide
1. Click INSERT tab.
2. Click Header & Footer button.
3. At Header and Footer dialog box with Slide tab selected, choose desired options.
4. Click Apply to All button.

Insert Header/ Footer in Notes and Handouts
1. Click INSERT tab.
2. Click Header & Footer button.
3. At Header and Footer dialog box, click Notes and Handouts tab.
4. Choose desired options.
5. Click Apply to All button.

In Addition

Using the Package for CD Feature

The safest way to transport a PowerPoint presentation from one computer to another is to use the Package for CD feature. With this feature, you can copy a presentation onto a CD or to a folder or network location and include all of the linked files, fonts, and the PowerPoint Viewer program in case the destination computer does not have PowerPoint installed on it. To use the Package for CD feature, click the FILE tab, click the *Export* option, click the *Package Presentation for CD* option, and then click the Package for CD button. At the Package for CD dialog box, type a name for the CD and then click the Copy to CD button.

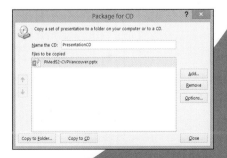

Activity 2.9

Changing Slide Size, Theme, Theme Colors, and Theme Fonts

By default, the slide size in PowerPoint 2013 is Widescreen (16:9), but you can change the slide size with options at the Slide Size button drop-down list in the Customize group on the DESIGN tab. Change the design theme applied to slides in a presentation or change the colors, fonts, effects, or background style of a theme with options on the DESIGN tab. Click the More button in the Variants group on the DESIGN tab to display options for changing the theme colors, fonts, effects, and background styles.

Project

You are not pleased with the design theme for the Vancouver presentation, so you decide to apply a different theme and then change the colors and fonts for the theme.

1. With **PMedS2-CVPVancouver.pptx** open, click the DESIGN tab.

2. Click the Slide Size button 🔲 in the Customize group and then click *Standard (4:3)* at the drop-down list.

3. At the Microsoft PowerPoint dialog box, click the Ensure Fit button.

   Clicking the Ensure Fit button scales down the contents of the slide to fit within the new slide size. Click the Maximize button to maximize the size of the content on the new slide.

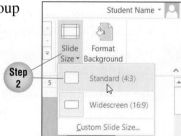

4. Run the presentation beginning with Slide 1 and notice any changes to the layout of the slides.

5. Click the Undo button on the Quick Access toolbar to return the presentation to the original slide size (Widescreen).

6. Click the More button at the right side of the themes thumbnails in the Themes group and then click the *Dividend* option at the drop-down gallery.

7. Click the More button in the Variants group, point to *Colors*, and then click *Blue Green* at the side menu.

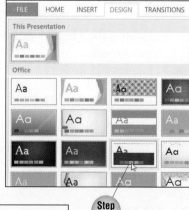

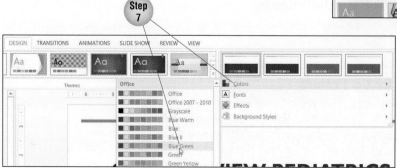

8 Click the More button in the Variants group, point to *Fonts*, and then click *Consolas-Verdana* at the side menu.

9 Apply a background style by clicking the More button in the Variants group, pointing to *Background Styles*, and then clicking the *Style 10* option at the side menu (second column, third row).

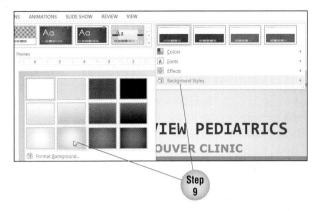

Step 9

10 With Slide 1 active, change the font of the title and subtitle to Constantia.

11 Make Slide 2 active. Notice that the title of the slide is difficult to see. Select the title *ABOUT VANCOUVER*, click the HOME tab, click the Font Color button arrow in the Font group, and then click the *Dark Blue* option at the drop-down gallery (ninth option from the left in the *Standard Colors* section).

12 Click once in the title *ABOUT VANCOUVER*, double-click the Format Painter button in the Clipboard group on the HOME tab, make Slide 3 active in the slide pane, and then select the title *POPULATION*. Apply the Dark Blue font color to the titles in Slides 4 through 9. Click the Format Painter button to turn off the feature.

13 Run the presentation beginning with Slide 1.

14 After running the presentation, remove the background style by clicking the DESIGN tab, clicking the More button in the Variants group, pointing to *Background Styles*, and then clicking the *Style 1* option at the side menu (first column, first row).

15 Make Slide 2 active and then move the text box placeholder so it is positioned in the center of the slide.

16 Make Slide 10 active and then move the shape so it is positioned in the center of the slide.

17 Save **PMedS2-CVPVancouver.pptx**.

In Brief

Change Slide Size
1. Click DESIGN tab.
2. Click Slide Size button.
3. Click desired slide size at drop-down list.

Change Theme
1. Click DESIGN tab.
2. Click More button at right side of theme thumbnails.
3. Click desired theme at drop-down gallery.

Change Theme Colors
1. Click DESIGN tab.
2. Click More button in Variants group.
3. Point to *Colors*.
4. Click desired option at side menu.

Change Theme Fonts
1. Click DESIGN tab.
2. Click More button in Variants group.
3. Point to *Fonts*.
4. Click desired option at side menu.

Change Slide Background
1. Click DESIGN tab.
2. Click More button in Variants group.
3. Point to *Background Styles*.
4. Click desired option at side menu.

In Addition

Customizing Theme Colors

Theme colors consist of four text colors, six accent colors, and two hyperlink colors. You can customize these theme colors with options at the Create New Theme Colors dialog box, shown at the right. Display this dialog box by clicking the More button in the Variants group on the DESIGN tab, pointing to *Colors* and then clicking *Customize Colors* at the side menu. Change a color by clicking the desired color option in the *Theme colors* section and then clicking the desired color at the color palette. Changes made to colors display in the *Sample* section of the dialog box. You can name a custom color theme with the *Name* option in the dialog box. Click the Reset button to return the colors to the default theme colors.

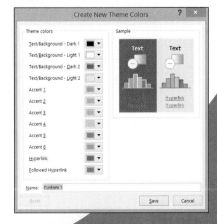

Activity 2.10

Inserting and Formatting Images

Add visual appeal to a presentation by inserting an image such as a logo, picture, or clip art in a slide. Insert an image from a drive or folder with the Pictures button in the Images group on the INSERT tab. If the slide layout contains a content placeholder, you can also insert a picture from a drive or folder by clicking the picture image in the content placeholder to display the Insert Picture dialog box. At this dialog box, navigate to the desired drive or folder and then double-click the image. To search for and insert clip art images from Office.com, click the Online Pictures button in the Images group on the INSERT tab to display the Insert Pictures window. At the window, type a search word in the *Office.com Clip Art* text box and then press Enter. In the list of clip art images and pictures that displays, double-click the desired image. Use buttons on the PICTURE TOOLS FORMAT tab to recolor an image, apply a picture style, arrange the image in the slide, and size the image. You can also size an image using the sizing handles that display around the selected image and move the image using the mouse.

Project

Dr. Severin has asked you to insert the clinic logo on the first slide and to enhance the visual appeal of some of the slides by inserting clip art images.

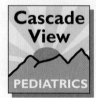

1. With **PMedS2-CVPVancouver.pptx** open, make sure Slide 1 is active.

2. Insert the clinic logo in the slide. To begin, click the INSERT tab and then click the Pictures button in the Images group.

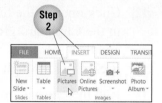

Step 2

3. At the Insert Picture dialog box, navigate to the PowerPointMedS2 folder on your storage medium and then double-click *CVPLogo.jpg*.

   The image is inserted in the slide, selection handles display around the image, and the PICTURE TOOLS FORMAT tab is selected.

4. Decrease the size of the logo by clicking in the *Shape Height* measurement box in the Size group on the PICTURE TOOLS FORMAT tab, typing **0.9**, and then pressing Enter.

   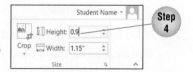

   Step 4

   When you change the height of the logo, the width automatically changes to maintain the proportions of the logo. You can also size an image using the sizing handles that display around the selected image. Use the middle sizing handles to increase or decrease the width of an image, use the top and bottom handles to increase or decrease the height, and use the corner sizing handles to increase or decrease both the width and height of the image at the same time.

5. Move the logo so it is positioned in the lower right corner of the slide (within the teal background). To do this, position the mouse pointer on the image until the pointer displays with a four-headed arrow attached, drag the image to the lower right corner, and then release the mouse button.

6. With the image selected, click the *Drop Shadow Rectangle* option in the Picture Styles group (fourth option from the left).

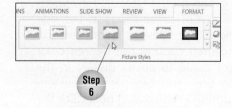

Step 6

7️⃣ Make Slide 4 active and then insert a clip art image. Begin by clicking the INSERT tab and then clicking the Online Pictures button 🖼️ in the Images group.

8️⃣ At the Insert Pictures window, click in the *Office.com Clip Art* text box, type **office building**, and then press Enter.

9️⃣ Double-click the image shown below and in Figure P2.2.

> If the building clip art shown below and in Figure P2.2 is not available, insert a building clip art image of your choosing.

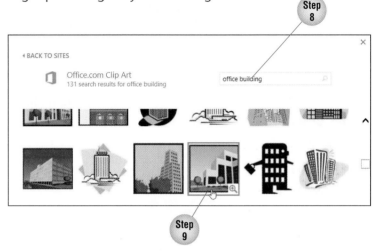

🔟 With the image selected, increase the size by clicking in the *Shape Height* measurement box, typing **3.6**, and then pressing Enter.

⑪ Move the clip art image so it is positioned as shown in Figure P2.2.

⑫ Make Slide 8 active, click the INSERT tab, and then click the Online Pictures button.

⑬ At the Insert Pictures window, click in the *Office.com Clip Art* text box, type **university**, and then press Enter.

⑭ Double-click the image shown in Figure P2.3 on page 420.

> If the university clip art shown in Figure P2.3 is not available, insert a university clip art image of your choosing.

⑮ Click in the *Shape Height* measurement box in the Size group on the PICTURE TOOLS FORMAT tab, type **2.4**, and then press Enter.

FIGURE P2.2 Slide 4

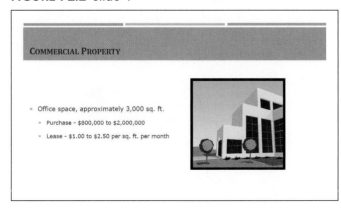

continues

16 Change the color of the image so it complements the color scheme of the presentation. To do this, click the Color button 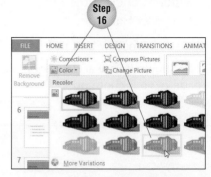 in the Adjust group and then click the *Aqua, Accent color 2 Light* option in the *Recolor* section (third column, third row).

17 Click the Corrections button 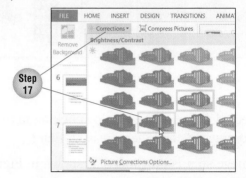 in the Adjust group and then click the *Brightness: -20% Contrast: +20%* option at the drop-down gallery (second column, fourth row).

18 Using the mouse, drag the image so it is positioned as shown in Figure P2.3.

19 Make Slide 2 active, click the INSERT tab, and then click the Online Pictures button.

20 At the Insert Pictures window, click in the *Office.com Clip Art* text box, type **mountain sun**, and then press Enter.

21 Double-click the image shown in Figure P2.4.

> If the mountain clip art shown in Figure P2.4 is not available, insert a mountain clip art image of your choosing.

FIGURE P2.3 Slide 8

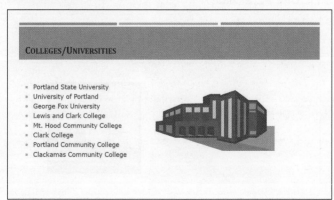

22 Click in the *Shape Height* measurement box, type **4.8**, and then press Enter.

23 Format the image as a watermark by clicking the Color button in the Adjust group on the PICTURE TOOLS FORMAT tab and then clicking the *Washout* option in the *Recolor* section (fourth column, first row).

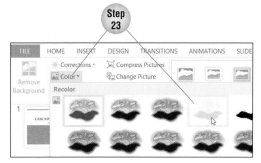

24 Click the Send Backward button arrow in the Arrange group on the PICTURE TOOLS FORMAT tab and then click *Send to Back* at the drop-down list.

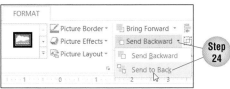

25 Using the mouse, drag the image so it is positioned as shown in Figure P2.4.

26 Save **PMedS2-CVPVancouver.pptx**.

FIGURE P2.4 Slide 2

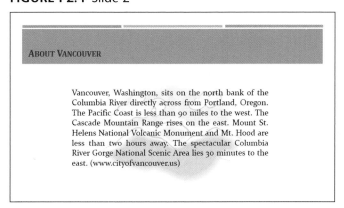

In Addition

Formatting with Buttons on the PICTURE TOOLS FORMAT Tab

You can format images in a slide with buttons and options on the PICTURE TOOLS FORMAT tab, shown below. Use buttons in the Adjust group to control the brightness and contrast of the image; change the image color; change to a different image; reset the image to its original size, position, and color; and compress the image. Compress a picture to save room on the hard drive or reduce download time. Use buttons in the Picture Styles group to apply a predesigned style, insert a picture border, or apply a picture effect. The Arrange group contains buttons for positioning the image, wrapping text around the image, and aligning and rotating the image. Use options in the Size group to crop the image and specify the height and width of the image.

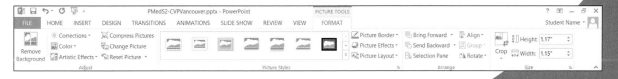

Activity 2.11

Inserting and Formatting WordArt

Use the WordArt feature to create text with special formatting that makes it stand out. You can format WordArt in a variety of ways, including conforming it to a shape. To insert WordArt, click the INSERT tab, click the WordArt button in the Text group, and then click the desired WordArt style at the drop-down gallery. When WordArt is selected, the DRAWING TOOLS FORMAT tab displays. Use options and buttons on this tab to modify and customize WordArt.

Project

To complete the presentation, Dr. Severin has asked you to insert a WordArt image containing the proposed opening date of the Vancouver clinic.

1 With **PMedS2-CVPVancouver.pptx** open, make Slide 9 active.

2 Click the New Slide button in the Slides group on the HOME tab.

3 Click the Layout button in the Slides group and then click the *Blank* option (first column, third row).

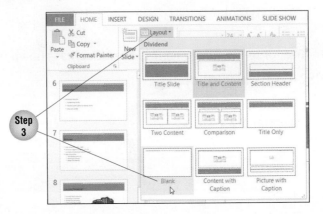

4 Insert WordArt by clicking the INSERT tab, clicking the WordArt button [A] in the Text group, and then clicking the *Fill - Aqua, Accent 2, Outline - Accent 2* option (third column, first row).

> This inserts a text box containing the words *Your text here* and also makes active the DRAWING TOOLS FORMAT tab.

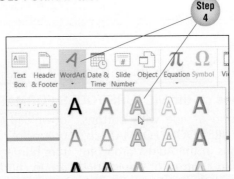

5 Type **Opening**, press the Enter key, and then type **September 2016**.

6 Select the text *Opening September 2016*, click the Text Effects button 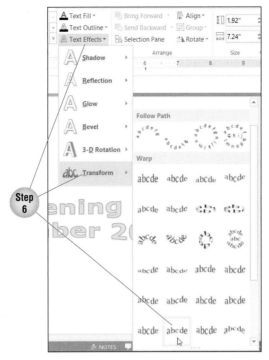 in the WordArt Styles group, point to *Transform* at the drop-down list, and then click the *Deflate* option at the drop-down gallery (second column, sixth row in the *Warp* section).

7 Click the Text Effects button, point to *Glow* at the drop-down list, and then click the *Aqua, 8 pt glow, Accent color 1* option at the drop-down gallery (first column, second row in the *Glow Variations* section).

8 Click in the *Shape Height* measurement box in the Size group, type **4**, and then press Enter.

9 Click in the *Shape Width* measurement box in the Size group, type **10**, and then press Enter.

Step 6

Step 8

Step 9

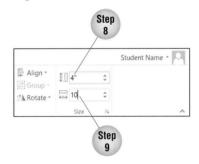

10 Drag the WordArt text so it is centered on the slide, as shown in Figure P2.5.

11 Save **PMedS2-CVPVancouver.pptx**.

FIGURE P2.5 Slide 10

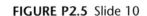

In Addition

Using Buttons and Options on the DRAWING TOOLS FORMAT Tab

When WordArt is selected in a slide, the DRAWING TOOLS FORMAT tab displays as shown below. You can draw a shape or text box with buttons in the Insert Shapes group. Apply a style, fill, outline, or effect to the WordArt text box with options in the Shape Styles group. Change the style of the WordArt text with options in the WordArt Styles group, specify the layering of the WordArt text with options in the Arrange group, and specify the height and width of the WordArt text box with options in the Size group.

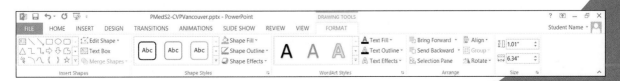

Activity 2.12

Inserting and Formatting an Organizational Chart with SmartArt

If you need to visually illustrate hierarchical data, consider creating an organizational chart with SmartArt. To display a menu of SmartArt options, click the INSERT tab and then click the SmartArt button in the Illustrations group. This displays the Choose a SmartArt Graphic dialog box. At this dialog box, click *Hierarchy* in the left panel and then double-click the desired organizational chart in the middle panel. This inserts the organizational chart in the slide. Some SmartArt graphics are designed to include text. You can type text in a graphic by selecting a shape and then typing text in the shape or you can type text in the *Type your text here* window that displays at the left side of the SmartArt graphic.

Project

As part of the presentation, Dr. Severin has asked you to insert an organizational chart identifying project personnel.

1 With **PMedS2-CVPVancouver.pptx** open, make Slide 9 active and then click the New Slide button in the Slides group on the HOME tab.

2 Create the organizational chart shown in Figure P2.6. To begin, click the INSERT tab and then click the SmartArt button in the Illustrations group.

> You can also click the Insert SmartArt Graphic option in the content placeholder.

3 At the Choose a SmartArt Graphic dialog box, click *Hierarchy* in the left panel and then double-click the first option in the middle panel, *Organization Chart*.

> This displays the organizational chart in the slide with the SMARTART TOOLS DESIGN tab selected. Use buttons on this tab to add additional boxes, change the order of the boxes, choose a different layout, apply formatting with a SmartArt style, and reset the formatting of the organizational chart.

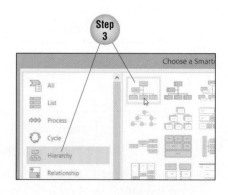

4 If a Type your text here pane displays at the left side of the organizational chart, close it by clicking the Text Pane button in the Create Graphic group.

> You can also close the window by clicking the Close button that displays in the upper right corner of the window.

5 Delete one of the boxes in the organizational chart by clicking the border of the first box from the left in the bottom row and then pressing the Delete key.

> Make sure that the selection border that surrounds the box is a solid line and not a dashed line. If a dashed line displays, click the box border again. This should change it to a solid line.

6 With the bottom left box selected, click the Add Shape button arrow in the Create Graphic group on the SMARTART TOOLS DESIGN tab and then click *Add Shape Below* at the drop-down list.

> This inserts a box below the selected box. Your organizational chart should contain the same boxes as shown in Figure P2.6.

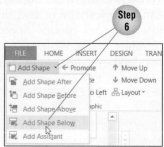

7 Click *[Text]* in the top box, type **Dr. Severin**, press the Enter key, and then type **Project Leader**. Click in each of the remaining boxes and type the text as shown in Figure P2.6.

8 Click the Change Colors button 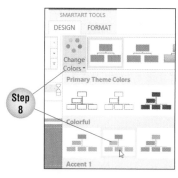 in the SmartART Styles group on the SMARTART TOOLS DESIGN tab and then click the *Colorful Range - Accent Colors 2 to 3* option (second option in the *Colorful* section).

9 Click the More button at the right side of the SmartArt Styles group.

10 Click the *Polished* option at the drop-down gallery (first column, first row in the *3-D* section).

11 Click the SMARTART TOOLS FORMAT tab.

12 Click inside the SmartArt graphic border but outside the SmartArt shapes.

13 Click in the *Shape Height* measurement box in the Size group, type **4.9**, and then press Enter.

14 Click the *CLICK TO ADD TITLE* placeholder and then type **Project Personnel**.

15 Make Slide 9 active and then click the HOME tab.

16 Click any character in the title *TOP EMPLOYERS* and then click the Format Painter button in the Clipboard group.

17 Make Slide 10 active and then select the title *Project Personnel*.

> This changes the font to 28-point Cambria, applies bold and small caps formatting, and changes the font color to *Dark Blue*.

18 Save **PMedS2-CVPVancouver.pptx**.

In Brief

Create SmartArt Organizational Chart
1. Click INSERT tab.
2. Click SmartArt button.
3. Click *Hierarchy* in left panel of Choose a SmartArt Graphic dialog box.
4. Double-click desired organizational chart.

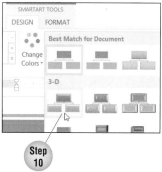

FIGURE P2.6 SmartArt Organizational Chart

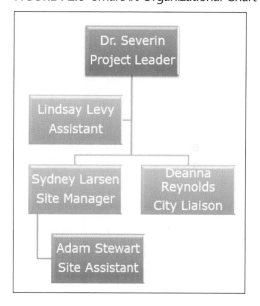

In Addition

Moving a SmartArt Graphic

Move a SmartArt graphic by positioning the arrow pointer on the border of the graphic until the pointer displays with a four-headed arrow attached, holding down the left mouse button, and then dragging the graphic to the desired location. You can increase the size of the graphic with the *Shape Height* and *Shape Width* measurement boxes or by dragging a corner of the graphic border. If you want to maintain the proportions of the graphic, hold down the Shift key while dragging the border to increase or decrease the size.

Activity 2.13

Inserting and Formatting a SmartArt Graphic

Use the SmartArt feature to create a variety of graphic diagrams including process, cycle, relationship, matrix, and pyramid diagrams. Click the INSERT tab and then click the SmartArt button to display the Choose a SmartArt Graphic dialog box. Click the desired graphic type in the left panel of the dialog box and then use the scroll bar at the right side of the middle panel to scroll down the list of choices. Double-click a graphic in the middle panel and the graphic is inserted in the slide. Use buttons on the SMARTART TOOLS DESIGN tab and the SMARTART TOOLS FORMAT tab to customize a graphic.

Project

Dr. Severin has asked you to include a graphic diagram identifying the major steps in the new clinic project.

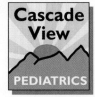

1. With **PMedS2-CVPVancouver.pptx** open, make Slide 10 active and then click the New Slide button in the Slides group on the HOME tab.

2. Click the Layout button in the Slides group and then click the *Blank* option at the drop-down list.

3. Create the SmartArt graphic shown in Figure P2.7. To begin, click the INSERT tab and then click the SmartArt button in the Illustrations group.

4. At the Choose a SmartArt Graphic dialog box, click *Relationship* in the left panel of the dialog box and then double-click the *Converging Radial* option.

5. If necessary, close the Type your text here pane by clicking the Close button that displays in the upper right corner of the window.

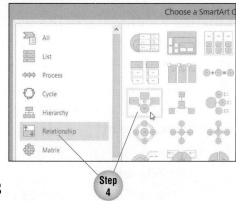

6. Click the Add Shape button in the Create Graphic group on the SMARTART TOOLS DESIGN tab.

7. Click in each of the shapes and type the text shown in Figure P2.7.

8. Click the Change Colors button in the SmartArt Styles group and then click the *Colorful - Accent Colors* option (first option from the left in the *Colorful* section).

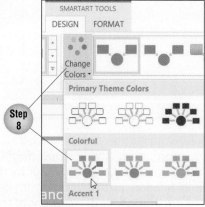

9 Click the More button at the right side of the SmartArt Styles group.

10 Click the *Inset* option (second column, first row in the *3-D* section).

11 Click the SMARTART TOOLS FORMAT tab.

12 Click inside the SmartArt graphic border but outside the SmartArt shapes.

> This deselects the shapes but keeps the graphic selected.

13 Click the More button at the right side of the thumbnails in the WordArt Styles group and then click the *Fill - White, Outline - Accent 2, Hard Shadow - Accent 2* option (fourth column, third row).

14 Position the arrow pointer on the SmartArt graphic border until the pointer displays with a four-headed arrow attached, hold down the left mouse button, and then drag the SmartArt graphic down so it is positioned as shown in Figure P2.7.

15 Save **PMedS2-CVPVancouver.pptx.**

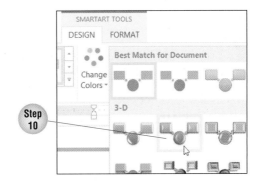

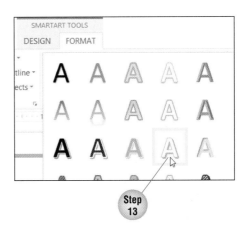

In Brief
Create SmartArt Graphic
1. Click INSERT tab.
2. Click SmartArt button.
3. Click desired category in left panel of Choose a SmartArt Graphic dialog box.
4. Double-click desired graphic.

FIGURE P2.7 SmartArt Relationship Graphic

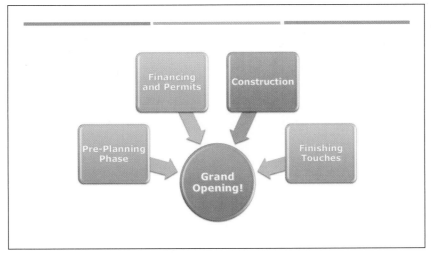

In Addition

Inserting Text in the Type Your Text Here Pane

You can enter text in a SmartArt shape by clicking in the shape and then typing the text. You can also insert text in a SmartArt shape by typing text in SmartArt's Type your text here pane. Display the pane by clicking the Text Pane button in the Create Graphic group on the SMARTART TOOLS DESIGN tab.

Activity 2.14

Applying Animation to Objects and Text

Animate individual objects and text in a slide with options on the ANIMATIONS tab. Click the ANIMATIONS tab to display a variety of animation styles and options for customizing and applying times to animations in a presentation. Click the More button at the right side of the thumbnails in the Animation group and a gallery of animation styles displays. You can apply these animations to objects and text as they enter a slide, exit a slide, or follow a motion path. You can also apply animations to emphasize objects in a slide. If you want to apply an existing animation to other objects in a presentation, use the Animation Painter button in the Advanced Animation group on the ANIMATIONS tab.

Project

Dr. Severin has asked you to apply animation effects to some of the slides in the presentation.

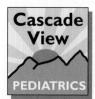

1. With **PMedS2-CVPVancouver.pptx** open, make sure Slide 11 is the active slide and that the SmartArt graphic is selected.

2. Click the ANIMATIONS tab and then click the *Fly In* option in the Animation group.

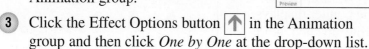

3. Click the Effect Options button ⬆ in the Animation group and then click *One by One* at the drop-down list.

4. Click twice on the up-pointing arrow at the right of the *Duration* measurement box in the Timing group.

   This displays *01.00* in the option box.

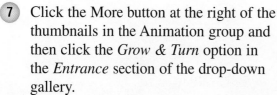

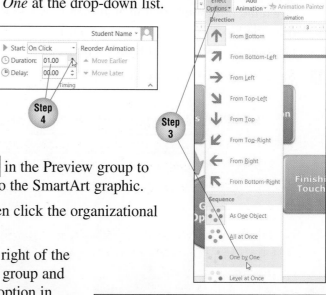

5. Click the Preview button ⭐ in the Preview group to view the animation applied to the SmartArt graphic.

6. Make Slide 10 active and then click the organizational chart to select it.

7. Click the More button at the right of the thumbnails in the Animation group and then click the *Grow & Turn* option in the *Entrance* section of the drop-down gallery.

8. Click the Effect Options button in the Animation group and then click *One by One* at the drop-down list.

9. Click Slide 3 to make it active and then click the bulleted text to select the placeholder.

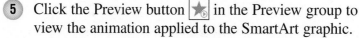
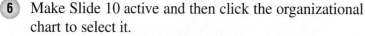

10. Click the *Fly In* option in the Animation group.

    Applying this animation creates a build for the bulleted items. A *build* displays the bullet points in a slide one by one and is useful for keeping the audience's attention focused on the point being presented, since it does not allow them to read ahead.

11 Click twice on the up-pointing arrow at the right of the *Duration* measurement box in the Timing group.

This displays *01.00* in the measurement box.

12 Apply the same animation to the bulleted text in Slides 4 through 8. To begin, click anywhere in the bulleted text to selected the placeholder and then double-click the Animation Painter button in the Advanced Animation group.

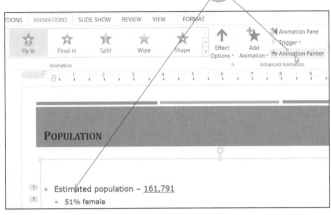

In Brief
Apply Animation to Object
1. Click desired object.
2. Click ANIMATIONS tab.
3. Click desired animation thumbnail.

13 Make Slide 4 active and then click anywhere in the bulleted text. (This selects the placeholder and applies the Fly In animation and the duration time.)

14 Make Slide 5 active and then click anywhere in the bulleted text.

15 Make Slide 6 active and then click in the bulleted text. Make Slide 7 active and then click in the bulleted text. Make Slide 8 active and then click in the bulleted text.

16 Click the Animation Painter button to turn off the feature.

17 Delete Slide 9.

The presentation should now contain 12 slides.

18 Make Slide 1 active and then run the presentation. Click the left mouse button to advance slides and to display the individual organizational chart boxes, bulleted items, and SmartArt graphic elements.

19 Print the presentation as handouts with six slides horizontally per page. To do this, click the FILE tab and then click the *Print* option.

20 At the Print backstage area, click the second gallery in the *Settings* category (contains the text *Full Page Slides*) and then click *6 Slides Horizontal* at the drop-down list.

21 Click the Print button.

22 Save and then close **PMedS2-CVPVancouver.pptx**.

In Addition

Applying a Custom Animation

Apply a custom animation to selected objects in a slide by clicking the Animation Pane button in the Advanced Animation group on the ANIMATIONS tab. This displays the Animation task pane at the right side of the screen. Use options in this task pane to control the order in which objects appear on a slide, choose animation direction and speed, and specify how objects will appear in the slide.

Features Summary

Feature	Ribbon Tab, Group	Button	Keyboard Shortcut
align left	HOME, Paragraph		Ctrl + L
align right	HOME, Paragraph		Ctrl + R
align vertically	HOME, Paragraph		
animation effect options	ANIMATIONS, Animation		
bold	HOME, Font	B	Ctrl + B
center	HOME, Paragraph		Ctrl + E
clip art	INSERT, Images		
copy selected text	HOME, Clipboard		Ctrl + C
cut selected text	HOME, Clipboard		Ctrl + X
decrease font size	HOME, Font		Ctrl + Shift + <
decrease list level	HOME, Paragraph		Shift + Tab
font	HOME, Font		
font color	HOME, Font		
Font dialog box	HOME, Font		Ctrl + Shift + F
font size	HOME, Font		
Format Painter	HOME, Clipboard		
header and footer	INSERT, Text		
hide slide	SLIDE SHOW, Set Up		
increase font size	HOME, Font		Ctrl + Shift + >
increase list level	HOME, Paragraph		Tab
italic	HOME, Font	I	Ctrl + I
justify	HOME, Paragraph		Ctrl + J
line spacing	HOME, Paragraph		
paste selected text	HOME, Clipboard		Ctrl + V
picture	INSERT, Images		
preview animation	ANIMATIONS, Preview		
replace font	HOME, Editing		Ctrl + H

Feature	Ribbon Tab, Group	Button	Keyboard Shortcut
shape	INSERT, Illustrations OR HOME, Drawing		
SmartArt	INSERT, Illustrations		
text box	INSERT, Text		
theme	DESIGN, Themes		
underline	HOME, Font	U	Ctrl + U
WordArt	INSERT, Text		

Knowledge Check

Completion: In the space provided at the right, write in the correct term, command, or option.

1. Save an existing presentation with a new name at this dialog box. _____
2. The Hide Slide button is located on this tab. _____
3. Increase the indent of text by clicking the Increase List Level button or by pressing this key on the keyboard. _____
4. Decrease the indent of text by clicking the Decrease List Level button or by pressing these keys on the keyboard. _____
5. The Cut button is located in this group on the HOME tab. _____
6. This group on the HOME tab contains two rows of buttons for changing fonts, font size, and font effects. _____
7. The Replace button is located in this group on the HOME tab. _____
8. Use this feature to apply the same formatting in more than one location within a slide or presentation. _____
9. Click this button in the Paragraph group on the HOME tab to apply right alignment to text. _____
10. Change the vertical alignment of text in a placeholder with options at this button's drop-down list. _____
11. Create a footer that displays at the bottom of all slides with options at this dialog box. _____
12. Click this tab to access the Themes group. _____
13. Use buttons on this tab to change the color of a selected picture, apply a picture style, and arrange and size the picture. _____
14. Use this feature to distort or modify text and to conform it to a variety of shapes. _____
15. Use this feature to create an organizational chart or choose from a variety of other graphic options. _____
16. The Effect Options button is located on this tab. _____

Skills Review

Review 1 Rearranging and Deleting Slides; Decreasing and Increasing Indents; Copying and Pasting Text

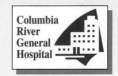

1. With PowerPoint open, open **CRGHComEd.pptx** from the PowerPointMedS2 folder on your storage medium.
2. Save the presentation with the name **PMedS2-R-CRGHComEd.**
3. Click the Slide Sorter button in the view area on the Status bar.
4. Select and then delete Slide 8 (contains the title *Pregnancy Exercise*).
5. Move Slide 3 (*Professional Education*) to the left of Slide 9 (*Course Offerings*).
6. Move Slide 4 (*Babysitting*) to the left of Slide 7 (*Support Groups*).
7. Click the Normal button in the view area on the Status bar.
8. Make Slide 4 (*Childbirth Preparation Refresher*) the active slide.
9. Increase the indent of the bulleted text *Breathing and relaxation* to the next list level.
10. Increase the indent of the bulleted text *Coach's role* to the next list level.
11. Make Slide 6 active and then decrease the indent of the bulleted text *Designed for boys and girls 11 to 13* to the previous list level.
12. Make Slide 3 (*Childbirth Preparation*) the active slide.
13. Select the text *Cost:* (including the space after the colon) and then click the Copy button.
14. Make Slide 4 (*Childbirth Preparation Refresher*) the active slide.
15. Move the insertion point immediately left of the dollar sign (located in the last bulleted item) and then click the Paste button.
16. Make Slide 5 (*Bringing up Baby*) the active slide, move the insertion point immediately left of the dollar sign, and then click the Paste button.
17. Make Slide 6 (*Babysitting*) the active slide, move the insertion point immediately left of the dollar sign, and then click the Paste button.
18. Make Slide 7 (*Support Groups*) the active slide, move the insertion point immediately left of the *F* in *Free* (located after the last bullet), and then click the Paste button.
19. Save **PMedS2-R-CRGHComEd.pptx**.

Review 2 Changing Theme Colors, Fonts, and Background Styles; Applying Fonts and Using Format Painter; Changing Alignment and Line Spacing

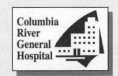

1. With **PMedS2-R-CRGHComEd.pptx** open, make Slide 1 the active slide and then click the DESIGN tab.
2. Click the More button in the Variants group, point to *Colors*, and then click *Blue Warm* at the side menu.
3. Click the More button in the Variants group, point to *Fonts*, and then click *Calibri Light-Constantia* at the side menu.
4. Click the More button in the Variants group, point to *Background Styles*, and then click the *Style 1* option at the side menu (first column, first row).
5. With Slide 1 active, select the text *Columbia River General Hospital*, change the font to 72-point Candara, change the font color to *Blue, Accent 2, Darker 50%*, and then apply bold formatting.

6. Make Slide 2 active, select the text *Community Education*, change the font to Candara, change the font color to *Blue, Accent 2, Darker 50%,* and then apply bold formatting.

7. Select the text *Class Offerings* and then change the font size to 32 points.

8. Make Slide 3 active, select the heading *Childbirth Preparation*, change the font to Candara, change the font color to *Teal, Accent 5, Darker 25%,* and then apply bold formatting.

9. Using Format Painter, apply the same formatting to the titles in Slides 4, 5, 6, 7, 9, and 10. (Skip Slide 8.)

10. Make Slide 2 active, click any character in the title *Community Education*, and then click the Format Painter button. Make Slide 8 active and then select *Professional Education*.

11. Select the subtitle text in Slide 8 and then change the font size to 32 points.

12. Make Slide 1 the active slide.

13. Click anywhere in the title and then click the Center button.

14. Make Slide 2 active and then center the title and subtitle.

15. Make Slide 8 active and then center the title and subtitle.

16. Make Slide 3 active, select the bulleted text, and then change the line spacing to *1.5*.

17. Make Slide 4 active, select the bulleted text, and then change the line spacing to *1.5*.

18. Make Slide 9 active, select the bulleted text, and then change the spacing after paragraphs to *12 pt*.

19. Make Slide 10 active, select the bulleted text, and then change the spacing before paragraphs to *18 pt*.

20. Print Slide 1.

21. Save **PMedS2-R-CRGHComEd.pptx**.

Review 3 Inserting and Formatting Images

Columbia
River
General
Hospital

1. With **PMedS2-R-CRGHComEd.pptx** open, delete Slide 1.

2. At the beginning of the presentation, insert a new slide with the Blank layout. *Hint: To insert a new slide at the beginning of the presentation, click immediately above the Slide 1 thumbnail in the slide thumbnails pane and then click the New Slide button arrow.*

3. Use the Pictures button in the Images group on the INSERT tab to insert **CRGHLogo.jpg** and then size and move the image so it displays as shown in Figure P2.8 on page 434.

4. Make Slide 3 active and then use the Insert Pictures window to search for clip art images related to pregnancy. Insert the image shown in Figure P2.9 on page 434 and then size and position it to match the figure. (If this particular image is not available, choose a similar clip art image related to pregnancy.)

5. Make Slide 6 active and then use the Insert Pictures window to search for clip art images related to babysitting. Insert the image shown in Figure P2.10 on page 434 and then size and position it to match the figure. (If this particular image is not available, choose a similar image related to babysitting or babysitter.) Change the color of the image to *Teal, Accent color 5 Light*. *Hint: Do this with the Color button on the PICTURE TOOLS FORMAT tab.*

6. Make Slide 9 active and then locate a clip art image using the search word *nurse*. You determine the clip art as well as the formatting, color, size, and positioning of the image.

7. Save **PMedS2-R-CRGHComEd.pptx**.

FIGURE P2.8 Review 3, Slide 1

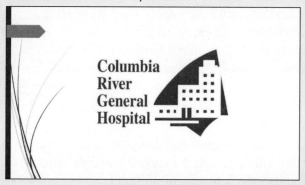

FIGURE P2.9 Review 3, Slide 3

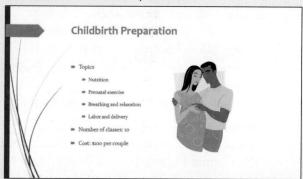

FIGURE P2.10 Review 3, Slide 6

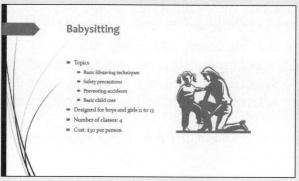

Review 4 Creating and Formatting SmartArt Graphics

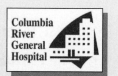

1. With **PMedS2-R-CRGHComEd.pptx** open, make Slide 10 active and then insert a new slide with the Blank layout.
2. Insert the SmartArt graphic shown in Figure P2.11 with the following specifications:
   - Click the *Hierarchy* option in the left panel at the Choose a SmartArt Graphic dialog box and then double-click *Hierarchy* in the middle panel.
   - To create the boxes in the order shown in the figure, click the outside border of the white inside box of the second box in the second row and then press the Delete key. Press the Delete key a second time and your boxes should display in the same order as the boxes in Figure P2.11.
   - With the SMARTART TOOLS DESIGN tab selected, change the colors to *Colorful Range - Accent Colors 3 to 4* and change the SmartArt style to *Polished*.
   - Type the text in the boxes as shown in Figure P2.11.
3. With Slide 11 active, insert a new slide with the Title Only layout. Click the *Click to add title* text and then type **Health Philosophy**. Select *Health Philosophy*, change the font to Candara, change the font color to *Teal, Accent 5, Darker 25%*, and then apply bold formatting.
4. Insert the SmartArt graphic shown in Figure P2.12 with the following specifications:
   - Click the *Relationship* option in the left panel at the Choose a SmartArt Graphic dialog box and then double-click *Basic Venn* in the middle panel.
   - With the SMARTART TOOLS DESIGN tab selected, change the colors to *Colorful Range - Accent Colors 4 to 5* and change the SmartArt style to *Polished*.
   - Type the text in the graphic as shown in Figure P2.12.
   - Decrease the size and then position the graphic so it displays as shown in Figure P2.12.
5. Save **PMedS2-R-CRGHComEd.pptx**.

FIGURE P2.11 Review 4, Slide 11

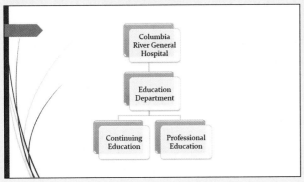

FIGURE P2.12 Review 4, Slide 12

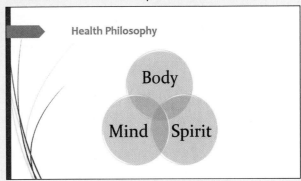

Review 5 Creating and Formatting WordArt; Applying Animation Schemes

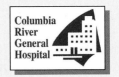

1. With **PMedS2-R-CRGHComEd.pptx** open, make active the last slide in the presentation, and then insert a new slide with the Blank layout.
2. Insert the WordArt shown in Figure P2.13 with the following specifications:
   - Click the *Fill - Blue, Accent 2, Outline - Accent 2* option at the WordArt button drop-down list.
   - Type the text shown in Figure P2.13.
   - Apply the Blue, Accent 3, Darker 50% text outline color. *Hint: Use the Text Outline button in the WordArt Styles group on the DRAWING TOOLS FORMAT tab.*
   - Click the Text Effects button on the DRAWING TOOLS FORMAT tab, point to *Transform*, and then click *Inflate Top* (first column, seventh row in the *Warp* section).
   - Increase the shape height to 4 inches and the shape width to 8.5 inches.
   - Position the WordArt as shown in Figure P2.13.
3. Make Slide 11 active and then animate the hierarchy graphic using options on the ANIMATIONS tab. (You determine the type of animation.)
4. Make Slide 9 active and then animate the bulleted items using options on the ANIMATIONS tab. (You determine the type of animation.)
5. Make Slide 1 active and then run the presentation.
6. Delete Slide 5.
7. Print the presentation as a handout with six slides horizontally per page.
8. Save and then close **PMedS2-R-CRGHComEd.pptx**.

FIGURE P2.13 Slide 13

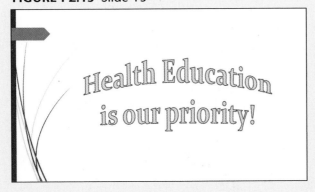

Skills Assessment

Assessment 1 Formatting a Presentation for Columbia River General Hospital

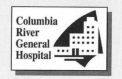

1. Open **CRGHCCPlan.pptx** and then save the presentation with the name **PMedS2-A1-CRGHCCPlan**.
2. Apply the Parallax theme and then change the theme colors to *Blue*, the theme fonts to *Garamond-TrebuchetMS*, and the background style to *Style 1*.
3. Make Slide 1 active and then center the title *"Community Commitment" Reorganization Plan*.
4. With Slide 1 active, insert **CRGHLogo.jpg**. *Hint: Do this with the Pictures button on the INSERT tab.* Change the shape width to 4 inches and then center the logo below the slide title.
5. Display the presentation in Slide Sorter view and then move Slide 3 (*Community Commitment*) to the left of Slide 2 (*Reorganization Factors*).
6. Move Slide 7 (*Changing Demographics*) to the left of Slide 3 (*Reorganization Factors*).
7. Change to Normal view, make Slide 4 active, and then demote (increase the indent of) the text *Medicare cost-cutting among doctors and hospitals* to the next list level.
8. Make Slide 5 active and then promote (decrease the indent of) the text *Reconfigure lobby and registration areas* to the previous list level.
9. Make Slide 3 active, select the bulleted text, and then change the line spacing to *1.5*.
10. Make Slide 4 active, select the bulleted text, and then change the line spacing before paragraphs to *12 pt*.
11. Make Slide 7 active, select the bulleted text, and then change the line spacing to *1.5*.
12. Insert a new slide after Slide 1 (the new slide will be Slide 2) and apply the Blank slide layout. Using the Text Box button on the INSERT tab, draw a text box in the slide and then type the text shown in Figure P2.14. Change the font size to 28 points, justify the paragraph of text, and right-align the name and title as shown in the figure.
13. Insert a new slide at the end of the presentation and then insert the Basic Target SmartArt graphic (located in the *Relationship* category) as shown in Figure P2.15. Add a shape to the graphic, change the colors to *Gradient Range - Accent 1*, and then apply the *Cartoon* SmartArt style. Type the text as shown in Figure P2.15 and then position the graphic as shown in the figure.
14. Insert a new blank slide at the end of the presentation and then insert WordArt that contains the text *Plan Completion* on one line and *May 2017* on the next line. You determine the style, shape, size, and position of the WordArt.
15. Print the presentation as handouts with six slides horizontally per page.
16. Save, run, and then close **PMedS2-A1-CRGHCCPlan.pptx**.

FIGURE P2.14 Slide 2

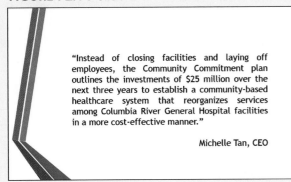

"Instead of closing facilities and laying off employees, the Community Commitment plan outlines the investments of $25 million over the next three years to establish a community-based healthcare system that reorganizes services among Columbia River General Hospital facilities in a more cost-effective manner."

Michelle Tan, CEO

FIGURE P2.15 Slide 9

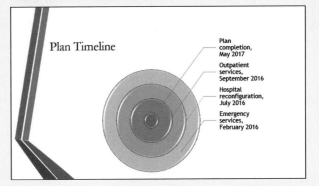

Plan Timeline

Plan completion, May 2017
Outpatient services, September 2016
Hospital reconfiguration, July 2016
Emergency services, February 2016

Assessment 2 Formatting a Presentation on Sickle Cell Anemia

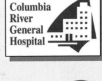

1. Open **SickleCell.pptx** and then save it with the name **PMedS2-A2-SickleCell**.
2. Apply any formatting you feel is necessary to improve the appearance of each slide. Insert at least one clip art image in the presentation.
3. Insert a new blank slide at the end of the presentation that contains WordArt text that reads *Thank you!* You determine the formatting, size, and positioning of the WordArt.
4. Apply an animation scheme of your choosing to the bulleted text in at least two of the slides in the presentation.
5. Run the presentation.
6. Print the presentation as handouts with six slides horizontally per page.
7. Save and then close **PMedS2-A2-SickleCell.pptx**.

Assessment 3 Drawing a Shape and Changing the Shape

1. Open **PMedS2-A2-SickleCell.pptx**.
2. Make Slide 9 active and then insert a new blank slide. Draw a shape of your choosing in the slide and then insert the following information in the shape. *Hint: Use the Symbol button on the INSERT tab to insert the á symbol and make sure the Font option is set to* (**normal text**) *in the Symbol dialog box.* You determine the formatting, size, and positioning of the text and shape:

   Dr. Maria Cárdenas
   North Shore Medical Clinic
   7450 Meridian Street, Suite 150
   Portland, OR 97202
   (503) 555-2330

3. Save **PMedS2-A2-SickleCell.pptx** and then print only Slide 10.
4. Use the Help feature to learn how to change a shape into another shape.
5. After learning how to change a shape, change the shape you created in Slide 10.
6. Save **PMedS2-A2-SickleCell.pptx** and then print only Slide 10.
7. Run and then close **PMedS2-A2-SickleCell.pptx**.

Assessment 4 Using an Office.com Design Theme Template

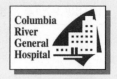

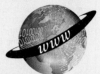

1. Office.com provides a number of design theme templates you can apply to a PowerPoint presentation. You decide to search for a design theme template related to healthcare. To do this, click the FILE tab and then click the *New* option. At the New backstage area, click the *Medical* option below the search text box. Scroll through the list of templates related to healthcare and then double-click the template named *Medical design presentation (widescreen)*.

2. Select and then delete all the slides in the slide thumbnails pane. (Only one gray, blank slide should display in the slide pane.)

3. Import a presentation into the blank design theme template. Begin by clicking the HOME tab, clicking the New Slide button, and then clicking *Reuse slides* at the drop-down list.

4. At the Reuse Slides task pane, click the Browse button and then click *Browse File* at the drop-down list.

5. At the Browse dialog box, navigate to the PowerPointMedS2 folder on your storage medium and then double-click *PMedS2-A1-CRGHCCPlan.pptx*.

6. Click each slide thumbnail in the Reuse Slides task pane, beginning with Slide 1, and then close the task pane.

7. Make Slide 1 active and then delete the hospital logo.

8. Check each slide and make any adjustments needed to make the presentation more attractive and easy to read.

9. Run the presentation.

10. Save the presentation with the name **PMedS2-A4-CRGHCCPlan.pptx**.

11. Print the presentation as handouts with six slides horizontally per page and then close the presentation.

Assessment 5 Locating Information on Support Groups

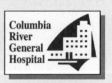

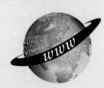

1. Using the Internet, search for support groups in your town or county for the following diseases or conditions: Alzheimer's, breast cancer, depression, diabetes, eating disorders, fibromyalgia, heart disease, and multiple sclerosis.

2. When you have gathered the information, prepare a presentation. Include your name and the name of the presentation on the first slide, and then prepare a specific slide for each support group that contains the name of the group and any other information you gathered, such as meeting dates and times, locations, telephone numbers, contacts, and so on.

3. On the final slide in the presentation, include the words *Thank you* as WordArt.

4. Apply an animation scheme of your choosing to all slides in the presentation.

5. Save the presentation with the name **PMedS2-A5-Support**.

6. Run the presentation.

7. Print the slides as handouts with six slides horizontally per page.

8. Save and then close **PMedS2-A5-Support.pptx**.

Assessment 6 Locating Information on Medical Front-Office Jobs

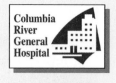

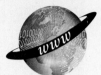

1. Using your local newspapers, employment agencies, and/or the Internet, locate information on medical front-office jobs such as medical office assistants.
2. Prepare a presentation with the information you find and include at least the following information: job titles, average wages, education requirements, required experience, and required knowledge of or training in specific software (if any).
3. Apply any formatting or enhancements you feel will improve the visual appeal of the presentation.
4. Save the presentation with the name **PMedS2-A6-Job**.
5. Run the presentation.
6. Print the slides as handouts with six slides horizontally per page.
7. Save and then close **PMedS2-A6-Job.pptx**.

Marquee Challenge

Challenge 1 Preparing a Presentation on Cholesterol

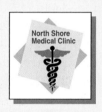

1. Prepare the presentation shown in Figure P2.16 on page 440 with the following specifications:
   - Apply the Ion Boardroom theme.
   - Change the theme colors to *Violet*.
   - Size and position the placeholders as shown in Figure P2.16.
   - Insert, size, and format at least two clip art images in the presentation.
   - Decrease the size of the title placeholder on Slide 1 so the title displays as shown in the figure.
   - Apply bold formatting to the titles in Slides 3 through 7.
   - Insert **NSMCLogo.jpg** in Slide 1 and then size and position the logo as shown in the figure. Apply a transparent background color to the logo. To do this, click the Color button in the Adjust group on the PICTURE TOOLS FORMAT tab and then click *Set Transparent Color* at the drop-down list. Move the mouse pointer to any white color in the logo background and then click the left mouse button.
   - Apply the Blank layout to Slide 2 and then create a text box for the title and another text box for the description. Make sure the font of the title is Century Gothic, change the font size to 36 points, change the font color to *Lavender, Accent 1*, and then apply bold formatting. Increase the size of the font in the description to 20 points and change the alignment to center.
   - Add 18 points of spacing before the bulleted text in Slides 3 through 7.
   - Apply the Blank layout to Slide 8 and then create a text box for the title. Apply the title formatting from Slide 2 to the title in Slide 8. Use WordArt to insert the telephone number (apply the Can Up transform text effect to the WordArt).
2. Save the completed presentation with the name **PMedS2-C1-NSMC**.
3. Print the presentation as handouts with four slides horizontally per page.
4. Close **PMedS2-C1-NSMC.pptx**.

North Shore Medical Clinic

GREATER PORTLAND HEALTHCARE WORKERS ASSOCIATION

What is Cholesterol?

Cholesterol is a type of fat (lipid) that is made by the body. Cholesterol is essential for good health and is found in every cell in the body. Too much cholesterol in the blood can raise the risk of heart attack or stroke.

Type of Cholesterol

▶ Low-density lipoproteins (LDL) – Deliver cholesterol to the body. About 70% of cholesterol is transported as LDL. Too much LDL is harmful to the body.

▶ High-density lipoproteins (HLD) – Removes cholesterol from the bloodstream. About 20% of cholesterol is transported as HDL.

LDL Cholesterol Levels

▶ Less than 130 is best

▶ Between 130 to 159 is borderline

▶ 160 or more means higher risk for heart disease

HDL Cholesterol Levels

▶ Less than 40 means higher risk for heart disease

▶ 60 or higher reduces the risk of heart disease

Improve Cholesterol Levels

▶ Do not smoke.

▶ Eat a healthy, low-fat diet that includes lots of fruits and vegetables.

▶ Exercise regularly.

▶ Limit alcohol consumption.

▶ Take medication.

Cholesterol Medications

▶ Statins (also called HMG-CoA reductase inhibitors)

▶ Resins (also called bile acid sequestrants)

▶ Fibrates (also called fibric acid derivatives)

▶ Niacin (also called nicotinic acid)

▶ Ezetimibe

Cholesterol Screening
Call for an Appointment

503-555-2330

Challenge 2 Preparing a Hospital Center Presentation

1. Prepare the presentation shown in Figure P2.17 on page 442 with the following specifications:
   - Apply the Facet theme and change the theme colors to *Marquee*.
   - Insert **CRGHLogo.jpg** in Slide 1 and then size and position the logo as shown in the figure.
   - Apply the Title Only layout to Slide 2 and then create a text box for the description of the disorder. Size and position the title and text box as shown in the figure.
   - Insert a Basic Venn SmartArt graphic in Slide 3, change the colors to *Colorful - Accent Colors*, apply the Polished SmartArt style, and then size and position the SmartArt as shown in the figure.
   - In Slide 5, use the Insert Pictures window to locate and insert a clip art image based on the search words *doctor bag*. Change the color of the picture to *Green, Accent color 2 Light* and then size and position the clip art as shown in the figure.
   - Insert an Organization Chart SmartArt graphic in Slide 6, change the colors to *Colorful - Accent Colors*, apply the Polished SmartArt style, and then size and position the SmartArt as shown in the figure.
2. Save the completed presentation with the name **PMedS2-C2-EatingDisorder**.
3. Print the presentation as handouts with six slides horizontally per page.
4. Close **PMedS2-C2-EatingDisorder.pptx**.

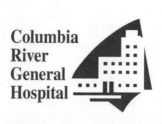

Columbia
River
General
Hospital

Eating Disorder Center

Eating disorders are a group of illnesses with a
biological basis modified and influenced by
emotional and cultural factors. People with
eating disorders often eat, or refuse to eat, to
satisfy psychological or emotional needs, rather
than a physical need.

Eating Disorder Components

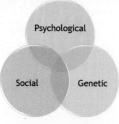

Psychological

Social   Genetic

Center Treatments

▶ Anorexia Nervosa
▶ Bulimia Nervosa
▶ Compulsive eating disorder
▶ Binge eating disorder
▶ Obesity

Center Specialists

▶ Amelia Halstead, MD
▶ Tyrone Larkin, MD
▶ Jo Burke, Dietician
▶ Kim Campanoli, NP
▶ Madeleine Fleming, RN
▶ Dolores Hernandez, MSW

Center Administrative Staff

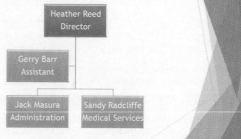

Heather Reed
Director

Gerry Barr
Assistant

Jack Masura
Administration

Sandy Radcliffe
Medical Services

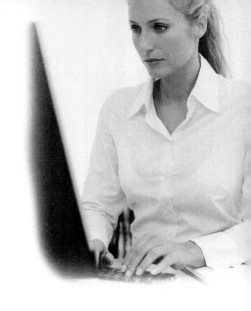

Integrating Programs
Word, Excel, and PowerPoint

Skills

- Export a PowerPoint presentation to a Word document
- Export a Word outline to a PowerPoint presentation
- Link an Excel chart with a Word document and a PowerPoint presentation
- Edit a linked object
- Embed a Word table in a PowerPoint presentation
- Edit an embedded object

Student Resources

Before beginning the activities in this section, copy to your storage medium the IntegratingMed2 folder from the Student Resources CD. This folder contains the data files you need to complete the projects in this section.

Projects Overview

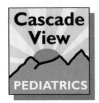

Create and format a Word document containing information on opening a clinic in Vancouver.

Prepare a presentation for the quarterly staff meeting using a Word outline; copy and link an Excel chart to the staff meeting presentation and to a Word document and then edit the linked chart; copy a Word table containing data on new patients, embed it in the staff meeting presentation, and then update the table; and copy a Word table containing information on quarterly equipment purchases and embed it in the staff meeting presentation.

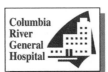

Export a PowerPoint presentation containing information on the Community Commitment plan to a Word document; copy and link an Excel chart containing information on class enrollments to an Education Department presentation and then edit the chart; and embed and edit a table containing information on department contacts into the Education Department presentation.

Activity 2.1

Exporting a PowerPoint Presentation to Word

You can send, or export, data from one program to another program within the Microsoft Office suite. For example, you can export Word data to a PowerPoint presentation, and vice versa. To export PowerPoint data to Word, click the FILE tab, click the *Export* option, click the *Create Handouts* option, and then click the Create Handouts button.

At the Send to Microsoft Word dialog box that displays, specify the layout of the data in the Word document and whether you want to paste or paste link the data and then click OK. One of the advantages of exporting presentation data to a Word document is that you can have greater control over the formatting of the data in Word.

Project

Dr. Severin has asked you to export the information from his presentation on opening a clinic in Vancouver to Word as a handout.

1. Open PowerPoint and then open **CVPVancouver.pptx**.

2. Save the presentation with the name **Int2Med-CVPVancouver**.

3. Click the FILE tab, click the *Export* option, click the *Create Handouts* option, and then click the Create Handouts button.

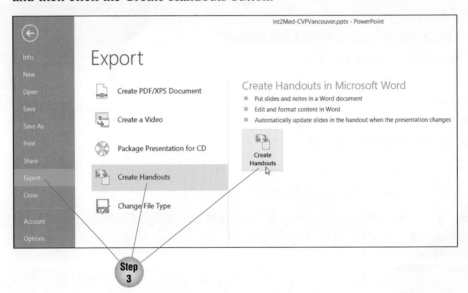

4. At the Send to Microsoft Word dialog box, click the *Blank lines next to slides* option.

5. Click the *Paste link* option at the bottom of the dialog box and then click OK.

   Click the *Paste link* option if you plan to update data in a PowerPoint presentation and want the data to update automatically in the Word document.

6. Click the Word button on the Taskbar.

   After a few moments, the slides display in a Word document as thumbnails followed by blank lines.

7. Save the Word document in the IntegratingMed2 folder on your storage medium and name it **Int2Med-CVPVanHandout**.

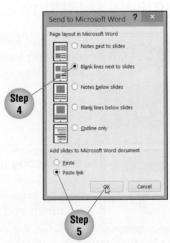

8 Print and then close **Int2Med-CVPVanHandout.docx**.

9 Click the PowerPoint button on the Taskbar.

10 Make Slide 2 active and then change *8.5%* to *9.6%*.

In Brief
Export PowerPoint Presentation to Word
1. Open presentation.
2. Click FILE tab.
3. Click *Export* option.
4. Click *Create Handouts* option.
5. Click Create Handouts button.
6. Choose desired options at Send to Microsoft Word dialog box.
7. Click OK.

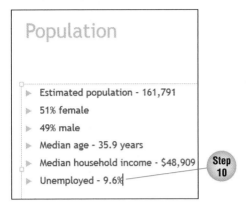

11 Make Slide 8 active, change *$199,300* to *$207,000*, and then change *$208,000* to *$216,800*.

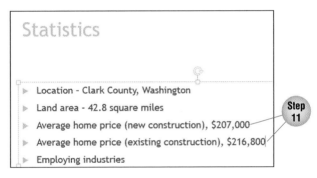

12 Save **Int2Med-CVPVancouver.pptx**.

13 Make Word the active program and then open **Int2Med-CVPVanHandout.docx**. At the message asking if you want to update the document with the data from the linked files, click the Yes button.

14 Scroll through the document and notice that the percentage in Slide 2 and prices in Slide 8 reflect the changes you made in the PowerPoint presentation.

15 Save, print, and then close **Int2Med-CVPVanHandout.docx**.

16 Make PowerPoint the active program and then close **Int2Med-CVPVancouver.pptx**.

In Addition

Pasting and Linking Data

At the Send to Microsoft Word dialog box, the *Paste* option is selected by default and is available for all of the page layout options. With this option selected, the data exported to Word is not connected or linked to the original data in the PowerPoint presentation. If you plan to update the data in the PowerPoint presentation and want the updated data to carry over to the Word document, select the *Paste link* option instead. This option is available for all of the page layout options except the *Outline only* option.

Activity 2.2

Exporting a Word Outline to a PowerPoint Presentation

As you learned in the previous section, you can export data from a PowerPoint presentation to a Word document. You can also export data from a Word document to a PowerPoint presentation. For example, you can create text for slides in a Word outline and then send that outline to PowerPoint. PowerPoint will create new slides based on the heading styles used in the Word outline. Paragraphs formatted with a Heading 1 style become slide titles. Heading 2 text becomes first-level bulleted text, Heading 3 text becomes second-level bulleted text, and so on. If styles are not applied to outline text in Word, PowerPoint uses tabs or indents to place text on slides. To export a Word document to a PowerPoint presentation, you need to add the Send to Microsoft PowerPoint button to the Quick Access toolbar.

Project

Lee Elliott has asked you to take the outline for the quarterly staff meeting and convert it to a PowerPoint presentation.

1. Make sure both Word and PowerPoint are open.

2. With Word the active program, open **NSMCOutline.docx**.

   Text in this document has been formatted with the Heading 1 and Heading 2 styles.

3. Add the Send to Microsoft PowerPoint button to the Quick Access toolbar. Begin by clicking the Customize Quick Access Toolbar button that displays at the right side of the Quick Access toolbar.

4. Click *More Commands* at the drop-down list.

5. At the Word Options dialog box, click the down-pointing arrow at the right side of the *Choose commands from* option box and then click *All Commands* at the drop-down list.

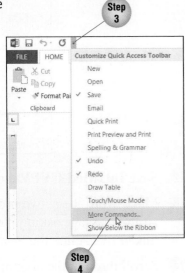

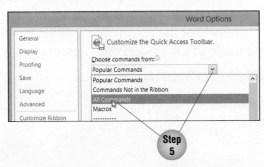

6. Scroll down the list box that displays below the *Choose commands from* option box and then double-click *Send to Microsoft PowerPoint*.

   Items in the list box display in alphabetical order.

7. Click OK to close the Word Options dialog box.

8. Send the outline to PowerPoint by clicking the Send to Microsoft PowerPoint button on the Quick Access toolbar.

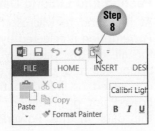

9 When the presentation displays on the screen, make sure Slide 1 is the active slide.

> The presentation is created with a blank design template.

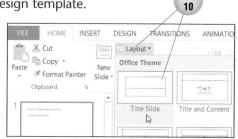

Step 10

10 Change the layout of Slide 1 by clicking the Layout button [⊞] in the Slides group on the HOME tab and then clicking *Title Slide* at the drop-down list.

11 Make Slide 4 active and then change the layout to *Title Only*. Make Slide 9 active and then change the layout to *Title Only*. Make Slide 10 active and then change the layout to *Title Only*.

12 Apply a theme by clicking the DESIGN tab, clicking the More button [⊽] at the right side of the theme thumbnails in the Themes group, and then clicking the *Parallax* option at the drop-down gallery.

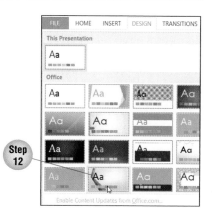

Step 12

13 Save the presentation in the IntegratingMed2 folder on your storage medium and name it **Int2Med-NSMCMeeting**.

14 Close **Int2Med-NSMCMeeting.pptx**.

15 Click the Word button on the Taskbar.

16 Right-click the Send to Microsoft PowerPoint button on the Quick Access toolbar and then click *Remove from Quick Access Toolbar* at the shortcut menu.

Step 16

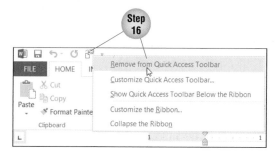

17 Close **NSMCOutline.docx** without saving the changes.

In Brief

Insert Send to Microsoft Office PowerPoint Button on Quick Access Toolbar
1. Click Customize Quick Access Toolbar button at the right side of Quick Access toolbar.
2. Click *More Commands*.
3. Click the down-pointing arrow at right side of *Choose commands from* option box.
4. Click *All Commands*.
5. Scroll down *Choose commands from* list box and then double-click *Send to Microsoft PowerPoint*.
6. Click OK.

Send Word Outline to PowerPoint Presentation
1. Open Word document.
2. Click Send to Microsoft PowerPoint button on Quick Access toolbar.

In Addition

Applying a Style in Word

Heading styles were already applied to the text in **NSMCOutline.docx**, so you did not need to complete that step, but if you create an outline in Word that you want to export to PowerPoint, you will need to know how to apply styles. Styles are available in the Styles group on the HOME tab in Word. To apply a style, select or position the insertion point within the desired text and then click the style in the Styles group. Word documents also contain a number of predesigned formats grouped into style sets. Click the DESIGN tab to display the available style sets in the Document Formatting group. Choose a style set and the available styles in the Styles group on the HOME tab change to reflect the set. To display additional available styles, click the More button that displays at the right side of the style thumbnails.

Activity 2.3

Linking an Excel Chart with a Word Document and a PowerPoint Presentation

You can copy and link an object, such as a table or chart, to files in other programs. For example, you can copy an Excel chart and link it to a Word document and/or a PowerPoint presentation. The advantage to copying and linking over just copying and pasting is that when you edit the object in the originating program, called the *source* program, the object is automatically updated in the linked files in the *destination* programs. When an object is linked, the object exists in the source program and is represented by a code in the destination program. Since the object is located only in the source program, changes made to the object in the source program are reflected in the destination program.

Project

To improve the readability of data, you will link an Excel chart to the quarterly staff meeting presentation and to a Word document.

North Shore
Medical Clinic

1 Open Word, Excel, and PowerPoint.

2 Make Word the active program and then open **NSMCQtrlyEx.docx**. Save the document with the name **Int2Med-NSMCQtrlyEx**.

3 Make PowerPoint the active program, open **Int2Med-NSMCMeeting.pptx**, and then make Slide 10 the active slide.

4 Make Excel the active program and then open **NSMCChart.xlsx**. Save the workbook with the name **Int2Med-NSMCChart**.

5 Copy and link the Excel chart to the Word document and the PowerPoint presentation. Begin by clicking once in the chart to select it.

> Make sure you select the entire chart and not a specific chart element. Try selecting the chart by clicking just inside the chart border.

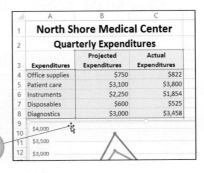

Step 5

6 With the chart selected, click the Copy button in the Clipboard group on the HOME tab.

7 Click the Word button on the Taskbar.

8 Press Ctrl + End to move the insertion point to the end of the document.

9 Click the Paste button arrow and then click *Paste Special* at the drop-down list.

10 At the Paste Special dialog box, click the *Paste link* option, click *Microsoft Excel Chart Object* in the As list box, and then click OK.

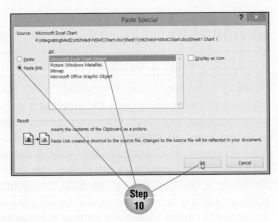

Step 10

11 Save, print, and then close **Int2Med-NSMCQtrlyEx.docx**.

12 Click the PowerPoint button on the Taskbar.

13 With Slide 10 the active slide, make sure the HOME tab is selected, click the Paste button arrow, and then click *Paste Special*.

14 At the Paste Special dialog box, click the *Paste link* option, make sure *Microsoft Excel Chart Object* is selected in the *As* list box, and then click OK.

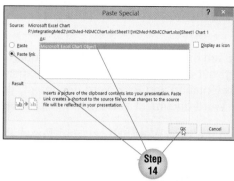

Step 14

15 Increase the size of the chart so it better fills the slide and then move the chart so it is centered on the slide below the title.

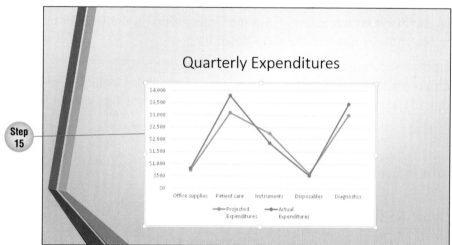

Step 15

Quarterly Expenditures

In Brief
Link Object between Programs
1. Open source program.
2. Open file containing object.
3. Select object and then click Copy button.
4. Open destination program.
5. Open file to which object will be linked.
6. Click Paste button arrow and then click *Paste Special*.
7. At Paste Special dialog box, click *Paste link* option.
8. Click OK.

16 Click outside the chart to deselect it.

17 Save the presentation with the same name (**Int2Med-NSMCMeeting.pptx**), print only Slide 10, and then close **Int2Med-NSMCMeeting.pptx**.

18 Click the Excel button on the Taskbar.

19 Click outside the chart to deselect it.

20 Save, print, and then close **Int2Med-NSMCChart.xlsx**.

In Addition

Linking an Object within a Program

In this section, you learned to link an object between programs using the Paste Special dialog box. You can also link an object between two files in the same program. For example, you can link an object between Word documents by using options at the Object dialog box. To do this, click the INSERT tab and then click the Object button. At the Object dialog box, click the Create from File tab. Type the desired file name in the *File name* text box or click the Browse button and then select the desired file from the appropriate folder. Click the *Link to file* check box to insert a check mark and then click OK.

Activity 2.4

Editing a Linked Object

The advantage to linking an object over simply copying it is that any changes you make to the object in the source program will automatically be applied to the object in the destination program(s). To edit a linked object, open the file containing the object in the source program, make the desired edits, and then save the file. The next time you open the file containing the linked object in the destination program, the object will be updated.

Project

As you are proofreading the text in the quarterly staff meeting presentation, you realize that you left out a category in the quarterly expenditures chart. Since you linked the Excel chart to the presentation and to a Word document, you decide to edit the chart in Excel. The charts in the Word document and PowerPoint presentation will update automatically.

1. Make sure Word, Excel, and PowerPoint are open.

2. Make Excel the active program and then open **Int2Med-NSMCChart.xlsx**.

3. Add a row to the worksheet by clicking once in cell A6 to make it the active cell. Click the Insert button arrow 📊 in the Cells group on the HOME tab and then click *Insert Sheet Rows* at the drop-down list.

4. Insert the following data in the specified cells:

   A6: **Respiratory**
   B6: **925**
   C6: **1200**

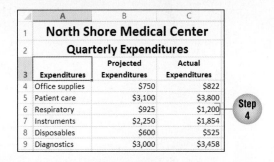

5. Click in cell A3.

6. Save, print, and then close **Int2Med-NSMCChart.xlsx**.

7. Make Word the active program and then open **Int2Med-NSMCQtrlyEx.docx**. At the message asking if you want to update the linked file, click the Yes button.

8. Notice how the linked chart is automatically updated to reflect the changes you made to the chart in Excel.

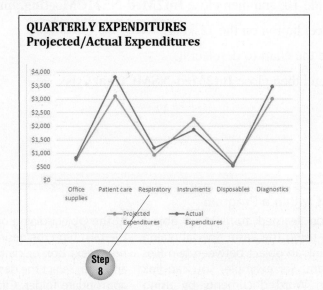

9 Save, print, and then close **Int2Med-NSMCQtrlyEx.docx**.

10 Make PowerPoint the active program and then open **Int2Med-NSMCMeeting.pptx**.

11 At the message telling you that the presentation contains links, click the Update Links button.

12 Make Slide 10 the active slide and then notice how the linked chart is automatically updated to reflect the changes you made to the chart in Excel.

In Brief
Edit Linked Object
1. Open source file.
2. Make desired changes to object.
3. Save and then close source file.
4. Open destination file(s) to check if linked object updated.

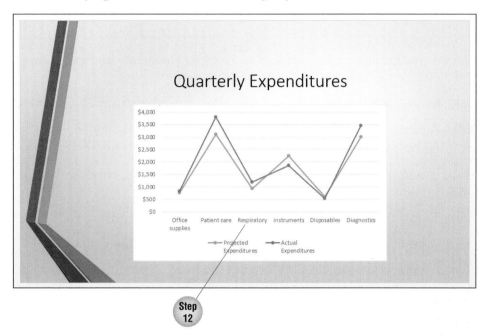

Step 12

13 Save the presentation and then print only Slide 10.

14 Close **Int2Med-NSMCMeeting.pptx**.

In Addition

Updating a Link Manually

If you want to control when linked data is updated, you can specify that you want to update a link manually in the destination program. To do this, open a Word document containing a linked object. Right-click the object, point to *Linked (type of object) Object*, and then click *Links*. At the Links dialog box, click the *Manual update* option and then click OK. With *Manual update* selected, a link will only be updated when you right-click a linked object and then click *Update Link*; or when you display the Links dialog box, click the link in the list box, and then click the Update Now button.

Activity 2.5

Embedding and Editing a Word Table in a PowerPoint Presentation

You can copy and paste, copy and link, or copy and embed an object from one file into another. A *linked object* resides in the source program and is represented by a code in the destination program. An *embedded object* resides in the source program as well as in the destination program. When you make a change to an embedded object in the source program, the change will not be made to the object in the destination program. The main advantage to embedding rather than simply copying and pasting is that you can edit an embedded object in the destination program using the tools of the source program.

Project To present information on new patients seen at the clinic, you decide to create a table in Word and then embed it in a slide in the staff meeting presentation.

1. Make sure Word and PowerPoint are open.

2. Make PowerPoint the active program and then open **Int2Med-NSMCMeeting.pptx**.

3. At the message telling you the presentation contains links, click the Update Links button.

4. Make Slide 4 the active slide.

5. Make Word the active program and then open **NSMCTable01.docx**.

6. Click in a cell in the table and then select the table. To do this, click the TABLE TOOLS LAYOUT tab, click the Select button ⟦⬚⟧ in the Table group, and then click *Select Table* at the drop-down list.

7. With the table selected, click the HOME tab and then click the Copy button in the Clipboard group.

8. Click the PowerPoint button on the Taskbar.

9. With Slide 4 the active slide, click the Paste button arrow and then click *Paste Special* at the drop-down list.

10. At the Paste Special dialog box, click *Microsoft Word Document Object* in the *As* list box and then click OK.

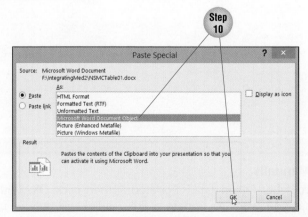

11 With the table selected in the slide, use the sizing handles to increase the size and change the position of the table as shown below.

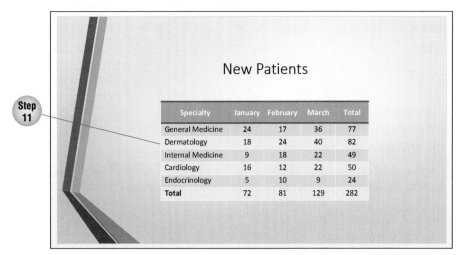

12 Click outside the table to deselect it.

13 Save **Int2Med-NSMCMeeting.pptx** and then print only Slide 4.

14 Make Slide 9 the active slide.

15 Click the Word button on the Taskbar and then close the document.

16 With Word the active program, open **NSMCTable02.docx**.

17 Click in a cell in the table and then select all cells in the table by clicking the table move handle that displays in the upper left corner of the table (a square with a four-headed arrow inside).

18 Click the HOME tab and then click the Copy button in the Clipboard group.

19 Click the PowerPoint button on the Taskbar.

20 With Slide 9 the active slide, click the Paste button arrow and then click *Paste Special* at the drop-down list.

21 At the Paste Special dialog box, click *Microsoft Word Document Object* in the *As* list box and then click OK.

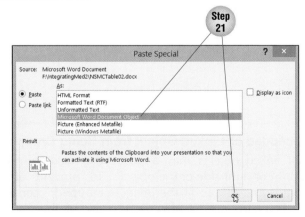

continues

In Brief

Embed Object
1. Open source program.
2. Open file containing object.
3. Select object and then click Copy button.
4. Open destination program.
5. Open file into which object will be embedded.
6. Click Paste button arrow and then click *Paste Special*.
7. At Paste Special dialog box, click object in *As* list box.
8. Click OK.

Edit Embedded Object
1. Open file containing embedded object.
2. Double-click object.
3. Make edits and then click outside object to deselect it.

22 Increase the size and change the position of the table in the slide so it displays as shown at the right.

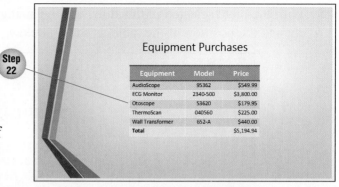

Step 22

23 As you look over the slide, you realize that the price of the otoscope is incorrect. Double-click the table to edit the amount.

Double-clicking the table displays the Word tabs and ribbon at the top of the screen. Horizontal and vertical rulers also display around the table.

24 Using the mouse, select *$179.95* and then type **$299.99**.

25 Recalculate the total by selecting *$5,194.94* and then pressing F9.

F9 is the keyboard shortcut to update a field. You could also update the formula by selecting the amount, clicking the TABLE TOOLS LAYOUT tab, clicking the Formula button in the Data group, and then clicking OK at the Formula dialog box.

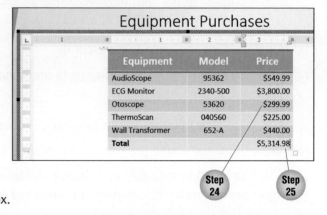

Step 24

Step 25

26 Click outside the table to deselect it.

Clicking outside the table also removes the Word tabs.

27 Print Slide 9 of the presentation.

28 Apply a transition and sound of your choosing to all slides in the presentation and then run the presentation.

29 Save and then close **Int2Med-NSMCMeeting.pptx**.

30 Click the Word button on the Taskbar and then close **NSMCTable02.docx**.

In Addition

Preventing an Embedded or Linked Object from Being Cropped

Large embedded or linked objects may appear cropped on the bottom or right side of the object even if enough room is available to fit the image on the page or slide. This is because Word converts embedded or linked objects into Windows metafiles (.wmf), which have a maximum height and width. If the embedded or linked object exceeds this maximum size, it appears cropped. To prevent an object from being cropped, consider reducing the size of the object by decreasing the font size, column size, line spacing, and so on.

Skills Review

Review 1 Exporting a PowerPoint Presentation to Word

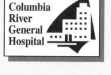

1. Open PowerPoint.
2. Open **CRGHCCRPlan.pptx** and then save it with the name **Int2Med-R-CRGHCCRPlan**.
3. Export the PowerPoint data to Word as slides with blank lines next to them. Click the *Blank lines next to slides* option and the *Paste link* option at the Send to Microsoft Word dialog box.
4. Save the Word document and name it **Int2Med-R-CRGHComPlan**.
5. Print and then close **Int2Med-R-CRGHComPlan.docx**.
6. Click the PowerPoint button on the Taskbar.
7. Make Slide 5 active and then delete the second bulleted item.
8. Make Slide 6 active and then insert a new bullet after (but at the same level as) the *Expand fitness center* bulleted item that reads *Implement community health education plan.*
9. Save and then print the presentation as handouts with four slides horizontally per page.
10. Make Word the active program, open **Int2Med-R-CRGHComPlan.docx**, and then click the Yes button at the message asking if you want to update the link.
11. Save, print, and then close the document.
12. Make PowerPoint the active program and then close **Int2Med-R-CRGHCCRPlan.pptx**.

Review 2 Linking and Editing an Excel Chart in a PowerPoint Slide

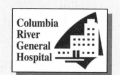

1. Open Excel and PowerPoint.
2. With PowerPoint the active program, open **CRGHEdDept.pptx**.
3. Save the presentation with the name **Int2Med-R-CRGHEdDept**.
4. Make Slide 6 active.
5. Make Excel the active program and then open **CRGHChart01.xlsx**. Save the workbook with the name **Int2Med-R-CRGHChart01**.
6. Click the chart once to select it (make sure you select the entire chart and not just a chart element) and then copy and link the chart to Slide 6 in the **Int2Med-R-CRGHEdDept.pptx** PowerPoint presentation. (Be sure to use the Paste Special dialog box to link the chart.)
7. Increase the size of the chart to better fill the slide and then center the chart on the slide.
8. Click outside the chart to deselect it.
9. Save the presentation with the same name (**Int2Med-R-CRGHEdDept.pptx**).
10. Print only Slide 6 of the presentation and then close **Int2Med-R-CRGHEdDept.pptx**.
11. Click the button on the Taskbar representing the Excel workbook **Int2Med-R-CRGHChart01.xlsx**.
12. Click outside the chart to deselect it.
13. Save and then print **Int2Med-R-CRGHChart01.xlsx**.
14. Insert another department in the worksheet (and chart) by making cell A6 active, clicking the Insert button arrow in the Cells group on the HOME tab, and then clicking *Insert Sheet Rows* at the drop-down list. (This creates a new row 6.) Type the following text in the specified cells:

   A6: **CPR**   C7: **105**
   B6: **85**   D7: **134**

15. Click in cell A3.
16. Save, print, and then close **Int2Med-R-CRGHChart01.xlsx** and then close Excel.
17. Click the PowerPoint button on the Taskbar and then open **Int2Med-R-CRGHEdDept.pptx**. At the message telling you that the presentation contains links, click the Update Links button. Display Slide 6 and then notice the change to the chart.
18. Save **Int2Med-R-CRGHEdDept.pptx** and then print only Slide 6.
19. Close **Int2Med-R-CRGHEdDept.pptx**.

Review 3 Embedding and Editing a Word Table in a PowerPoint Slide

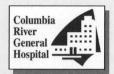

1. Open Word and PowerPoint.
2. Make PowerPoint the active program, open **Int2Med-R-CRGHEdDept.pptx**, and then make Slide 7 the active slide. (At the message asking if you want to update links, click the Cancel button.)
3. Make Word the active program and then open **CRGHContacts.docx**.
4. Select the table and then copy and embed it in Slide 7 in **Int2Med-R-CRGHEdDept.pptx**. (Make sure you use the Paste Special dialog box.)
5. With the table selected in the slide, use the sizing handles to increase the size and change the position of the table so it better fills the slide.
6. Click outside the table to deselect it and then save **Int2Med-R-CRGHEdDept.pptx**.
7. Double-click the table and then click in the text *Christina Fuentes*.
8. Insert a row below by clicking the TABLE TOOLS LAYOUT tab and then clicking the Insert Below button.
9. In the new row, type John Shapiro in the *Contact* column, type Sterling Health Services in the *Agency* column, and then type (503) 555-4220 in the *Telephone* column.
10. Click outside the table to deselect it.
11. Print Slide 7 of the presentation.
12. Apply a transition and sound of your choosing to all slides in the presentation.
13. Run the presentation.
14. Save and then close **Int2Med-R-CRGHEdDept.pptx** and then close PowerPoint.
15. Close the Word document **CRGHContacts.docx** and then close Word.

INDEX